2nd edition
psychiatry

The National Medical Series for Independent Study

2nd edition
psychiatry

EDITORS

James H. Scully, M.D., F.A.P.A.
Donald W. Bechtold, M.D.
Jon A. Bell, M.D.
Steven L. Dubovsky
Gordon L. Neligh, M.D.
Janice L. Petersen, M.D.

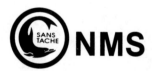 **NMS**

National Medical Series from Williams & Wilkins
Baltimore, Hong Kong, London, Sydney

Harwal Publishing Company, Malvern, Pennsylvania

Williams & Wilkins

Library of Congress Cataloging-in-Publication Data

Psychiatry/editor, James H. Scully.—2nd ed.
   p.   cm.—(The National medical series for independent study)
(A Williams & Wilkins publication)
  Includes bibliographies and index.
  ISBN 0-683-06264-6
  1. Psychiatry—Examinations, questions, etc.
I. Scully, James H. II. Series. III. Series: A Wiley
medical publication.
  [DNLM: 1. Psychiatry—examination questions.
2. Psychiatry—outlines. WN 18 P9765]
RC457.P77   1989
616.89'0076—dc20
DNLM/DLC
for Library of Congress   89-2210
                         CIP

10 9 8 7 6 5 4

Contents

Contributors

Donald W. Bechtold, M.D.
Assistant Professor of Psychiatry
Director of Training in Child Psychiatry
University of Colorado Health Sciences
    Center School of Medicine
Denver, Colorado

Jon A. Bell, M.D.
Professor of Psychiatry and Medicine
Director, Anxiety and Mood Disorders Clinic
Associate Director, Emergency
    Psychiatric Service
University of Colorado Health Sciences
    Center School of Medicine
Denver, Colorado

Steven L. Dubovsky, M.D.
Professor of Psychiatry and Medicine
Vice Chairman, Department of Psychiatry
University of Colorado Health Sciences
    Center School of Medicine
Denver, Colorado

Gordon L. Neligh, III, M.D.
Assistant Professor of Psychiatry
Director, Program for Public Psychiatry
University of Colorado Health Sciences
    Center School of Medicine
Denver, Colorado

Janice L. Petersen, M.D.
Assistant Professor of Psychiatry
Director, Medical Student Education
    in Psychiatry
University of Colorado Health Sciences
    Center School of Medicine
Denver, Colorado

James H. Scully, M.D., F.A.P.A.
Associate Professor of Psychiatry
Director, Residency Training Program
Vice Chairman for Education
Department of Psychiatry
University of Colorado Health Sciences
    Center School of Medicine
Denver, Colorado

Preface to Second Edition

Since the publication of the first edition, there have been a number of changes in the field of psychiatry that are now reflected in the second edition. The third edition of the *Diagnostic and Statistical Manual of Mental Disorders (DSM-III)* has been revised to become the *DSM-III-R*. This revised edition continues to advance the abilities of clinicians to diagnose psychiatric disorders in a consistent and reliable way. The second edition of *Psychiatry* takes into account the changes in the *DSM-III-R* classification.

Research in the function of the brain is one of the frontier areas of medicine. The chapter on schizophrenia has been completely revised to include the recent advances in research on the function of the brain in mental illness.

A new chapter on the clinical examination of the patient has also been added. This chapter includes the approaches to taking a psychiatric history from a patient as well as how to conduct a thorough mental status examination. Additionally, recent epidemiologic data have been added that better illustrate the extent of mental illness in our population.

Lastly, 200 new questions have been added to the second edition, and hopefully, these will continue to be of use to the reader.

James H. Scully

Preface to First Edition

This book is designed to outline the major clinical areas of psychiatry, and the current understanding of the diagnosis and treatment of psychiatric illness is presented in outline form. While only a few physicians specialize in the area of mental illness, almost every physician sees patients with psychiatric disorders in his or her clinical practice. Many surveys of practice patterns reveal that nearly one-half of the patients with psychiatric illness receive most, if not all, of their care from nonpsychiatric physicians. It is clearly necessary then for all physicians to know something about the diagnosis and treatment of psychiatric illness.

A recent major advance in our ability to diagnose mental illness has been achieved by a publication of the American Psychiatric Association, the *Diagnostic and Statistical Manual of Mental Disorders*, third edition, which is known as the *DSM-III*. Although psychiatric illnesses have been described for thousands of years, particular mental disorders have been subject to interpretation. The *DSM-III* attempts to bring descriptive and observable criteria to the diagnosis of psychiatric illness.

A great deal of research is under way in our attempt to understand the brain and behavior. Research in psychiatry is now at a point comparable to where it was in general medicine about 20 years ago. The future looks promising for better understanding of the basic mechanisms of mental illness as well as for improving the treatment of those who suffer.

James H. Scully

Acknowledgments

We would like to express our deepest appreciation to Matt Harris of Harwal Publishing Company who has taken on the project of the National Medical Series and to Jane Edwards, the project editor, for her editorial guidance and patience during the preparation of this second edition. Special thanks are also due Ann Spera for her help in preparing the manuscript in addition to her duties as secretary of the Residency Training Program in Psychiatry at the University of Colorado School of Medicine.

Introduction

Psychiatry, 2nd edition, is one of six clinical science review books in the *National Medical Series for Independent Study*. This series has been designed to provide students and house officers, as well as physicians, with a concise but comprehensive instrument for self-evaluation and review within the clinical sciences. Although *Psychiatry*, 2nd edition, would be most useful for students preparing for the National Board of Medical Examiners examinations (Part II, Part III, FLEX, and FMGEMS), it should also be useful for students studying for course examinations. These books are not intended to replace the standard clinical science texts, but, rather, to complement them.

The books in this series present the core content of each clinical science area using an outline format and featuring approximately 500 study questions. The questions are distributed throughout the book at the end of each chapter and in a challenge examination at the end of the text. In addition, each question is accompanied by the correct answer, a paragraph-length explanation of the correct answer, and specific reference to the outline points under which the information necessary to answer the question can be found.

We have chosen an outline format to allow maximum ease in retrieving information, assuming that the time available to the reader is limited. Considerable editorial time has been spent to ensure that the information required by all medical school curricula has been included and that the question format parallels that of the National Board examinations. We feel that the combination of the outline and Board-type study questions provides a unique teaching device.

We hope you will find this series interesting, relevant, and challenging. The authors and the staff at Harwal/Wiley welcome your comments and suggestions.

The Clinical Examination

James H. Scully

I. OVERVIEW

A. Psychiatric evaluation

1. The psychiatric evaluation differs from a routine medical examination in that it is a mental status examination rather than a physical examination (although a physical examination may also be included). Furthermore, the examiner inquires about the patient's feelings and relationships, not just historical facts. The psychiatric evaluation consists of:
   a. Gathering data from a careful history of the patient's problems
   b. Conducting an examination of the patient
   c. Developing a differential diagnosis for further study
   d. Constructing a treatment plan

2. Special skill is needed in taking a psychiatric history because of the potential embarrassment patients feel about disclosing emotional problems. Most people are less open about discussing psychiatric symptoms as compared to physical symptoms.
   a. While most patients are not psychotic, even confused and disorganized patients can be helped by the physician to give accurate details of their history.
   b. Confidentiality is important in all physician–patient interactions but even more so when psychiatric issues are discussed. Physicians should not discuss their patients in hallways or elevators.
   c. In teaching programs, case material must be presented; however, it is important to maintain anonymity, and the participants in any conference are bound by confidentiality.
   d. Exceptions to the rule of confidentiality are made when the need for safety becomes paramount, such as in cases of child abuse or when threats are made to harm others.

B. Interview

1. The patient must be helped to feel comfortable enough to give information.

2. Nonverbal communication, such as facial expressions and posture, is as important as verbal communication. Also of note is *how* the story is told (i.e., the tone of voice or the feelings expressed by the patient).

3. During the first few minutes of the interview, the physician should allow the patient to talk about his or her chief complaint.

C. History of present illness. The interviewer should obtain information about:

1. The onset, deviation, or change over time of the symptoms

2. Stressful events, especially losses, including death, job loss, or financial loss

3. The patient's perception of any change in him- or herself or another individual's perception of the patient, such as his or her spouse or supervisor at work

4. Past psychiatric illness or treatment, including medications, hospitalizations, or other therapy

5. Legal issues with respect to the present illness (e.g., lawsuits, arrests, or jail) or any problems in school, such as truancy or suspension

6. Any secondary gain—that is, is anything to be gained by the patient from the current problem, such as monetary compensation or relief from responsibilities at home, school, or work

D. Personal history

1. Developmental milestones

a. Information about the patient's early development is important, including details about the pregnancy and delivery. Information may be obtained from the patient, family members, or hospital records.

b. It is important to determine the patient's temperament as a child as well as any important family events, such as death, separation, or divorce, that may have influenced the development of this temperament.

c. School (i.e., grades or delinquency), friends, family stability, early sexual experiences, and neglect or abuse are all issues that must be addressed. The patient's relationships as a child with his or her parents, siblings, or friends can be important barometers.

2. Social history

a. It is important to determine the breadth of the patient's social life; for example, is he or she a loner and how hard or easy is it for the patient to make or keep friends.

b. Determine if there have been any changes in personality noted by the patient or by his or her family or friends.

c. Determine the marriage status and the current level of sexual functioning.

d. Employment history is also important, including the number of jobs the patient has had and the reasons the jobs were terminated, noting any problems with alcoholism or antisocial behavior.

e. Military service history should include the highest rank attained and a history of any disciplinary problems or combat experience.

3. Family history

a. The physician should ask about psychiatric hospitalizations or any other kind of mental health treatment of a family member, including suicide attempts, problems with alcohol, or other psychiatric problems. Families tend to deny significant history.

b. A good family history will also include the genetic risk factors as well as family attitudes toward mental illness and treatment.

c. The physician should also determine if any psychotropic medication is being used successfully by a family member for the same illness. If so, there is a good chance that this medication will be helpful to the present patient.

4. Psychiatric history.
Any previous problem should be noted in the history of the present illness. The physician should note the previous treatment, including the name and address of the therapist, medications, and outcome of treatment.

5. Use and abuse of substances.
Screening questions for alcohol and drug problems should always be asked, including whether or not family or friends ever objected to the patient's drinking or drug problem or whether the patient ever felt that he or she had a problem with alcohol or drugs (legal or illegal), including tobacco.

II. PSYCHIATRIC EXAMINATION.
The approach to the assessment of a patient with a psychiatric disorder should always include the psychiatric interview and the mental status examination. It may also include, as necessary, a physical examination, laboratory studies, and psychological tests.

A. Psychiatric interview

1. Physician–patient relationship

a. Patients are often anxious about a psychiatric evaluation. They may be self-referred, but most often they are referred by another health care professional and, thus, are ambivalent about the psychiatric examination. The physician must be courteous and respectful and acknowledge the patient's feelings about being interviewed.

b. The environment can influence the difficulty of the evaluation. The setting of the evaluation can range from a private office to a busy, noisy intensive care unit in a general hospital.

c. Family (or others) may provide important information. However, permission to question family members must always be obtained from the patient.

d. Interruptions from pagers or phones must be minimized. Time to complete the interview must be sufficient. While classically the interview is 50–60 minutes long, 20 minutes may be enough.

e. The physician should always sit down to be at eye level with the patient.

2. The informal mental status examination
begins immediately and includes an evaluation of the patient's:

    a. Appearance
    b. Manner of relating
    c. Use of language
    d. Mood and affect
    e. Content of discussion

3. Interview technique
    a. The interviewer must lead the interview, using both open-ended and specific questions.
        (1) Open-ended questions allow the patients to use their own language; for example, "Tell me about your home life," or "Tell me how your hospital stay has been."
        (2) Direct, specific questions are also important; for example, "Have you ever consulted a mental health professional before," or "Are you thinking about killing yourself?"
    b. It is crucial to communicate to the patient that you are listening.
        (1) Attentive silence. Allowing the patient to talk is important but not sufficient. The physician must establish eye contact and convey the message that he or she is interested in what the patient is saying.
        (2) Facilitation. Comments, such as "Tell me more about it," help the patient to focus while relating the history.
        (3) Summarization. The interviewer should briefly sum up portions of the patient's story; for example, "So you have been increasingly sad for 3 weeks during which time you have lost 7 lb and have been waking up at 4:00 A.M." This lets the patient know that the physician has been listening and also allows the patient to correct any misunderstandings.
        (4) Clarification. Clarifying statements are similar to summary statements but also include connections of which the patient may not be aware; for example, "Your difficulty sleeping and your crying spells began in mid-September. Was this after your youngest child left for college?"

B. Mental status examination. In contrast to the psychiatric history, which is a record of the patient over the course of his or her entire life, the mental status examination is an evaluation of the patient at one point in time. During the interview, the physician should make observations about the following:

    1. Appearance. Interviewers should note overall appearance, dress, grooming, and any unusual features or gestures, particularly what makes the patient unique or different.

    2. Attitude. It is important to note how the patient relates to the physician and to being interviewed, including whether the patient is cooperative, uncooperative, bored, seductive, hostile, and so on.

    3. Behavior and psychomotor activity. The physician should note gait, position, and overall level of activity, noting any twitches, mannerisms, agitation, or psychomotor retardation. Manic patients may be unable to sit still, whereas schizophrenic patients may exhibit bizarre postures or be abnormally stiff and awkward.

    4. Speech. The physician should describe how the patient speaks, noting:
        a. Rate of speech (e.g., rapid, slow, pressured, or halting speech)
        b. Amount of speech (e.g., taciturn, lacking spontaneity, or grandiose speech)
        c. Tone of speech (e.g., monotone, emotional, sing-song, or slurred speech)
        d. Speech impairments (e.g., dysarthria, stuttering, or echolalia). Also, note accents, dialects, or any other unusual speech pattern.
        e. Aphasia, which is a disorder of speech and language due to neurologic illness. The patient is either unable to speak normally or unable to comprehend speech properly. It is important for the clinician to distinguish aphasia from disorders of speech and language due to psychiatric illness.

    5. Mood and affect. The emotional state of the patient that is experienced internally is **mood**. The outward expression of the patient's internal emotional state is **affect**.
        a. It is important to note whether mood and affect are the same; for example:
            (1) A patient who has a depressed mood is likely to appear sad and quiet and speak softly and slowly. However, some depressed patients have an agitated and anxious affect.
            (2) A schizophrenic individual may act silly or unconcerned while discussing a very sad event, such as the death of a loved one. This inappropriate "split" between affective feeling and thought content has led to the use of the term "schizophrenia" or split mind; it does not mean "split personality."
        b. It is important also to note the depth and range of emotional expression.

      (1) **Labile affect** describes sudden shifts in emotional state. The patient may laugh one minute and cry the next without a clear stimulus.

      (2) **Flat affect** describes a shallow and blunted emotional state. Facial expression and voice are lacking spontaneity.

6. Perception. The presence of a perceptual problem should be noted in the mental status examination or in the history. Perceptual abnormalities involve the sensory nervous system and include:

  a. Hallucinations. Hallucinations are false perceptions of a sensory stimulus in the absence of a sensory stimulus. Any sensory modality can be involved.

    (1) **Auditory hallucinations** are seen in psychosis. The hallucinations contain voices, not just sounds, that criticize, comment on the patient's actions, or give commands.

    (2) **Visual hallucinations** are often seen with organic psychosis, especially toxic or drug-related states.

    (3) **Gustatory (taste) and olfactory (smell) hallucinations** should alert the physician to a disorder of the temporal lobe.

    (4) **Tactile hallucinations** are also seen in organic states, such as alcohol withdrawal or cocaine and amphetamine abuse. **Formication** is the tactile hallucination of insects crawling over the skin.

    (5) **Kinesthetic hallucinations** include feeling movement when none occurs. "Out of body" experiences described in near-death situations may be examples of kinesthetic hallucinations. This phenomenon is usually described as floating above one's body and looking down on the scene.

    (6) Hallucinations of any sort that occur while falling asleep (**hypnagogic**) or awakening (**hypnopompic**) are not necessarily considered serious or pathologic and are seen in normal individuals.

  b. Illusions. An illusion is the misinterpretation of a true sensory stimulus. For example, a patient in the hospital may misperceive the movement of the bed curtain as a person and become frightened. Illusions can be present in schizophrenia but are most common in delirium.

  c. Depersonalization and derealization are alterations in the perception of one's reality. With depersonalization, the patient feels detached and views him- or herself as strange and unreal. Derealization involves a similar alteration in the sense of reality of the outside world. Objects in the outside world may seem altered in size and shape, and people appear dead or mechanical.

7. Thinking process. The pattern of a patient's speech allows the examiner to note the quality of the thought process, including its flow, logic, and associations. Abnormalities of the thinking process include:

  a. Loose associations. This involves the shifting of ideas from one to another with no logical connection, accompanied by a lack of awareness on the part of the patient that these ideas are not connected. The patient's thoughts are difficult for the examiner to follow.

  b. Tangential thinking. The patient wanders off the subject as new but related words are spoken. The associations are not totally loose, that is, the examiner can usually follow the patient, but the patient often loses track of the question.

  c. Circumstantiality. The patient loses the point of what he or she is trying to say as with tangential thinking; however, with circumstantiality, the patient stays in the general topic area. Irrelevant details cause digressions in conversation, which can be mild if the patient is merely anxious but can be severe if the patient is delirious and distractible.

  d. Blocking occurs when the thinking process stops altogether. The mind goes blank. Blocking can occur in states of acute anxiety as well as in schizophrenia.

  e. Perseveration is the repetition of the same words or phrases over and over again despite the interviewer's direction to stop.

  f. Echolalia is the direct repetition of the interviewer's words, like a parrot.

  g. Flight of ideas, as seen in mania, involves rapid speech with quick changes of ideas that may be associated, such as by the sound of the words, but may also involve loose associations.

8. Content of thought. Disturbances in the thought content include:

  a. Delusions, which are fixed, false beliefs that are outside the patient's culture. For example, the belief that thoughts are being broadcast outside one's head is a delusion, but a belief in Santa Claus is not. Delusions can be paranoid (or persecutory), grandiose, nihilistic, somatic, or bizarre. **Delusions of reference** involve the belief by the patient that some person or object has special significance or power, such as being convinced that a radio disk jockey is sending the patient special commands.

      (1) Because delusions are fixed, false beliefs, they are not amenable to correction by the physician. Contradicting the patient's delusional belief may cause the patient to get angry and stop the interview.

      (2) The physician should not pretend to agree with the delusion but rather should take a neutral stance and continue the examination.

  b. Obsessions, which are intrusive thoughts, ideas, or impulses that are persistent. The patient recognizes that the ideas do not make sense and are not being imposed from outside (a delusion). An example is a patient who is always fighting an impulse to run down the hall of the office building through a plate glass window at the end. He knows that it is potentially life-threatening and does not want to hurt himself but still cannot stop thinking about it and feeling anxious. Other obsessions commonly seen are fears of contamination or obsessive unrealistic fears about physical health as seen in hypochondriasis (see Chapter 7).

  c. Suicidal and homicidal thoughts. Every mental status examination should include questions about violence towards the self or others. The interviewer must exercise judgment and tact in discussing these issues, but the questions must be asked.

9. Judgment. The clinician should assess the social judgment of the patient during the examination by determining whether the patient understands the consequences of his actions; for example, asking the patient a judgment question, such as "What would you do if you were stranded at Kennedy Airport with only $1.00 in your pocket," can help with this determination. The examiner must, however, recognize differences in cultural values when assessing judgment.

10. Cognition and sensorium. The ability of the brain to function is also measured by the mental status examination. A formal mental status examination, a number of which are available, is necessary to examine adequately the patient's orientation, concentration, and memory. Although all mental status examinations are somewhat limited in scope as compared to extensive neuropsychological tests, the Mini-Mental State examination shown in Figure 1-1 is a useful bedside clinical examination.

C. Clinical laboratory studies. The clinical laboratory has become increasingly important in the diagnosis and treatment of psychiatric illness. The three main functions of the laboratory include: screening patients for any underlying medical ("organic") condition that might be causing the psychiatric symptom, monitoring blood levels of psychotropic medications, and identifying biologic markers in the diagnoses and treatment process. This last area is one of the most exciting new areas of psychiatric research.

  1. Screening tests for organic illness
    a. Suggested studies
      (1) Complete blood count
      (2) Blood chemistry
        (a) Serum glucose
        (b) Electrolytes, including calcium and phosphorus
        (c) Liver function tests, SGOT, SGPT, and bilirubin
        (d) Blood urea nitrogen
      (3) Urine analysis
      (4) Screening for syphilis   T P H A
      (5) Electrocardiogram
      (6) Thyroid function tests
      (7) Chest x-ray
      (8) Vitamin B_{12} and folate levels
    b. Additional procedures when clinically indicated (i.e., when routine laboratory studies are negative but an organic etiology is still suspected) include:
      (1) Arterial blood gas analysis
      (2) Blood alcohol level
      (3) Urine drug screen
      (4) Lumbar puncture and examination of the cerebrospinal fluid
      (5) Thyroid function tests
      (6) Heavy metal screen
      (7) Antinuclear antibodies
      (8) Serum and urine copper levels
      (9) Urine for uroporphyria
      (10) Pregnancy test
      (11) Human immunodeficiency virus (HIV) test
      (12) Mono spot test for infectious mononucleosis

Patient _____
Examiner _____
Date _____

MINI-MENTAL STATE

Maximum
Score   Score

ORIENTATION

5   ( ) What is the (year) (season) (date) (day) (month)?
5   ( ) Where are we: (state) (country) (town) (hospital) (floor)?

REGISTRATION

3   ( ) Name 3 objects (1 second to say each). Then ask the patient all 3 after you have said them. Give 1 point for each correct answer. Then repeat them until he learns all 3. Count trials and record.

Trials_____

ATTENTION AND CALCULATION

5   ( ) Serial 7's: Give 1 point for each correct answer. Stop after 5 answers. Alternatively spell "world" backwards.

RECALL

3   ( ) Ask for the 3 objects repeated above. Give 1 point for each correct answer.

LANGUAGE

9   ( ) Name a pencil and watch (2 points).
Repeat the following: "No ifs, ands, or buts" (1 point).
Follow a 3-stage command: "Take a paper in your right hand, fold it in half, and put it on the floor" (3 points).
Read and obey the following:
Close your eyes (1 point).
Write a sentence (1 point).
Copy design (1 point).

_____ Total score

ASSESS level of consciousness along a continuum _____

Alert Drowsy Stupor Coma

INSTRUCTIONS FOR ADMINISTRATION OF
MINI-MENTAL STATE EXAMINATION

ORIENTATION

(1) Ask for the date. Then ask specifically for parts omitted (e.g., "Can you also tell me what season it is?") Give 1 point for each answer.
(2) Ask in turn, "Can you tell me the name of this hospital?" (town, country, etc.). Give 1 point for each correct answer.

Figure 1-1. The mini-mental state examination. (Reprinted with permission from Folstein MF, Folstein SE, McHugh PR: Mini-mental state, a practical method for grading the cognitive state of patients. *Psych Res* 12:189–198, 1975.)

REGISTRATION

Ask the patient if you may test his memory. Then say the names of 3 unrelated objects, clearly and slowly (1 second to say each). After you have said all 3, ask patient to repeat them. This first repetition determines the score (0–3), but keep saying them until he can repeat all 3 (up to 6 trials). If the patient does not eventually learn all 3, recall cannot be meaningfully tested.

ATTENTION AND CALCULATION

Ask the patient to begin with 100 and count backwards by 7. Stop after 5 subtractions (93, 86, 79, 72, 65). Score the total number of correct answers.

If the patient cannot or will not perform this task, ask him to spell the word "world" backwards. The score is the number of letters in correct order (e.g., dlrow = 5, dlorw = 3).

RECALL

Ask the patient to recall the 3 words previously asked (score 0–3).

LANGUAGE

Naming: Show the patient a wrist watch and ask what it is. Repeat for pencil (score 0–2).

Repetition: Ask the patient to repeat the sentence after you. Allow only 1 trial (score 0 or 1).

Three-stage command: Give the patient a piece of plain blank paper and repeat the command. Give 1 point for each part correctly executed.

Reading: On a blank piece of paper print the sentence, "Close your eyes," in letters large enough for the patient to see clearly. Ask the patient to read it, and do what it says. Give 1 point if the patient actually closes his eyes.

Writing: Give the patient a blank piece of paper and ask him to write a sentence for you. Do not dictate a sentence; it is to be written spontaneously. It must contain a subject and verb and be sensible. Correct grammar and punctuation are not necessary.

Copying: On a clean piece of paper, draw 2 intersecting pentagons (each side about 1 in), and ask the patient to copy them exactly as they are. All 10 angles must be present, and 2 must intersect to score 1 point. Tremor and rotation are ignored.

Estimate the patient's level of sensorium along a continuum, from alert on the left to coma on the right.

Figure 1-1. Continued.

c. **Electroencephalography (EEG)**
   (1) The EEG can be used to diagnose a variety of seizure disorders. The behavior associated with temporal lobe seizure (partial complex seizure) is sometimes difficult to distinguish from "functional" psychiatric disorders.
   (2) In delirium, due to metabolic problems, the EEG generally shows high voltage slow wave activity and can be helpful in the differential diagnosis.
d. **Neuroendocrine tests**
   (1) **Dexamethasone suppression test (DST).** This test has limited value in diagnosing mental illness but can be used to follow the response of a depressed patient to treatment. The patient is given 1 mg of dexamethasone orally at 11:00 P.M. Plasma cortisol levels are measured at 8:00 A.M. and 4:00 P.M. (rarely also 11:00 P.M.). The dexamethasone should ordinarily suppress the patient's cortisol response. Plasma cortisol levels above 5 μg/dl are considered abnormal. Unfortunately, a number of conditions, such as dehydration, alcohol abuse, hypertension, diabetes, weight loss, and several drugs, can give a false-positive result.
   (2) **Thyrotropin-releasing hormone (TRH) stimulation test.** Some depressed patients have a subclinical hypothyroid condition that causes depression. Other patients may have a lithium-induced hypothyroidism. The TRH stimulation test involves the intravenous injection of 500 mg of TRH. Thyroid-stimulating hormone (TSH) is measured at 15, 30, and 90 minutes. Normally, plasma TSH levels will rise sharply 10–20 μg/ml above baseline. An increase of less than 7 μg/ml is considered suppressed and may correlate with the diagnosis of depression.

e. Sleep studies: polysomnography. Several medical problems associated with psychiatric symptoms, such as sleep apnea, seizure disorders, headaches, sexual dysfunction, and insomnia can be evaluated by the sleep laboratory. In addition, patients with major depression also have abnormal sleep patterns. The sleep laboratory uses the EEG, ECG, and the electromyogram (EMG) along with (as needed) the penile tumescence plethysmograph, oxygen saturation, and movement measuring devices. In depression, findings have included:
   (1) Hyposomnia
   (2) Rapid eye movement (REM)–latency, that is, a shortened time between the onset of sleep and the onset of the first REM period
   (3) Greater proportion of REM sleep early in the night

2. Monitoring plasma levels of psychotropic drugs. In general, the judgment of the clinician remains the most important aspect of monitoring therapeutic efficiency. However, it is becoming increasingly useful to monitor blood levels of certain psychotropics.
   a. Lithium. Because of the potential toxicity of lithium at blood levels very close to therapeutic levels, monitoring lithium levels is mandatory. Plasma samples should be drawn 10–12 hours after the last dose of lithium.
      (1) Therapeutic levels range between 0.6–1.5 mg/L.
      (2) Toxicity usually occurs at levels above 2.0 mg/L but may occur at lower levels.
   b. Cyclic antidepressants. Plasma levels of tricyclic antidepressants can be useful in adjusting dosages, checking on compliance, and minimizing toxic side effects. The drugs most often studied are nortriptyline, amitriptyline, imipramine, and desipramine.
      (1) Nortriptyline has a therapeutic window* at plasma levels between 50–175 ng/ml.
      (2) Amitriptyline has a therapeutic window* between 150–250 ng/ml.
      (3) Imipramine has a linear response curve (i.e., the favorable response correlates with plasma levels beginning at about 150 ng/ml). Above 300 ng/ml, side effects outweigh therapeutic effects. A sample should be taken 10–12 hours after the last dose.
      (4) Desipramine is similar to imipramine but has not been as well studied. Plasma levels below 145 ng/ml may be therapeutic.
   c. Neuroleptics. Therapeutic levels for antipsychotic medications have not been as well established as therapeutic levels for antidepressants. Blood levels may be used to check compliance or nonabsorption.

3. Identifying biologic markers by brain imaging
   a. Computed tomography (CT). The CT scan can visualize lesions larger than 0.5 cm on cross section. Additionally, increased ventricle size associated with loss of brain cells can be demonstrated. This may have some usefulness in demonstrating type II schizophrenia as well as dementia. Type II schizophrenia is characterized by chronicity, poor response to medications, negative symptoms, and neurologic signs.
   b. Magnetic resonance imaging (MRI). This technique is based on measuring radio frequencies emitted by nuclei when a strong magnetic field is applied. Detailed anatomy can be seen. Lesions not seen by CT scan, such as demyelinating diseases (e.g., multiple sclerosis), can be demonstrated.
   c. Positron emission tomography (PET) demonstrates specific areas of brain activity. Organic compounds, such as glucose, are labeled by short-lived positron-emitting elements of oxygen, carbon, and nitrogen. A cyclotron is required to produce the labeled glucose, which limits widespread use of this technique. The prepared compound can be localized in the brain, thus demonstrating the biochemical activity of specific brain areas. For example, decreased activity in the frontal cortex has been demonstrated in patients with schizophrenia. PET does not demonstrate detailed anatomy or lesions less than 0.5 cm.

D. Psychological tests. These tests provide a relatively standardized objective measurement of certain aspects of the patient, such as intelligence and personality.

1. Intelligence tests. Most of these tests measure what is called the intelligence quotient (IQ), which is arbitrarily defined as mental age/chronologic age × 100. An individual's test score is compared to a standard or norm established by giving the same tasks to a large group of people. These tests are influenced by culture and do not measure the entire intellectual capacity of the individual being tested. By definition, an average IQ is 100 (rage 90–110). The **Wechsler Adult Intelligence Scale (WAIS)** is the most widely used intelligence test.

---

*The therapeutic effect of this drug increases as blood levels increase until an upper limit of the blood level is reached.

   a. It has six verbal and five performance subjects, including information, comprehension, arithmetic, similarities, digit span, vocabulary, picture completion, block design, picture arrangement, object assembly, and digit symbol.
   b. This test generates a verbal IQ, a performance IQ, and a full-scale or combined IQ. A difference between the verbal and performance IQ scores of greater than 10 points is suggestive of an organic brain syndrome.

2. Personality tests
   a. Minnesota Multiphasic Personality Inventory (MMPI). The MMPI consists of 550 yes or no questions answered by the patient. The results are given as scores in 10 scales: hypochondriasis, paranoia, masculinity–femininity, psychopathy, depression, hysteria, psychasthenia, schizophrenia, hypomania, and social introversion. The pattern of scores is interpreted comparing the patient's score (and subscores) against standardized data. Although a relatively objective test, a trained psychologist should interpret the MMPI test results.
   b. Rorschach Test. This is the famous inkblot test. Ten standard ambiguous inkblots are shown to the patient in a set order. The patient's responses are then explored. This is a "projective" test in which the patient demonstrates his or her thinking and association patterns.
   c. Thematic Apperception Test (TAT). Also a projective test, TAT consists of 30 pictures, not all of which are shown. The psychologist chooses a specific picture, depending on the psychological area to be examined. For example, one of the pictures shows a seated young woman looking up at an older man. The patient is asked to make up a story about the picture. This requires that the patient indirectly reveal his or her fantasies, fears, and conflicts. The test is not particularly useful in developing a descriptive diagnosis.
   d. Sentence Completion Test (SCT). Like TAT, this test is used to elicit the patient's associations. The test consists of a series of incomplete sentences that the patient is asked to complete. Examples are, "I am afraid . . . ," "I feel guilty . . . ," and "My mother is . . . ." The psychologist notes the themes and feeling tone in the responses of the patient as well as subject areas that the patient avoids.
   e. Draw-a-Person Test (DAP). Originally used only with children, this test can also be used with adults. The patient is asked to "draw a picture of a person." Then the patient is asked to draw a person of the sex opposite from the person in the first drawing. This test assumes that the drawing represents to some degree the patient's view of him- or herself. The test can also be used to detect brain damage.

3. Neuropsychological tests. Specific aspects of brain functioning can be tested by neuropsychological tests, which are usually given in a battery. Expertise is required to conduct these tests. Neuropsychological tests can be used to detect subtle cognitive defects in patients who are not known to be demented and to assess strengths and weaknesses to aid in the rehabilitation of patients with brain damage.
   a. The Halstead-Reitan battery is a series of tests.
   (1) The trail-making test asks the patient to connect alternating numbers and letters, thereby assessing the patient's visuomotor perception.
   (2) The rhythm test asks the patient to identify pairs of rhythmic beats, thereby assessing auditory perception, attention, and concentration.
   (3) With the other subtests, the neuropsychologist is able to test a variety of brain functions, such as perception, sensation, concept formation, visuomotor–motor integration, and abstract thought.
   b. Luria-Nebraska Neuropsychological battery and **Bender-Gestalt** are also used in diagnosing brain damage.

III. CLASSIFICATION OF MENTAL DISORDERS

A. Problems with definitions. Although the term "mental disorder" does not have a precise definition, it can be defined as a "significant clinical syndrome with behavioral and psychological symptoms, causing distress or impairment in functioning." Historically, mental disorders have been dealt with either as organic, physical problems or as spiritual or cultural phenomena.

1. The cause of a mental disorder may be:
   a. Organic
   b. Psychological
   c. Environmental

2. "Normal reactions" to stressful events, such as the death of a loved one, are not considered mental disorders.

3. Socially unacceptable behavior, such as crime, is not necessarily indicative of a mental disorder.

4. Few diagnostic systems consider mental disorders to involve the brain *and* the mind, but this split has impaired the development of a comprehensive, integrated understanding of mental disorders.

B. **An atheoretical approach to classifying mental disorders** has been undertaken in recent years. *The Diagnostic and Statistical Manual of Mental Disorders*, 3rd edition, revised (*DSM-III-R*) uses a multiaxial evaluation system based as much as possible on phenomenology rather than etiology.

1. **Axis I: Clinical syndromes.** These include organic mental disorders, schizophrenia, depression, and substance abuse.

2. **Axis II: Personality disorders in adults and developmental disorders in children**

3. **Axis III: Physical disorders.** These physical disorders do not have to be causes of the psychiatric symptoms, but they are relevant to the treatment.

4. **Axis IV: Severity of psychosocial stressors.** Stressors can be either acute (less than 6 months' duration) or chronic (greater than 6 months). The physician has to decide how much stress an "average" person would experience given the same stressor as the patient. The severity of the psychological stressors is rated on a scale of 1, which is equal to none, and 6, which is equal to catastrophe. A catastrophic stressor might be the death of a child or being held hostage. Examples of stressors include:
   a. **Marital**, such as engagement, marriage, separation, and divorce
   b. **Parenting**, such as birth, illness of a child, or a problem with a child
   c. **Interpersonal problems**, such as with friends or neighbors
   d. **Occupational**, such as problems at school or work, including retirement
   e. **Living circumstances**, such as moving
   f. **Financial**, such as any change in status, especially loss
   g. **Legal**, such as arrest, lawsuit, or trial
   h. **Developmental milestones**, such as puberty or menopause
   i. **Physical illness or injury.** When related to development of an Axis I disorder, it is listed in Axis III
   j. **Other** includes natural or man-made disaster, rape, or unwanted pregnancy

5. **Axis V: Global assessment of functioning.** The physician is asked to rate the patient's level of social and occupational functioning at the time of the evaluation and during the past year. Axes IV and V can be very helpful in understanding the content of a psychiatric disorder in an individual. They are not, however, diagnoses themselves.

IV. PREVALENCE OF PSYCHIATRIC DISORDERS.
Incidence rates of mental illness are rarely studied because of the difficulty in fixing the time of onset of psychiatric disorders as well as the high likelihood of recurrence. The best study of the prevalence of psychiatric disorders is the Epidemiologic Catchment Area (ECA) study. Fifteen *DSM-III-R* diagnostic categories were studied in three cities (i.e., New Haven, Baltimore, and St. Louis) in the early 1980s (Table 1-1). Since only 15 disorders were studied, the true prevalence for all psychiatric disorders is undoubtedly higher. A cross section of the general population was interviewed.

A. About 15%–20% of the population studied had 1 of the 15 disorders in the past 6 months.

B. Approximately 25%–40% of the general population had one of the disorders sometime during their lifetime.

C. Overall, the rates for men and women were about the same, but there were very different rates between the sexes for specific disorders.

1. Men had higher rates of substance abuse and antisocial personality.

2. Women had higher rates of depression, phobias, and dysthymic disorder.

3. In this study, only women had somatization disorder.

Table 1-1. Results of the Epidemiologic Catchment Area Study

	Males*		Females*	
	6 Months	**Lifetime**	**6 Months**	**Lifetime**
Any *DSM-III-R* disorder	15% – 20%	30% – 40%	15% – 25%	25% – 36%
Substance abuse	10% – 13%	25% – 36%	2% – 4%	8% – 10%
Mood				
Mania	0.5% – 1%	1%	0.5% – 1%	0.5% – 1.5%
Major depressive episode	1% – 2%	2% – 5%	3% – 5%	5% – 9%
Dysthymia	1% – 2%	1% – 2%	3% – 5%	3% – 5%
Schizophrenia	1%	1%	0.5% – 1.5%	1% – 2.5%
Anxiety				
Agoraphobia	1% – 3%	1.5% – 5%	4% – 8%	5% – 12%
Simple phobia	2% – 8%	4% – 14%	6% – 15%	8% – 26%
Panic	0.3% – 0.8%	0.6% – 1.2%	1%	1% – 3%
Obsessive–compulsive	1% – 2%	1% – 2%	2%	2% – 3%
Somatization	0%	0%	3%	3%
Antisocial personality	1% – 2%	4% – 5%	0.3% – 1%	0.5% – 1%
Severe cognitive impairment	1%	1%	1%	1%

*Approximate percentage of the general population.

STUDY QUESTIONS

Directions: Each question below contains five suggested answers. Choose the **one best** response to each question.

1. Special skill is needed in conducting a psychiatric interview because

(A) psychiatric patients usually do not tell the truth
(B) patients may be embarrassed about their symptoms
(C) patients usually cannot remember all the details
(D) patients may be afraid of the legal consequences of their answers
(E) patients are usually too psychotic to give accurate details

2. A history of being fired from jobs or leaving them for any reason on multiple occasions is a clue to the diagnosis of

(A) depression
(B) schizophrenia
(C) schizoid personality
(D) antisocial personality
(E) none of the above

3. The examination of a patient with a psychiatric disorder should always include

(A) a physical examination
(B) laboratory studies
(C) psychological tests
(D) a mental status examination
(E) screening tests for organic illness

4. The psychiatric interview should always be conducted

(A) in a quiet office
(B) with family members
(C) for at least 45 minutes
(D) with complete confidentiality
(E) at eye level

5. The informal mental status examination includes an observation of all of the following factors EXCEPT

(A) the patient's appearance
(B) recent memory
(C) mood and affect
(D) manner of relating
(E) use of language

6. The condition in which a person is unable to provide normal language due to a neurologic condition is

(A) dysarthria
(B) stuttering
(C) echolalia
(D) pressured speech
(E) aphasia

7. A person who laughs one minute and cries the next without any clear stimulus is said to have

(A) flat affect
(B) euphoria
(C) labile mood
(D) labile affect
(E) "split personality"

8. A false perception of a sensory stimulus in the absence of a stimulus is

(A) hallucination
(B) illusion
(C) delusion
(D) derealization
(E) depersonalization

9. A condition in which the patient feels detached from him- or herself as though an outside observer is called

(A) derealization
(B) depersonalization
(C) illusion
(D) hallucination
(E) detachment

10. Circumstantiality is a disorder of

(A) mood
(B) affect
(C) speech
(D) behavior
(E) thinking

11. If a patient presents with a paranoid delusion about the Federal Bureau of Investigation (FBI) bugging the phones, the physician should

(A) explain to the patient what a delusion is
(B) call the FBI to prove that the idea is false
(C) go along with the patient to establish rapport
(D) listen without agreeing or disagreeing
(E) stop the examination and hospitalize the patient

12. A decrease in rapid eye movement (REM)–latency, that is, the period between the onset of sleep and the onset of the first REM period, is seen in

(A) dementia
(B) delirium
(C) schizophrenia
(D) depression
(E) alcoholism

13. An example of a catastrophic stress is

(A) moving
(B) loss of job
(C) puberty
(D) death of child
(E) retirement

14. In the Epidemiologic Catchment Area (ECA) study, the most prevalent disorder in all three cities studied was

(A) depression
(B) schizophrenia
(C) alcoholism
(D) phobias
(E) dementia

Directions: Each question below contains four suggested answers of which **one or more** is correct. Choose the answer

A if **1, 2, and 3** are correct
B if **1 and 3** are correct
C if **2 and 4** are correct
D if **4** is correct
E if **1, 2, 3, and 4** are correct

15. A complete psychiatric examination must include an investigation of

(1) suicidal thoughts
(2) homicidal thoughts
(3) delusional thoughts
(4) hallucinations

16. In conducting a psychiatric interview, it is important to

(1) spend at least an hour with the patient
(2) address the patient's feeling about the evaluation
(3) see the family to obtain information about the patient
(4) minimize interruptions from pagers or phones

17. Developmental milestones that should be reviewed in evaluating a patient's history include

(1) school performance (e.g., grades)
(2) number of marriages
(3) death of a parent
(4) employment record

18. In taking a family history from a patient, it is important to

(1) realize that families tend to deny mental illness
(2) learn about potential genetic risks for the patient
(3) obtain information about suicide attempts in family members
(4) inquire about effective psychotropic medications used by family members

19. A patient suffering from a serious depression may be likely to demonstrate

(1) silly and unconcerned affect
(2) agitated and anxious affect
(3) flat or restricted affect
(4) sad and unhappy affect

20. Hallucinations that are generally considered symptoms of serious mental disorders include

(1) auditory
(2) hypnopompic
(3) visual
(4) hypnagogic

21. Examples of delusional thinking include

(1) a belief that one's internal organs are rotting away from disease
(2) viewing people as either dead or mechanical
(3) a belief that co-workers are organizing a plot to get one fired
(4) an intrusive impulse to scream obscenities in church

22. Disorders of the thinking process that may be observed during the informal mental status examination include

(1) circumstantiality
(2) lability
(3) blocking
(4) derealization

23. If someone is said to be disoriented, it is likely that they do not know

(1) the date
(2) where they are
(3) what time it is
(4) who is President

24. The dexamethasone suppression test has limited usefulness in the diagnosis of depression because

(1) the difficulty in conducting the test has led to patient noncompliance
(2) plasma control levels have a diurnal variation
(3) the test is too expensive for routine use
(4) many medical conditions give false-positive results

25. Measuring blood levels of tricyclic antidepressants in the laboratory can be useful to

(1) adjust dosages
(2) check on patient compliance
(3) minimize toxic side effects
(4) minimize tolerance and addiction

26. Blood levels of neuroleptic medications are useful to check

(1) therapeutic levels
(2) noncompliance
(3) toxicity
(4) nonabsorption

27. Computerized tomography of the brain has been useful in

(1) visualizing lesions larger than 0.5 cm
(2) demonstrating loss of brain cells
(3) demonstrating abnormalities seen in type II schizophrenia
(4) visualizing biochemical activity in the brain

28. Intelligence tests, which measure the intelligence quotient (IQ), have which of the following characteristics?

(1) they compare an individual against a large group
(2) they are influenced by culture
(3) they do not measure an individual's entire intellectual capacity
(4) they define as average an IQ of 100

29. Scales used in the Minnesota Multiphasic Personality Inventory (MMPI) include

(1) block design
(2) masculinity–femininity
(3) vocabulary
(4) schizophrenia

30. The Thematic Apperception Test has which of the following characteristics?

(1) it uses pictures of scenes and people
(2) it asks the patient to "project" his or her fantasies and conflicts
(3) it uses specific pictures, depending on the areas to be examined
(4) it is useful in developing a descriptive diagnosis

ANSWERS AND EXPLANATIONS

1. The answer is B. (*I A 2*) Patients who have psychiatric problems are often embarrassed about disclosing their symptoms to the physician. Stigma regarding psychiatric illness is still prevalent in our society. However, patients do not usually lie when asked in a sensitive manner by the physician. Unless they have a memory deficit, they can generally give accurate details. Occasionally, some patients may be afraid of the legal consequences of their answers, but this is unusual. Most psychiatric patients are not psychotic, and even many psychotic patients can give accurate details of their history.

2. The answer is D. (*I D 2 d*) History of work performance is important in understanding a patient's stability in terms of important life functions. Patients who are depressed sometimes do not function well but generally do not have a long history of multiple job losses. The same is true for patients with schizophrenia who are often underemployed and do not have good work records but do not have a history of being fired from many jobs. Schizoid personalities tend to avoid changes. Patients with antisocial personality disorder, however, often have a long history of multiple job firings. This history can be a clue to the diagnosis.

3. The answer is D. (*II*) When a patient with a psychiatric disorder is examined for the first time, a mental status examination should always be conducted. Physical examination, psychological tests, and laboratory tests, including screening tests for organic illness, are very important but are not always necessary as are the psychiatric interview and the mental status examination. For example, a patient who complains of anxiety along with headache and a tremor should at least have his or her blood pressure checked as well as laboratory studies of thyroid function evaluated.

4. The answer is E. (*II A 1 b–e*) The psychiatric interview should always be conducted at eye level with the patient. This can be very important when interviews are conducted in medical settings, such as a general hospital. It is not always possible to conduct an interview in a quiet office, although this is obviously helpful when possible. Family members may be interviewed when they can provide helpful information, but issues of confidentiality need to be considered. Psychiatric interviews do not have a specific time limit, and while generally confidential, there are aspects of psychiatric interviews, such as when threats are made against another individual, where confidentiality is not absolute.

5. The answer is B. (*II A 2*) The *informal* mental status examination begins when the physician first observes the patient. It should include the patient's appearance, manner of relating, use of language, mood and affect, and content of the discussion. Assessment of recent memory requires a *formal* mental status examination.

6. The answer is E. (*II B 4 e*) Disorder of speech and language due to neurologic illness is called aphasia. The patient is unable to speak normally or to comprehend speech properly. It is important to distinguish aphasia from other psychiatric problems, such as echolalia, pressured speech, or stuttering. In dysarthria, the patient has difficulty enunciating but can produce normal language.

7. The answer is D. (*II B 5*) The person who laughs one minute and cries the next without a clear stimulus from the environment is said to have a labile affect. Mood is considered an emotional state of the patient as experienced by the patient, and since it is unclear what the patient experiences at this time, a labile mood is not correct. For example, a patient might be depressed with a depressed mood (feel sad inside) but demonstrate an anxious affect to the interviewer. Flat affect involves little or no demonstration of emotion, and split personality defines a split between affective feeling and thought content.

8. The answer is A. (*II B 6 a–c, 8 a*) Hallucination is defined as a false perception of a stimulus in the absence of any stimulus. An illusion occurs when there is a misperception of a true stimulus, and a delusion is a fixed, false belief. Depersonalization and derealization are alterations in the perception of reality. They usually occur together. In derealization, the immediate environment is perceived as somehow unreal or changed. In depersonalization, the experience is of being detached or outside one's body.

9. The answer is B. (*II B 6 c*) Depersonalization is the condition in which a patient feels detached from him- or herself as though an outside observer. One's reality is distorted and misperceived. Derealization involves an alteration in the sense of reality of the outside world. Illusion is a misperception of a sensory stimulus, and hallucination is a false perception of a sensory stimulus where one is not present. Detachment is not a technical term used in psychiatry to describe a mental phenomenon.

10. The answer is E. (*II B 7 c*) Circumstantiality is a problem in a patient's thinking, which manifests in the pattern of speech. The patient wanders around a given subject without totally losing track of the subject but often losing the point of what he or she is trying to say. It is not a disorder of mood or affect. While it is sometimes called circumstantial speech, it is a problem of thinking rather than speech.

11. The answer is D. (*II B 8 a*) Because a delusion is a fixed, false belief, it is not useful to try to correct the patient's belief, especially during the evaluation interview. It is best to take a neutral stance and continue the interview. Also, it is not helpful to agree with the patient to something that obviously is not true. While a patient may need to be hospitalized at some point, it is again important to continue the interview to find out more information.

12. The answer is D. [*II C 1 e (2)*] A decrease in rapid eye movement (REM)–latency is seen in the sleep electroencephalograms of depressed patients. No evidence of this has been detected in such conditions as dementia, delirium, schizophrenia, or alcoholism.

13. The answer is D. (*III B 4*) Catastrophic stressors are such things as the death of a child or being held hostage. To determine the severity of a stressor, the physician must decide how much stress an average person would experience given the same stressor as the patient. Therefore, loss of a job or moving, while high stressors, are not generally seen as catastrophic. Puberty and retirement are life-phase stressors, and the normal person does not experience these as catastrophic.

14. The answer is C. (*IV; Table 1-1*) The Epidemiologic Catchment Area study reported that the highest prevalence of illness in three cities was alcohol abuse, after which came phobias. Depression, schizophrenia, and dementia were significantly less common. Alcohol abuse has a lifetime prevalence of 25%–36% of men and 8%–10% of women. Simple phobias were present in 4%–14% of men and 8%–26% of women over a lifetime. These disorders were far more common than any other in the study, but alcoholism was overall the most prevalent condition.

15. The answer is E (all). (*II B 6 a, 8 a, c*) Every psychiatric examination must evaluate a patient's suicidal and homicidal potential. In addition, questions must be asked about the content of thought, including delusions and hallucinations. While hallucinations and delusions are not usually present in the normal mental status examination, they still must be ruled out by questions from the physician.

16. The answer is C (2, 4). (*II A 1 a–e*) Most patients are ambivalent about a psychiatric evaluation. They are concerned that they are going crazy or are seen as bad, especially when they are referred by other health care professionals. It is important to address the patient's feelings about being evaluated early in the interview. It is also important to minimize interruptions from pagers and phones. The amount of time needed for the interview should be sufficient but may be as short as 20 minutes or so. While the family can provide very important information, it is always important to see a patient first and discuss any potential interaction with family members.

17. The answer is B (1, 3). (*I D 1*) Developmental milestones that should be reviewed in a patient's history include early childhood problems, especially a death or separation from a parent, and school performance, including grades, friends, and delinquency. The number of times a patient has been married and his employment record are part of the social rather than developmental history.

18. The answer is E (all). (*I D 3*) Family histories are increasingly important in the evaluation of a psychiatric patient. The physician should realize that families tend to minimize or deny mental illness and do not talk about it easily. It is important, however, to learn about family mental illness because of the increased genetic risk in patients. If a psychotropic medication has been used successfully in a family member, it is more likely to be useful in the patient because of genetic factors.

19. The answer is C (2, 4). (*II B 5*) Generally speaking, depressed patients are expected to exhibit a sad and unhappy affect; however, they may also exhibit an agitated and anxious affect. A silly and unconcerned affect and a flat or restricted affect are more likely to be seen in schizophrenia.

20. The answer is B (1, 3). [*II B 6 a (1)–(6)*] Hypnopompic and hypnagogic hallucinations, which occur either while the patient is awaking or falling sleep, are seen in normal individuals. Auditory and visual hallucinations are generally considered signs of serious mental disorders, including schizophrenic and organic psychoses.

21. The answer is B (1, 3). (*II B 6 c, 8 a, b*) Delusions are fixed, false beliefs that are not amenable to reality testing. Examples are a belief that one's internal organs are rotting (somatic delusion) or that co-workers are organizing to get one fired (paranoid delusion). Perceiving people as dead or mechanical is a perceptual abnormality called derealization. An intrusive impulse to scream obscenities in church is an obsession, not a delusion.

22. The answer is B (1, 3). (*II B 7 c, d*) Disorders of the thinking process can be observed by following the pattern of the patient's speech, which allows the examiner to note the quality of the thought process. Disorders include circumstantiality where the patient loses the point of what he or she is trying to say and blocking where the patient's thinking stops altogether. Lability refers to quickly changing mood, and derealization is a perceptual abnormality where there is an alteration or loss of the sense of reality of the outside world.

23. The answer is A (1, 2, 3). (*II B 10; Figure 1-1*) Orientation is the ability of the patient to know the date, time, and place. Also, the patient should know who he or she is. Knowing who is President is a question of memory rather than orientation.

24. The answer is D (4). [*II C 1 d (1)*] The dexamethasone suppression test has limited usefulness because a number of conditions, such as dehydration, alcohol abuse, hypertension, diabetes, and weight loss can give false-positive results. The test is not difficult to perform, and patient compliance is not a problem. The timing of the test reconciles the plasma cortisol variation throughout the day, and the test is not particularly expensive in comparison to other biologic tests.

25. The answer is A (1, 2, 3). (*II C 2 b*) The measurement of blood levels of tricyclic antidepressants can be useful in adjusting doses, checking on compliance, and minimizing toxic side effects. Tricyclic antidepressants are not drugs to which patients develop a tolerance or become addicted.

26. The answer is C (2, 4). (*II C 2 c*) Therapeutic blood levels of antipsychotic medications have not been well established, but they can be monitored for noncompliance or nonabsorption. Toxicity is not generally tested by blood levels because therapeutic levels of neuroleptic medications are often toxic.

27. The answer is A (1, 2, 3). (*II C 3 a, c*) Computerized tomography (CT scan) of the brain has been useful in visualizing lesions of the brain larger than 0.5 cm in cross section. Increased atrophy associated with the loss of brain cells as seen in type II schizophrenia can be demonstrated. Biochemical activity is measured by positron emission tomography, not CT scan.

28. The answer is E (all). (*II D 1*) Intelligence tests measure what is called the intelligence quotient (IQ). These tests compare an individual against the standard or norm established by giving the test to a large number of people. The tests are influenced by culture and do not measure the entire intellectual capacity of an individual. By definition, the average IQ is 100 with a range of 90–110.

29. The answer is C (2, 4). (*II D 2 a*) The Minnesota Multiphasic Personality Inventory is a personality inventory study with 10 scales, including hypochondriasis, schizophrenia, masculinity–femininity, paranoia, psychopathy, depression, hysteria, psychasthenia, hypomania, and social introversion. Block design and vocabulary are tested by the Wechsler Adult Intelligence Scale, the most widely used intelligence test.

30. The answer is A (1, 2, 3). (*II D 2 c*) The Thematic Apperception Test consists of a number of pictures, showing various scenes. The patient is asked to project his or her fantasies, fears, and conflicts by telling a story about the picture. Psychologists choose specific pictures to show to individual patients, depending on which psychological area is to be examined. Projective tests, in general, are not useful in developing descriptive diagnoses because they do not focus on phenomenology of symptoms but upon the patient's psychological life.

2

Schizophrenic Disorders

Gordon L. Neligh*

I. **DEFINITION.** Schizophrenia is a disorder, or a group of disorders, characterized by positive and negative symptoms. Positive symptoms are those symptoms that are *added* to the clinical picture, including delusions, hallucinations, and agitation. Negative symptoms are characteristics of the patient that are *subtracted* from the clinical picture, including affective flattening, social withdrawal, apathy, anhedonia, and poverty of thought and content of speech. Current criteria for the diagnosis of schizophrenia require that symptoms be present for at least several months, although the course varies widely among individuals. The etiology of schizophrenia is unknown. The prognosis is highly variable, depending, at least in part, on the diagnostic criteria used to define the disorder. Modern treatment includes a combination of pharmacologic, psychotherapeutic, and psychosocial interventions, the responses to which are also highly variable.

II. **DIAGNOSIS.** For over a century, researchers and clinicians have attempted to define the syndrome of schizophrenia in a way that would help to predict its course, treatment, and prognosis. Diagnostic advances have made possible the identification of genetic, biochemical, psychological, and social factors that contribute to the course and treatment of schizophrenia. Efforts to define the diagnostic criteria for schizophrenia continue. An historical perspective of the dilemma of the diagnosis of schizophrenia is given below.

A. **Emil Kraepelin** (1855–1926) combined catatonia, hebephrenia, and dementia paranoides into a single syndrome of **dementia praecox**, or dementia of early life.

1. He differentiated this condition from conditions caused by stress, manic-depressive insanity, and other mental illnesses.

2. He identified a number of symptoms as being characteristic of dementia praecox, including hallucinations, delusions, thought disorder, abnormalities of speech, and automatic obedience.

3. He identified this illness as having an onset early in life and a progressively deteriorating course in intellectual abilities and emotional functioning.

4. This diagnostic approach lost favor because it was found that patients, even in Kraepelin's group, did not, in fact, share an inevitable deterioration in course and prognosis.

B. **Eugen Bleuler** (1857–1939) noted that patients suffering from dementia praecox did much better as a group than was noted by Kraepelin. Without a uniformly poor prognosis to define the syndrome, Bleuler turned his attention to psychological processes to define the syndrome which he called **schizophrenia** or "split mind."

1. He believed that schizophrenics could improve over time, but he did not believe they could recover fully to their premorbid functioning.

2. He identified disturbances of **association, affect, autism,** and **ambivalence** (known as the **four A's**) as being more characteristic of schizophrenia than a deteriorating course or hallucinations and delusions.

3. As a colleague of Carl Jung, Bleuler's ideas and treatment approaches were strongly influenced by psychoanalytic theory, and as a result, his focus was on the psychological processes of schizophrenia instead of specific behavioral features.

*The author wishes to thank Mark Pecevich, M.D., of the Colorado State Hospital for his comments and suggestions on this chapter.

4. This diagnostic approach has lost favor because of poor interrater reliability in identifying these symptoms and because none of the symptoms is specific to schizophrenia.

C. Kurt Schneider, more recently (1957), has defined diagnostic criteria for schizophrenia on the basis of clustering and frequency of symptoms.

1. He designated a group of the most common or **first rank symptoms,** which include:
   a. Auditory hallucinations (i.e., audible thoughts, voices heard arguing, or voices commenting upon one's actions)
   b. Thought insertion and thought withdrawal
   c. Somatic passivity symptoms
   d. Diffusion of thought
   e. Delusional perception of feelings
   f. Perceptions that impulses and actions are due to the influences of others

2. He cautioned that the diagnosis of schizophrenia can in some cases be made in the absence of first rank symptoms and in the presence of only the less common second rank symptoms.

3. While the first rank symptoms are common among schizophrenics, they are not individually specific to schizophrenia and can be found in other disorders, such as organic mental syndromes and mood disorders.

D. The *Diagnostic and Statistical Manual of Mental Disorders*, 3rd ed., revised (*DSM-III-R*) has taken elements from all of the above diagnostic systems and from studies of the frequency of symptoms in different populations and formulated diagnostic criteria for schizophrenia.

1. Characteristic psychotic symptoms must be present in the active phase for at least 1 week (unless the symptoms are successfully treated). These symptoms include:
   a. Bizarre delusions (i.e., involving a phenomenon that is totally implausible, such as thought broadcasting or being controlled by someone who is deceased)
   b. Prominent hallucinations that have the following characteristics:
      (1) They last for more than a few brief moments.
      (2) They occur over several days or several weeks.
      (3) They consist of voices:
         (a) Speaking without any relation to depression or elation
         (b) Keeping a running commentary on the person's behavior or thoughts
         (c) Conversing together
   c. Incoherence or marked loosening of associations
   d. Catatonic behavior
   e. Flat or grossly inappropriate affect

2. Functioning in work, social relations, and self-care is markedly below the highest level achieved before the onset of the disturbance. When the onset is in childhood or adolescence, there is a failure to achieve an expected level of social development.

3. Schizoaffective disorder and mood disorder with psychotic features must be ruled out (i.e., if present, the duration of all episodes of a major depressive or manic syndrome must be brief relative to the duration of the active disturbance).

4. Continuous signs of the disturbance for at least 6 months. The 6-month period must include an active phase of at least 1 week (or less if symptoms have been successfully treated) during which there were psychotic symptoms characteristic of schizophrenia (see section II D 1) with or without a prodromal or residual phase as defined below.
   a. Prodromal phase consists of a clear deterioration in functioning before the active phase of the disturbance that is not due to a disturbance in mood or to a psychoactive substance use disorder and that involves at least two of the symptoms listed in section II D 4 c.
   b. Residual phase, which follows the active phase, entails the persistence of at least two of the symptoms listed in section II D 4 c, provided these are not due to a disturbance in mood or to a psychoactive substance use disorder.
   c. Prodromal or residual symptoms include the following:
      (1) Marked social isolation or withdrawal
      (2) Marked impairment in role functioning as wage earner, student, or homemaker
      (3) Markedly peculiar behavior (e.g., collecting garbage, talking to self in public, or hoarding food)
      (4) Marked impairment in personal hygiene and grooming
      (5) Blunted or inappropriate affect

(6) Digressive, vague, overelaborate, or circumstantial speech, poverty of speech, or poverty of content of speech

(7) Odd beliefs or magical thinking that influence behavior and that are inconsistent with cultural norms (e.g., superstitiousness, belief in clairvoyance, telepathy, and a "sixth sense"), overvalued ideas, or ideas of reference

(8) Unusual perceptual experiences (e.g., recurrent illusions or sensing the presence of a force or person not actually present)

(9) Marked lack of initiative, interests, or energy

  d. **The durational criteria** of the *DSM-III* and the *DSM-III-R* have been both praised and criticized. Researchers have viewed the narrowing of the diagnostic criteria as a positive step that permits greater accuracy in diagnosis. However, some clinicians feel that the 6-month symptom requirement excludes patients whom they believe to be schizophrenic but who do not fit this diagnostic criterion.

5. **Organic factors cannot be established as initiating and maintaining the disturbance.**

6. **With a history of autistic disorder, the diagnosis of schizophrenia is made only if prominent delusions or hallucinations are also present.**

E. **The International Pilot Study of Schizophrenia** was an attempt by the World Health Organization (WHO) to discover reliable methods of diagnosing schizophrenia across different cultures and national boundaries. Using psychiatric interviews and the Present State Examination (PSE), the most common symptoms were noted (see below). However, the most common symptoms were not necessarily as specific to the diagnosis of schizophrenia as were the less commonly observed symptoms; that is, the most common symptoms are also commonly found in other disorders, such as organic mental disorders and mood disorders.

1. **The most frequently found symptoms** (in descending order) include:
  a. Lack of insight
  b. Auditory hallucinations
  c. Verbal hallucinations
  d. Ideas of reference
  e. Suspiciousness
  f. Flatness of affect
  g. Voices speaking to the patient
  h. Delusional mood
  i. Delusions of persecutions
  j. Inadequate description of problems
  k. Thought alienation
  l. Thoughts spoken aloud

2. **Highest reliability of symptoms** was observed in patients who reported symptoms, such as:
  a. Suicidal ideation
  b. Elated thoughts
  c. Ideas of reference
  d. Delusions of grandeur
  e. Hearing thoughts aloud
  f. Derealization
  g. Lack of concentration
  h. Hopelessness
  i. Delusions of persecution and reference

3. **Lowest reliability of symptoms** was noted in observed data, such as:
  a. Negativism
  b. Perseveration
  c. Stereotyped behavior

4. **Disadvantages.** This diagnostic approach is of limited use with individual patients as it does not propose minimal or threshold criteria for the diagnosis in individual cases. Rather, it has been a basis for other diagnostic systems, such as the *DSM-III-R* and the *International Classification of Diseases*, 9th ed. (*ICD-9*).

III. **EPIDEMIOLOGY.** Because of problems in defining the diagnosis of schizophrenia and difficulties in sampling methods, precise epidemiologic data on schizophrenia have been difficult to obtain.

A. **Incidence, prevalence, and costs**

1. **Incidence** rates reflect the number of new cases of a disorder in a population over a given

time. The incidence of schizophrenia has been reported to range from 0.030%–0.120% a year for individuals over 15 years of age with the greatest incidence rates appearing among the industrialized nations and among groups suffering from high levels of cultural disruption.

2. **Prevalence** is the number of cases in a population at a given time. **Point prevalence** is the number of cases at one instant in time, and **period prevalence** is the number of cases within a specific time period, such as a 6-month prevalence or lifetime prevalence As with the incidence of schizophrenia, developing countries generally have lower prevalence rates of schizophrenia, reflecting lower incidence rates and better prognostic expectations than in the industrialized world (e.g., schizophrenics in the Third World tend to recover from their illness at a higher rate than schizophrenics in the industrialized nations).

   a. **Point prevalence** of schizophrenia has been estimated to be from below 0.010% to as high as 3.0% in different populations, as a result of both varying diagnostic criteria and true differences.

   b. **Lifetime prevalence** of schizophrenia in the United States is estimated to be somewhat less than 1.0%.

3. **Costs.** In the United States, the indirect costs of schizophrenia have been estimated to be between $10 and $20 billion annually.

B. **The sex ratio** of schizophrenia is roughly equal in the Western World; however, men tend to develop schizophrenia earlier than women. In the Third World countries, men appear to suffer from schizophrenia at a rate that may be several times that for women. Perhaps because of the difference in age of onset, men with schizophrenia tend to be single, whereas women with schizophrenia tend to be divorced or separated. Perhaps because of a later onset, women tend to have a better prognosis for schizophrenia in many parts of the world.

C. **Onset** of schizophrenia usually occurs in late adolescence or early adulthood, although cases continue to appear with decreasing frequency throughout adult life.

   1. Onset tends to be earlier for men than women.

   2. Early onset cases tend to have more disorganized features and a worse prognosis for recovery and preservation of function than late onset cases.

   3. Late onset cases tend to have more paranoid features and a better prognosis and preservation of function than early onset cases.

   4. About 25% of schizophrenics have an identifiable schizoid personality, which includes:
      a. Social withdrawal
      b. Passivity
      c. Daydreaming
      d. Few friends before the onset of psychotic symptoms

D. **Course and prognosis** vary widely, depending upon a variety of social, economic, and treatment factors as well as the diagnostic criteria used to define the population. Social recovery (i.e., return to independent living and social and occupational functioning) is often more common than complete remission of symptoms.

   1. Kraepelin's dementia praecox patients experienced only a 12% improvement in symptoms.

   2. In other studies, schizophrenics experienced 10%–35% complete recovery rates.

   3. Recovery rates are better for schizophrenics:
      a. With a late onset of illness
      b. From the Third World countries
      c. In times of economic prosperity

   4. The Vermont Longitudinal Study and several other studies suggest that over a very long period (15 or more years) over two-thirds of schizophrenics experience complete or "social" recovery with adequate treatment.

E. **Socioeconomic status** is correlated with the prevalence and incidence of schizophrenia as well as its course.

   1. **In the United States**, the highest rates of schizophrenia are found in the lower socioeconomic classes, suggesting that either socioeconomic factors produce or precipitate schizophrenia or that schizophrenics tend to drift downward (**drift hypothesis**) in socioeconomic status.

2. In India, the highest rates of schizophrenia occur in the upper castes, suggesting that social stress on a class of people, rather than drift, may be a major factor in precipitating schizophrenia.

3. In the Great Depression, the outcome of schizophrenia in the United States and Great Britain was worse than either before or after.

4. In cities with populations over 100,000, the incidence of schizophrenia increases in proportion to the size of the city, although this relationship does not hold true in rural areas and smaller cities.

F. Familial patterns of incidence of schizophrenia reveal that biologic relatives of schizophrenics have an increased risk for developing this illness. However, recent studies with narrower diagnostic criteria than used previously suggest lower rates of risk among biologic relatives of schizophrenics found in earlier studies.

1. Monozygotic twins raised together have a concordance rate of 91%, while monozygotic twins raised apart are concordant at a 78% rate in one study. Other studies of twins reveal a concordance rate of 40%–50% for monozygotic twins and about 10%–14% for dizygotic twins.

2. If both parents are schizophrenic, the child's risk for developing schizophrenia is between 15% and 55%.

3. Some studies show high rates of mental illness (not necessarily schizophrenia) or, in some cases, positive traits, such as creativity, in relatives of schizophrenics.

4. Patterns of transmission of schizophrenia in families do not fit any known pattern of pure genetic transmission, and current theories suggest a pattern of transmission that may be activated through as yet unknown biologic, social, and psychological factors.

5. Recent findings suggest that in some families a specific gene is associated with schizophrenia. In other families, this gene was absent. Based on these results, it appears that at least two mechanisms may be etiologic for schizophrenia, one of which is genetic.

G. Season of birth appears to be correlated with the risk for developing schizophrenia. In both the northern and southern hemispheres, the risk for developing schizophrenia is greatest for individuals born in the late winter and early spring.

H. Mortality risks for young schizophrenics are several times those of the general population. As schizophrenic individuals age, their risk of mortality approaches that of the general population. The risk of mortality is significantly increased among schizophrenics by suicides, accidents, and respiratory diseases.

IV. CLINICAL FEATURES of schizophrenia vary, according to diagnostic criteria used to define the population and, to some extent, the etiologic models of the clinician or researcher. There are no established biologic markers or pathognomonic clinical features that define the diagnosis of schizophrenia, and it must be emphasized that any single clinical feature of schizophrenia may also be associated with other mental and physical illnesses. Also, agreement among clinicians about the presence or absence of a particular clinical feature is not always good. In general, features of schizophrenia reported by patients (e.g., hallucinations) tend to be more reliable than those observed by clinicians (e.g., poverty of thought content).

Symptoms of schizophrenia usually include disruptions in areas of psychological and social functioning. However, even in cases of severe disruption, some areas of functioning may be preserved; for example, a hospitalized patient with chronic schizophrenia who exhibits bizarre behavior and severe disruptions of speech and thinking may retain the skills of a concert pianist. Symptoms of schizophrenia, the descriptions of which follow, may change and become less severe over the course of the illness.

A. Form of thought refers to the structure of thought as experienced by the patient and displayed through verbal communication. These disturbances are defined as **formal thought disorder**, (i.e., a disturbance of the *form* of thought), which may manifest as:

1. **Loosening of associations,** which is observed in speech when connections among ideas are absent or obscure. The flow of ideas is not coherent and does not proceed toward a goal. This symptom may be contrasted with tangentiality and flight of ideas that is typical of mania and anxiety disorders in which ideas are coherent, but the patient may lose the point of a string of ideas. In "loosening of associations," the listener may feel as if his or her

attention had wavered and a critical transition to understanding the patient's thought had been lost. Examples of loosening of associations follow.

   a. **Word use may be highly idiosyncratic and individualized.** Words may be created (neologism) or selected by the patient, according to an internal logic and special symbolism that are the patient's own.

   b. **Abnormal concept formation is a perceptual defect** in schizophrenics in which patients are unable to exclude irrelevant or competing ideas from their consciousness; thinking becomes overinclusive, incorporating extraneous items and unimportant details into thoughts and ideas that have specific meanings to the patient but are difficult for the outside observer to follow.

   c. **Logic in schizophrenia may follow a primitive pattern** (in the piagetian sense). Logical errors of reasoning from the specific to the universal, exclusion of important information from the reasoning process, and frank distortion of logical connections are all present in schizophrenia. Ideas may be connected, according to "magical" processes in which parts stand for the whole, and causal connections are assumed to exist when no connections can be perceived by others. The symbolic content of ideas may be highly individualized and magical, and symbols may be treated as if they were actual objects or inappropriately substituted for other logical elements.

   d. **Concreteness may substitute for abstraction.** The ability to form abstract ideas may be severely impaired. The ability to discern abstractions within ideas may become limited, and concrete interpretations of abstract ideas may become predominant. The ability to understand metaphors and similies may be lost. In general, patients with early onset schizophrenia may experience greater deterioration of abstraction ability than patients with late onset disease as measured by psychological tests. Simultaneous preoccupation with symbols and abstractions and the loss of the ability to process these symbols and abstractions are features commonly seen among schizophrenics.

   e. **Language structural problems** are seen in schizophrenia, but many of these problems are quite rare; however, unusual, stilted language is commonly seen.

   (1) **Neologisms** are new words created out of elements of other words or de novo.

   (2) **Verbigeration** is the persistent repetition of words or phrases.

   (3) **Echolalia** is a repetition of the words or phrases of the examiner, which is seen in severely disorganized psychotic states.

   (4) **Mutism** is a functional inhibition of speech and vocalization, which is seen in a variety of nonpsychotic and psychotic illnesses.

   (5) **Word salad** is a complete lack of language, which is seen in psychosis and several very specific central nervous system lesions.

2. **Poverty of content and speech** is seen in several of the schizophrenic spectrum disorders. Speech may be complex, concrete, or limited in overall productivity, but generally lacks specific information content.

3. **Thought blocking** is an internal interruption in a patient's speech and flow of thought. It may appear as though the patient were being interrupted by an hallucination, although the patient may or may not be able to identify the interruption.

B. **Content of thought.** Among the most characteristic features of schizophrenia are **delusions**, which are defined as fixed, false beliefs. Delusions cannot be changed by reasoning and are not consistent with the cultural beliefs of the patient's cultural group. However, they may have a culturally based content, such as Americans believing that they are the targets of influence by the Central Intelligence Agency. In some cases, delusions may be so individualistic that no cultural connections can be made. Delusions may be relatively circumscribed or may pervade all aspects of the patient's life and thinking. In some cases, delusions may appear relatively trivial to the patient, but more commonly, they become an organizing force in the patient's life. Delusions may be simple in their organization or may be highly complex and systematized. Sexual, religious, and philosophical content of delusions are common.

1. **Delusions of persecution** are ideas that others are trying to harm, spy on, or otherwise influence or humiliate the patient, or interfere in his or her affairs. Persecutory delusions are frequently very pervasive and actively incorporate features of the patient's life as evidence of persecution.

2. **Delusions of reference** are beliefs on the part of the patient that random events in the environment have special meaning and are directed specifically at the patient. For example, delusions of reference frequently involve the belief that strangers, television, or radio are talking about the patient or that random events, such as accidents, have been designed to harm or influence the patient. **Ideas of reference** differ from delusions of reference in intensity rather than form.

3. **Delusions of influence** are beliefs on the part of the patient that their thoughts and actions are controlled by outside forces. In extreme cases, patients feel as if they were robots without thoughts and actions of their own; they feel like passive vehicles for the control and intentions of these outside forces. Patients may feel that body parts, frequently the genitals, are manipulated by unseen forces. Likewise, patients may feel as if their thoughts have been removed and then replaced by alien thoughts.

4. **Thought broadcasting** is experienced by patients as thoughts leaving their head and going directly to objects in the environment. This may be experienced by patients as a physical sensation. Thought broadcasting is a symptom that is difficult to understand by those who have not experienced this phenomenon.

5. **Grandiose delusions** are more common in patients with mania than those with schizophrenia. However, schizophrenic patients may feel as if they are central figures in the complex delusional systems in the environment. The patient's feelings of having special knowledge, special relationships with important figures, or of posing a special threat to conspiracies may all be considered grandiose. These grandiose delusions can be differentiated from the expansive and positive grandiose delusions that are typical of mania.

6. **Somatic delusions** in schizophrenia typically include feelings that the body has been manipulated or altered by outside forces. These somatic delusions must be differentiated from the somatic delusions of other disorders, such as delusions of having cancer or a decaying body, which are typical of major depression with melancholic features. Patients with somatic delusions may feel that:
   a. An electronic device has been placed in their bodies.
   b. Their bodies are under the control of others.
   c. Portions of their bodies are not their own.

7. **Other types of delusions.** A variety of other delusional states have been described in schizophrenia. In their extreme forms, these delusional states are rarely seen in modern psychiatry.
   a. **Delusional love** in which the patient believes that he or she has a special romantic relationship, often with a public figure, is a rare symptom in clinical practice but is reportedly common in the lives of public figures, particularly in the broadcast media.
   b. **Nihilism** in which the delusional system of imagined loss or destruction centers around the self and the world may attain the extreme form of **Cotard's syndrome** in which the patient believes that the self, the world, and even time has been lost or destroyed. (This syndrome may be more common in mood disorders and parietal lobe lesions.)
   c. **Capgras' syndrome** is a delusional belief system in which the patient believes that important people in the environment have been taken away, and duplicates have been substituted for them.

C. **Perceptual disorders** in schizophrenia include a variety of distortions of sensory experiences and their interpretation. Almost any aspect of the self and the environment may be involved in perceptual distortions of schizophrenia, although some patterns of sensory distortion appear to be more common to schizophrenia than to other disorders. Recent data suggest that the fundamental perceptual defect in schizophrenia is the inability to habituate and suppress extraneous environmental stimuli or internal thought processes. However, it must be emphasized that no perceptual disturbance is pathognomonic of schizophrenia. Perceptual distortions may occur in normal subjects, mood disorders, organic mental syndromes, and a variety of other conditions.

1. **Hallucinations** are sensory experiences that occur without corresponding environmental stimuli.
   a. **Auditory hallucinations** range from unformed buzzing sounds to complex voices holding conversations. Hearing voices holding conversations about the patient in the third person, saying negative and derogatory things, or a single voice, telling the patient to commit some action, are the auditory hallucinations most characteristic of schizophrenia. The voices may be muffled or distinct, familiar or unfamiliar, single or multiple, and of either sex. Patients may hear their own voice spoken aloud.
   b. **Command hallucinations** are a special form of auditory hallucination in which voices tell the patient to commit some action. In some cases, these hallucinations are so persistent that they become difficult to resist. When the command hallucinations tell the patient to harm him or herself or someone else, they must be considered dangerous.
   c. **Visual hallucinations.** Although more common to other disorders, particularly organic mental disorders, visual hallucinations are also experienced by schizophrenic patients. These hallucinations may be simple, but they are most characteristic of schizophrenia

when they are complex and related to the patient's delusional system, such as a visitation from aliens.

   d. Other hallucinations may be **tactile, gustatory, olfactory** (frequently an unpleasant and indescribable odor), or **somatic.** Like the visual hallucinations, these hallucinatory experiences occur in other disorders (e.g., olfactory hallucinations in complex partial seizures); in schizophrenia, they are frequently connected to delusional systems.

2. **Illusions** are misperceptions or misidentifications of identifiable environmental events or objects. Illusions are common to a variety of disorders, as well as occurring in normal individuals. They may occur in any sensory modality and in schizophrenia, may be variants of a normal experience given a delusional explanation.

   a. Déjà vu feelings are defined as those in which unfamiliar situations feel strangely familiar. In addition to occurring in schizophrenia, these occur as a normal phenomenon and in several forms of epilepsy.

   b. Jamais vu feelings are defined as those in which familiar situations are experienced as novel and unfamiliar. These occur in epilepsy as well as schizophrenia.

   c. Hypersensitivity to light, sound, or smell is common to schizophrenia and to other disorders, such as migraine headaches.

   d. Distorted perceptions of time occur in a variety of conditions, such as dissociative states and anxiety, as well as schizophrenia.

   e. Misperceptions of movement, perspective, and size are typical of organic conditions and anxiety but also occur in schizophrenia.

   f. Changes in body perceptions, one's own or the bodies of others, also occur.

D. Affect is defined as the observable manifestations of mood and emotion. Affective findings in schizophrenia may be, in some cases, unreliable due to the parkinsonian effects of the neuroleptics and to cultural differences in body language. Affective disturbances in schizophrenia include the following:

1. **Blunted affect** refers to the reduction of the range of emotional response on the part of the patient. This phenomenon may be perceived by others as a lack of depth of feeling, hostility, depression, or a lack of social responsiveness. Severe blunting of affect is suggestive of substantial deterioration of personality, while a full range of emotional responsiveness is considered a good prognostic sign. There is evidence to suggest that restrictions of affective expression are adaptations to chronic institutionalization in some cases.

2. **Flat affect** represents an extreme form of affective blunting in which body language associated with emotion is almost entirely lost. Facial expressiveness, changes in voice tone, gestures, body posture changes reflecting mood, and other nuances of nonverbal expression are almost entirely absent. Patients with flat affect may also feel that internal emotions are absent.

3. **Inappropriate affect** is a mismatching of thought or speech content and affective expression. For example, a patient may grin while describing a violent or traumatic event or express sadness while describing a pleasant event. Like other affective findings, this is not pathognomonic of schizophrenia and is found in a number of other conditions, including personality disorders, organic mental syndromes, and depression. Normal individuals may also exhibit inappropriate affect.

4. **Unusual emotions** include the extreme fear that often accompanies acute psychotic experiences, the global negativism that accompanies some catatonic states, or the feelings of cosmic and religious rapture that are experienced by some schizophrenic individuals. For clinical purposes, these states cannot be considered diagnostic features of schizophrenia.

E. Sense of self is the perception of one's individuality, separateness from others, and continuity in space and time. The erosion of the sense of self may lead to the delusions of reference and influence found in schizophrenia.

1. **In normal individuals,** a solid sense of self is thought to be the basis of good self-esteem and an ability of the individual to weather losses, disappointments, and slights from others. In addition, a well-integrated sense of self permits the perception of the self and others as whole and continuous in individuals in whom negative and positive features are integrated.

2. **In schizophrenic individuals,** as well as other conditions, a disrupted sense of self may manifest as:

   a. Loss of self-esteem

   b. Confusion about sexual identity
   c. An inability to separate oneself from events in the environment (i.e., feeling that one's thoughts have harmed another person)
   d. Projection of the patient's own fears or suspicions onto others
   e. Experiencing the self and others as dichotomous opposites (i.e., all good or all bad) with little integration of the opposing features

F. Volitional symptoms of schizophrenia are among the most persistent and intractable. Difficulties initiating and maintaining purposeful and goal-directed activity and interest in the environment may account for the difficulties many schizophrenics experience in maintaining work and stable living situations.

   1. Interest on the part of schizophrenics in the environment may be difficult to generate and maintain. This difficulty may be related to ambivalence, resulting from conflicting wishes or desires, or to an inability to generate interest internally.

   2. Initiative, or the ability to begin goal-directed activity, is often lacking in advanced cases of schizophrenia. Patients may experience difficulty finding housing, financial support, and other survival needs as a consequence of this symptom and may be unable to initiate spontaneous movement without direction from others.

   3. Drive is the ability to pursue goal-directed activity after it has been started. Although not unique to schizophrenia, difficulties in maintaining goal-directed behavior appear to be quite common in schizophrenia, possibly as a result of:
   a. The cognitive symptoms experienced by these patients
   b. The inability to sustain thoughts amid the perceptual and cognitive disturbances of schizophrenia
   c. A lack of drive, which may be an independent feature of this disorder

   4. Ambition may be preserved in the absence of drive and initiative, as in the case of patients whose grandiose wishes are to be film or music stars, or may be absent. Unrealistic ambitions in combination with the patient's delusions may be an organizing principle for complex dysfunctional patterns of behavior.

G. Relationship to the external world. The tendency for patients to become increasingly preoccupied with internal events and decreasingly influenced by external events is characteristic of schizophrenia. Preoccupation with delusional and hallucinatory symptoms and difficulty in communicating with others may lead to withdrawal from the world, which in its extreme form is called **autism.**

H. Motor activity in schizophrenia may present as a variety of unusual features, none of which are unique to schizophrenia. Some alterations in motor activity and behavior may be associated with the pharmacologic treatment of schizophrenia.

   1. Quantitative changes. The amount of activity and its "driven" quality ranges from the extremes of agitation in excited catatonic states and acute psychotic exacerbations to the withdrawn and inactive states associated with catatonic stupor and chronic institutionalization. It should be noted that catatonia is a syndrome that is caused by mood disorders and organic syndromes more frequently than by schizophrenia. **Akathisia**, a condition associated with high levels of motor agitation, **bradykinesia**, a condition associated with difficulty in initiating motor activity, and **tardive dyskinesia**, a condition associated with unusual facial expressions and generalized choreoathetotic movements, are commonly associated with the effects of the neuroleptic medications rather than with schizophrenia.
   a. Catatonic stupor is a state of dramatic motor inactivity in which patients may, if untreated, be immobile for weeks or months at a time. Patients may be unable to initiate eating, drinking, or elimination functions. As patients recover, it is clear that they have been aware of events in the environment. Patients in this state may require aggressive medical care to avoid dehydration, electrolyte disturbances, and infections. Catatonic stupor may change abruptly to catatonic excitement in some cases.
   b. Catatonic excitement is a psychiatric emergency. The patient's activity and speech may be excessive, driven, and purposeless. Patients in this state may be very violent and, before pharmacologic and electroconvulsive treatments, frequently died of acute hyperthermia. Catatonic excitement may also be caused by organic conditions (e.g., by drugs like phencyclidine) and mania. This hypermetabolic state requires aggressive psychiatric intervention to prevent the patient's exhaustion, violence, and hyperthermia.

   2. Qualitative changes. Patients with schizophrenia may show a variety of movement abnormalities even without treatment. Psychopharmacologic interventions frequently confuse the clinical picture of movement abnormalities by adding features of parkinsonian movement difficulties and the choreoathetotic movements of tardive dyskinesia. Even without treatment, however, patients with schizophrenia may exhibit increased flexor muscle tone, unusual mannerisms, and bizarre gestures.

   a. Catatonic posturing is demonstrated by patients who assume strange postures and hold them for very long periods.

   b. Catatonic rigidity is demonstrated by patients who resist being moved from their unusual rigid postures.

   c. Waxy flexibility. Patients' limbs may be moved like wax, and they will hold the newly assumed position for long periods of time.

   d. Echopraxia is the behavioral equivalent of echolalia. Patients involuntarily mimic the movements of another person.

   e. Automatic obedience refers to the finding in some patients of unquestioningly following orders or directives in a robot-like manner.

   f. Mannerisms and grimacing. The manner of schizophrenic individuals may appear artificial and stilted. Inappropriate silliness is seen, particularly in hebephrenic patients and patients with frontal lobe damage, and is frequently accompanied by unusual mannerisms. Particular mannerisms may have special meanings that are connected to delusions or hallucinations. Grimacing movements may be subtle or pronounced but may be mistaken for the orofacial dystonias of tardive dyskinesia.

   g. Stereotyped behaviors (stereotypy). Purposeless repetitive movements (or verbalizations) are seen in a variety of conditions, including schizophrenia. These movements may involve the entire body, such as rocking movements, or may involve repetition of complex gestures. The movements may have magical significance or may be purposeless to the patient.

   h. Perseveration involves the involuntary repetition of a task; for example, patients who are asked to copy a series of circles may continue to copy the figures until they run off the page, or patients may repeat an answer to a question until asked to stop. This symptom is also seen in organic mental syndromes, particularly in patients with damage to premotor areas.

I. Social behavior. In early and severe cases of schizophrenia, there may be a loss of social skills, body language, and empathic abilities that permit patients to interact successfully with others and to pursue social and vocational functioning. Schizophrenic individuals frequently are perceived by others as bizarre, hostile, or socially inappropriate. Impairment of social skills may be a primary problem or the result of disturbances of thinking, perception, speech, and behavior or of long-term institutionalization. Schizophrenics who are severely socially debilitated may live on the fringe of society as severely dysfunctional "street people," while in the past, these same individuals may have been long-term institutionalized patients.

V. DIAGNOSTIC SUBTYPES OF SCHIZOPHRENIA

A. *DSM-III-R* **diagnostic subtypes.** The diagnosis of the particular type of schizophrenia depends upon the clinical picture at the time of the evaluation. The clinical picture for a single patient may vary, encompassing several types of schizophrenia over the course of a lifetime. Because of the variations in the symptom clusters associated with schizophrenia, diagnostic subtypes have changed significantly over time. The current *DSM-III-R* diagnostic subtypes of schizophrenia include the following (after meeting basic diagnostic criteria for schizophrenia):

1. Catatonic schizophrenia. The schizophrenic symptoms are dominated by any of the following:

   a. Catatonic stupor or mutism

   b. Catatonic negativism, which is an apparently motiveless resistance to all instructions or attempts to be moved

   c. Catatonic rigidity

   d. Catatonic excitement

   e. Catatonic posturing

2. Disorganized schizophrenia does not involve organized delusions or catatonic features, although fragmentary, unsystematized delusions are common. It is marked by the following features:

   a. Incoherent speech and marked loosening of associations

   b. Grossly disorganized behavior

   c. Flat or grossly inappropriate affect

   d. Absence of diagnostic criteria for catatonic schizophrenia

3. **Paranoid schizophrenia** may have the best prognosis of any type of schizophrenia. Hallucinatory and delusional symptoms are often organized around a single theme. Social and occupational functioning may be well preserved. Diagnostic criteria are as follows:
   a. Complete absorption with systematized delusions or with auditory hallucinations organized around a single theme
   b. Absence of:
      (1) Incoherence or grossly disorganized behavior
      (2) Marked loosening of associations
      (3) Flat or grossly inappropriate affect
      (4) Catatonic behavior

4. **Undifferentiated schizophrenia.** This diagnostic category is used for patients whose symptoms do not meet any of the first three categories or who have symptoms of several types of schizophrenia. Diagnostic criteria are as follows:
   a. Prominent delusions and hallucinations
   b. Incoherence or grossly disorganized behavior
   c. Absence of diagnostic criteria for paranoid, catatonic, or disorganized schizophrenia.

5. **Residual schizophrenia.** This diagnostic category is applied to patients who have experienced at least one psychotic episode but who are without prominent psychotic symptoms at the time of the evaluation; however, they continue to experience disability from symptoms. Criteria include the following:
   a. Absence of:
      (1) Prominent delusions or hallucinations
      (2) Incoherence or grossly disorganized behavior
   b. Ongoing evidence of the disturbance as evidenced by two or more symptoms, such as:
      (1) Marked social isolation or withdrawal
      (2) Marked impairment of role functioning
      (3) Marked peculiar behavior
      (4) Marked impairment in personal hygiene and grooming
      (5) Blunted or inappropriate affect
      (6) Digressive, vague, circumstantial, or overelaborative speech
      (7) Odd beliefs or magical thinking
      (8) Unusual perceptual experiences
      (9) Marked lack of initiative, interest, or energy

B. **Non–*DSM-III-R* diagnostic subtypes.** Although not used in the *DSM-III-R*, a number of other diagnostic categories for schizophrenia are used in the literature, such as those in the *International Classification of Diseases*, 9th ed. (*ICD-9*). These categories were not included in the *DSM-III-R* for a variety of reasons, including overlapping categories and lack of diagnostic reliability. Some of these diagnostic categories are as follows:

1. **Schizoaffective disorder** is listed in the *DSM-III-R* as a disorder "not classified elsewhere." In the past, it was considered to be a type of schizophrenia. It involves both schizophrenic and mood symptoms. The patient must exhibit concurrent mood and schizophrenic symptoms of a major type (i.e., hallucinations, delusions, catatonic behavior, flat or grossly inappropriate affect, or bizarre or grossly inappropriate behavior). For a diagnosis of schizoaffective disorder, the *DSM-III-R* requires that there be a period of at least 2 weeks of schizophrenic symptoms without mood disturbance and that schizophrenia and organic mental syndromes have been ruled out. Patients may exhibit either **manic** or **depressive** symptom patterns.

2. **Hebephrenic schizophrenia** is generally considered to be equivalent to the *DSM-III-R* category of **disorganized schizophrenia.**

3. **Pseudoneurotic schizophrenia** is a term applied to patients who manifest primarily neurotic symptoms but who demonstrate abnormal thinking patterns, pananxiety, and an unusual preoccupation with sexual issues. This diagnostic category is being supplanted by borderline personality disorder and other diagnostic groupings, because the diagnostic reliability is poor. This category was rarely used outside of North America.

4. **Oneiroid schizophrenia** is a term applied to schizophrenic individuals who feel and behave as if they were living in a dream. They may follow routines of daily life, while believing and experiencing life in the dream world. Because oneiroid states are usually of a transient nature in the course of schizophrenia, they are currently considered to be more of a phase in the development of schizophrenia than as a specific type.

5. **Paraphrenia** is roughly equivalent to paranoid schizophrenia as the term is used in the

ICD-9. It refers to a condition with well-systematized paranoid or grandiose delusions in which there is no deterioration of the personality over time (suggesting an overlap with delusional disorder in the *DSM-III-R*). Social and occupational functioning may be well preserved, and patients are fairly comfortable with their delusions. In a variant of this condition, **late paraphrenia** is a condition that occurs primarily in women in late middle age or early old age, and frequently involves persecutory delusions, somatic hallucinations, marked suspiciousness, and hostility. The significance of this syndrome remains unclear.

6. **Simple schizophrenia** is characterized by slow insidious loss of drive, interest, ambition, and initiative. Hallucinations and delusions are rare, but social impairment is the hallmark of this condition. In current diagnostic thinking, most of the people who fit this category are probably now considered to have schizoid or schizotypal personalities.

VI. **PATHOGENESIS.** According to current diagnostic criteria, there is always an active phase with psychotic symptoms during the course of schizophrenia. In addition, there must be a 6-month persistence of symptoms and a temporary deterioration of functioning to below pre-illness levels. The course of schizophrenia may be highly variable, including a prodromal phase, remission between episodes, and a downward deteriorating course, ending in full or social recovery.

A. **Premorbid personality.** Although certain personality features seem to antedate the development of schizophrenia in about 25% of cases, research has not demonstrated specific personality features that reliably predict the development of schizophrenia. Studies have revealed different histories in some schizophrenics of:

1. Extreme dependency (e.g., sharing bedrooms with parents until late adolescence and experiencing panic when away from home)

2. Shyness, withdrawal, social awkwardness, and an inability to form close relationships

3. An asocial premorbid personality pattern

4. A pattern of overcompliance and conformity

5. Schizotypal and schizoid personality features in family members who do not develop schizophrenia

B. **Family interactional patterns** are thought by some investigators to be potential predisposing factors to the development of schizophrenia. Whatever the premorbid interactive pattern between children who develop schizophrenia and their parents, the relationship between the initial onset of schizophrenia to parental interactive styles is unclear. This should not be confused with findings that high expressed emotionality in families may precipitate relapses in schizophrenic patients.

1. Some studies suggest that children predisposed to schizophrenia do not exhibit the same responsiveness to mothers as do other children, and mothers of these children react to this lack of responsiveness with frustration and disappointment.

2. Other studies suggest that mothers of schizophrenics are overly anxious, rejecting, aggressive, and indifferent.

3. Recent studies suggest that parents' relatively normal reactions to certain cognitive and interactive patterns of preschizophrenic children may be associated with the eventual development of schizophrenia.

C. **Initiating factors** do not appear to be specific to schizophrenia but represent specific stresses that interact with a predisposing trait to precipitate schizophrenia.

1. **Time of onset.** The peak time of onset of schizophrenia is in late adolescence and early adulthood. This is a time of multiple stresses related to leaving home, choosing a career, and developing relationships. A smaller peak occurs in the fourth decade, particularly among women.
   a. It has been proposed that separation from parents unmasks psychotic features that have been present since childhood.
   b. Others suggest that these intense stresses are responsible for activating the processes that result in schizophrenia.

2. **Precipitating events**
   a. **Psychosocial stressors.** Cultures experiencing social and economic stress are associated with high rates of schizophrenia. However, it cannot yet be determined which stressors produce schizophrenia in vulnerable individuals and which do not.

   b. Traumatic events. On a case by case basis, specific traumatic events that appear to precipitate schizophrenic symptoms can be isolated. It is not clear, however, that either the level of stress or loss for the schizophrenic individual is different than might be experienced by a normal individual.
   c. Drug and alcohol abuse. Certain drugs, such as amphetamines, cocaine, hallucinogens, phencyclidine, and alcohol, may precipitate schizophrenic symptoms. It is not clear whether these drugs cause syndromes that resemble schizophrenia or whether these drugs precipitate schizophrenia in vulnerable individuals. In some cases, use of these drugs may represent an attempt at self-treatment in individuals who are developing schizophrenia.

D. Clinical course
   1. Onset. The onset of schizophrenia is variable and has prognostic significance.
      a. Acute. Schizophrenia may present abruptly with confusion, agitation, affective involvement, hallucinations, and delusions, following an identifiable stressor. This clinical picture may develop in a period as short as a day or two; however, relatively few of these patients develop schizophrenia with the chronic course required for a *DSM-III-R* diagnosis and instead meet the criteria for **brief reactive psychosis** or **schizophreniform disorder**, which has a somewhat longer but less than 6-month course.
      b. Trema (German term for stage fright) is characterized by anxious, irritable, and depressed feelings that may last for a few days to a month or more. These feelings may be a reaction to perceptions that something is going wrong. As this condition progresses, the patient may feel as though the environment is odd and ominous.
      c. An insidious prodromal phase portends a bad prognosis when psychotic features eventually appear. In general, the prognosis is worse if the patient experiences substantial deterioration in functioning without ever having achieved a high level of psychosocial functioning prior to the onset of psychotic symptoms. Symptoms observed in patients with this pattern of onset include:
      (1) Social withdrawal
      (2) Impairment in role functioning (e.g., as a student, parent, or spouse)
      (3) Peculiar behavior
      (4) Neglect of grooming and personal hygiene
      (5) Blunted or inappropriate affect
      (6) Vague, digressive, overelaborative, or circumstantial speech, or poverty of speech or content of speech
      (7) Odd beliefs or magical thinking influencing behavior. These beliefs are not consistent with the cultural group of which the patient is a member, although this may be difficult to determine in individuals with a counterculture life-style.
      (8) Unusual perceptual experiences, such as recurrent illusions, "telepathy," or recurrent déjà vu experiences.
      (9) Marked lack of initiative, drive, ambition, interest, or energy
   2. Active phase. Schizophrenia cannot be diagnosed without an active phase, involving active hallucinations, delusions, catatonic behavior, or grossly inappropriate affect and behavior. By definition, this phase must last at least 1 week and may remit in part or completely or continue as the central feature of the clinical course.
   3. Residual phase. Symptoms of the residual phase are largely those of the prodromal phase. Negative symptoms of schizophrenia may be prominent, and difficulty recovering previous levels of psychosocial functioning may be a major part of the clinical picture. A variety of different lifetime courses have been described, and recovery of social function is more common than complete recovery from residual symptoms. Recent studies suggest that over several decades, about two-thirds of schizophrenics achieve full or social recovery.
   4. Duration. By definition, symptoms of schizophrenia must be present for at least 6 months for a diagnosis of schizophrenia to be made. This durational criterion has been incorporated into the diagnostic criteria for schizophrenia to separate patients with good prognoses and a high probability of complete recovery from those with poor prognoses. It was also hoped that this criterion would create a narrow and homogeneous group of patients to whom the diagnosis of schizophrenia could be properly applied.
      a. For patients without symptoms for 6 months, a variety of other diagnoses may be appropriate, including schizophreniform disorder, brief reactive psychosis, and atypical psychosis.
      b. If there is no episode of acute psychosis, diagnoses of schizoid or schizotypal personality disorders, delusional disorder, paranoid personality disorder, or borderline personality disorder may be appropriate.

5. **Deterioration from a previous level of functioning** is a key diagnostic feature. Role performance in relationships, work, self-care, or school performance is impaired, and residual symptoms may interfere with social functioning. However, recent studies challenge the assumption that this deterioration is uniform and lifelong. The Vermont Longitudinal Study, for example, found that 10 years following the initiation of a deinstitutionalization project for chronic schizophrenics, 70% of the patients were recidivists or were socially isolated. However, 25 years after deinstitutionalization, 50%–70% of these patients had achieved either complete remission or considerable improvement. All of these patients participated in a comprehensive rehabilitation program. These findings are supported in the literature concerning major heterogeneity of outcome in patients, even those who met the *DSM-III-R* criteria for schizophrenia.

30 %

   a. Patterns of long-term courses. A large number of courses for individual schizophrenic patients has been described. Onset may be acute or insidious. The course may involve a single continuous episode of symptoms, may be episodic, or may evolve from an episodic to a continuous course. Outcome may range from eventual severe impairment to complete recovery. Almost all combinations of these elements are possible. About 25% of schizophrenics experience the insidious onset of symptoms, continuous course, and eventual severe impairment described by Kraeplin.

   b. Patterns of recovery. Different measures of recovery produce very different outcome estimates.

     (1) Social recovery is often defined as economic and residential independence with low disruption in social relationships. Errors in this measurement are possible because it is tied to the status of the economy and to the level of tolerance for social deviance in the culture. These rates tend to be higher than those for complete recovery.

     (2) Complete recovery implies complete remission of psychotic symptoms and return to previous levels of social and occupational functioning.

     (3) Hospitalization rates have been used to measure failures in recovery. Although easiest to measure, it is probably the least accurate measure of the course of schizophrenia. Rates of rehospitalization may depend upon a variety of factors, ranging from the health care resources and service delivery systems available to community acceptance of deviant behavior.

   c. Deteriorating courses. Although there are currently doubts about the uniformity of the course and inevitability of deterioration in schizophrenia, psychiatry early in this century categorized stages in the deterioration of schizophrenics who were untreated with modern medications and in institutions of the time. Silvano Arieti, for example, defined four stages of deterioration:

     (1) The development of psychotic symptoms, progressing through loss of anxiety

     (2) The development of routine stereotyped behaviors

     (3) The loss of psychotic symptoms

     (4) The development of bizarre behaviors, such as hoarding useless objects, strange self-decoration and food habits, and incontinence

   d. Neurologic deterioration

     (1) It has been reported that computerized tomography (CT) demonstrates anatomic changes in the brain of long-term schizophrenics, including enlarged lateral ventricle size and loss of normal hemispheric asymmetries.

     (2) Positron emission tomography (PET) demonstrates unusual blood flow patterns in the brains of schizophrenics.

     (3) Many of the neurologic studies are flawed, and the identification of specific neuropathology in schizophrenia has yet to be established.

E. Prognosis. Much of the data on the prognosis of schizophrenia is based upon observations of the disease courses of less than 10 years or of patients whose behaviors may represent adaptations to institutionalized life. In addition, the prognosis of schizophrenia may depend upon socioeconomic factors and the availability of adequate psychosocial interventions. Many of the factors listed below may be seen as intermediate-term prognostic factors. Much remains to be learned about the long-term prognosis of schizophrenia.

   1. Statistics

     a. Kraeplin reported that 13% of his dementia praecox patients recovered from the first schizophrenic episode, although many of these patients relapsed later, resulting in a 2.6% lasting recovery rate.

     b. Modern treatment methods in the United States make it possible for about 90% of schizophrenics to recover sufficiently to live outside the hospital most of the time.

     c. Some studies suggest that about 25% of individuals who meet the diagnostic criteria for schizophrenia will not experience substantial or complete recovery 20–25 years (or longer) after the onset of illness.

2. **Prognostic variables.** Prognostic variables in schizophrenia fall into several groups. Early in the course of schizophrenia, a number of variables have been identified that predict a short to intermediate course in schizophrenia. Long-term prognostic factors have not been identified. Positive symptoms (i.e., hallucinations, delusions, and formal thought disorder) carry much less ominous prognostic implications than the negative symptoms (i.e., affective flattening, social withdrawal, apathy, anhedonia, and poverty of thought and speech content).

    a. **Separation of good from poor prognostic factors.** Patients who presented with an acute onset of psychotic symptoms with obvious precipitating factors, confusion, and verbal aggression of a short duration were considered to be schizophrenic under the old diagnostic systems. However, because these individuals very often did not develop further psychotic episodes or residual symptoms, the 6-month durational criterion was added to the *DSM-III* and *DSM-III-R* in the belief that these patients represent different illnesses from those in which a longer course and negative symptoms predominate. As a result, patients currently fitting *DSM-III-R* diagnostic criteria for schizophrenia are a group that has been selected for poor prognostic features in the short- or intermediate-term.

        (1) Acute psychotic disorders are now considered to be schizophreniform disorder or brief reactive psychosis if they do not go on to the 6-month course required for a diagnosis of schizophrenia.

        (2) Patients with mood disorders in addition to psychotic symptoms are now diagnosed as having schizoaffective disorder, major depression with melancholic features, or bipolar mood disorder.

        (3) Many patients previously considered to be schizophrenic are now included in diagnostic categories of delusional disorder and borderline personality disorder.

    b. **Poor prognostic factors.** Patients with a predominance of negative symptoms, poor cognitive performance on neuropsychological testing, and abnormalities on CT and PET scans are reported to have poor outcomes.

F. Complications

1. **Network size.** As compared to normal individuals, chronic schizophrenics tend to have small social networks. While the social networks of normal individuals may be comprised of 20–30 individuals, chronic schizophrenics may have networks as small as 3–5 people.

2. **Impaired educational achievement.** Despite normal or high intelligence, many schizophrenics are unable to complete educational plans after the onset of illness.

3. **Impaired work performance.** Schizophrenics may have significant difficulties finding employment, particularly during economic depressions. Schizophrenics often are employed at lower skilled jobs than their educations and intelligence would suggest.

4. **Sexual relationships.** Marriage rates for schizophrenics are lower than rates for the general population. Schizophrenic men tend to be married less frequently than schizophrenic women.

5. **Crime.** Schizophrenics are not more violent than the average person in the population, in spite of the frequent publicity for bizarre and violent crimes committed by schizophrenics. There is evidence that when services are not provided to schizophrenics through the mental health service delivery system, they may enter the criminal justice system, often for relatively minor crimes. This process is often referred to as the **criminalization of the mentally ill**.

6. **Premature death.** Schizophrenics risk premature death from suicide, homicide, and medical illnesses, such as infectious diseases and neoplasms.

VII. DIFFERENTIAL DIAGNOSIS. The diagnosis of schizophrenia is made after a complete clinical and historical evaluation of the individual case. Patients who fit the *current* diagnostic criteria for schizophrenia are unlikely to be confused with other diagnostic groups. However, symptoms suggestive of schizophrenia may be found in a number of conditions, which must be ruled out (Table 2-1).

    A. **Organic mental disorders and syndromes.** An acute organic mental syndrome, which may present with psychotic symptoms, is called a **delirium**. Long-term, supposedly irreversible organic mental syndromes are called **dementias**.* Dementia often mimics the negative symptoms of schizophrenia. To differentiate schizophrenia from organic mental syndromes,

---

*The literature suggests that a large number of cases of dementia can be treated or reversed with adequate diagnosis.

Table 2-1. Partial Differential Diagnosis of Schizophrenia

Organic mental disorders	Toxic
Vascular	Sympathomimetics
Cerebral vasculitis	Sedatives
Perfusion problems	Steroids
Autoimmune	Anticholinergics
Systemic lupus erythematosus	Hallucinogens
Nutritional	Environmental toxins
B_{12} deficiency	Traumatic
Folate deficiency	Subdural hematoma
Nicotinic acid deficiency	Localized bleeds
Thiamine deficiency	Trauma to brain tissue
Pyridoxine deficiency	Endocrine
Metabolic	Thyroid abnormalities
Electrolyte problems	Pituitary adenomata
Wilson's disease	Neoplastic
Acute intermittent porphyria	Tumors in brain tissue
Organ system diseases	Paraneoplastic effects
Alcoholic	
Withdrawal syndromes	**Mood disorders**
Long-term dementing changes	Manic episodes
Sleep disorders	Major depressive episodes
Kleine-Levin syndrome	with melancholic features
Sleep apnea	
Hydrocephalus	**Other psychotic illnesses**
Obstructive	Schizoaffective disorder
Normal pressure	Brief reactive psychosis
Epilepsy	Atypical psychosis
Complex partial seizures	
Degenerative	**Personality disorders**
Multiple sclerosis	Borderline personality disorder
Huntington's chorea	Paranoid personality disorder
Congenital/hereditary	Schizoid personality disorder
Infections	Schizotypal personality disorder
Bacteria	Avoidant personality disorder
Viruses	
Parasites	**Culture-bound religious and belief systems**
Fungi	

the psychiatrist must rely upon a high index of suspicion, an exacting mental status examination, physical and neurologic examinations, and sometimes neuropsychological examination.

Organic mental syndromes may produce **focal** abnormalities, resulting primarily from localized damage to the brain that can mimic a variety of cognitive, behavioral, and even linguistic findings found in schizophrenia. **Nonfocal** or generalized alterations in brain function can present with acute confusion and psychotic symptoms suggestive of schizophrenia, although visual hallucinations are somewhat more common, and auditory hallucinations less common in organic mental syndromes. Causes of organic mental disorders that should be considered when evaluating schizophrenic individuals include the following:

1. **Vascular disorders.** Arteriosclerosis, arteriovenous malformations, aneurysms, cerebrovascular accidents, and perfusion problems must be considered in the differential diagnosis of schizophrenia, particularly in older patients. Cerebral vasculitis from autoimmune disease is particularly apt to mimic schizophrenia.

2. **Autoimmune diseases** are those in which the body generates immune responses to some of its own tissues. Although a relatively rare group of illnesses, it must be considered. Systemic lupus erythematosus (SLE), scleroderma, polyarteritis nodosa, Wegener's granulomatosis, and thromboangiitis obliterans as well as other autoimmune vasculitides must be considered as contributory or causative of organic mental disorders. Steroids used to treat these conditions may also cause organic mental syndromes. Lupus is particularly notorious for mimicking schizophrenia, sometimes producing an insidious onset and hallucinations and delusions in a clear sensorium before physical symptoms appear.

3. **Nutritional deficiencies.** Thiamine, pyridoxine, B_{12}, folate, and nicotinic acid deficiencies all produce characteristic syndromes that include organic mental disorders. Overdoses of vitamins, such as vitamin A and pyridoxine, must also be suspected in patients who advocate "megavitamin therapy."

4. **Metabolic disturbances.** Both diseases of internal organ systems and general metabolic and electrolyte disturbances can produce organic mental disorders. Electrolyte problems involve calcium (both too high and too low) and potassium levels. Rare diseases, such as Wilson's disease and acute intermittent porphyria, can be mistaken for schizophrenia. Sarcoidosis and polycythemia vera should also be considered in this group.

5. **Alcoholism.** Alcohol withdrawal syndromes and other organic mental disorders associated with alcohol are sufficiently common in medical practice that they merit inclusion as a separate category. The major alcohol withdrawal syndrome, **delirium tremens** (DTs) must be differentiated from the minor withdrawal syndrome and alcoholic hallucinosis. DTs and alcoholic hallucinations are frequently mistaken for acute schizophrenia. Likewise, nutritional deficiencies, such as thiamine and folate deficiencies, that are frequently associated with alcoholism may produce symptoms that may be mistaken for schizophrenia.

6. **Sleep disorders**
   a. Patients with **sleep apnea** usually present as if they suffered from depression, but illusions caused by fatigue and rapid eye movement (REM) sleep deprivation may, in theory, be mistaken for schizophrenia. These patients may also suffer from excessive daytime sleepiness, symptoms of hypertension, and right heart failure.
   b. **Kleine-Levin syndrome** is an episodic sleep disorder, usually found among adolescent boys, characterized by episodes of excessive sleep, eating binges, hypersexuality, and personality changes. Clinicians who do not believe hallucinations and delusions are necessary for the diagnosis of schizophrenia might mistake this condition for the insidious onset of schizophrenia or for a preschizophrenic condition.
   c. Other sleep disorders, such as **narcolepsy**, are less likely to present with findings of schizophrenia or organic mental syndromes than of depression.

7. **Hydrocephalus.** Two types of hydrocephalus should be considered in patients with organic mental syndromes.
   a. **Obstructive hydrocephalus** is usually found in children but may be found in adults who have an obstruction of the normal flow of cerebrospinal fluid following an accident or a tumor.
   b. **Normal pressure hydrocephalus**, which manifests as gait disturbance, "dementia," and often incontinence, is often found in older individuals. It may occur after an accident or in association with other diseases, such as Parkinson's or Alzheimer's diseases, or may be "idiopathic." Because of the behavioral features of normal pressure hydrocephalus, it may be mistaken for "terminal" stage schizophrenia in chronic, institutionalized populations.

8. **Epilepsy.** Seizure phenomena may manifest as psychiatric disorders, including a variety of organic mental syndrome findings. Personality changes in persons suffering from epilepsy have been widely described and should be considered in the differential diagnosis of organic personality syndromes as well as schizophrenia.
   a. **Complex partial seizures** (also called partial complex and temporal lobe seizures) may present with a variety of psychiatric symptoms, including hallucinations, nontargeted aggression, and unusual stereotyped acts. Automatisms may include chewing, eating movements, scratching, disrobing, rubbing, fumbling, running, or walking.
   b. **Absence seizures** in children, if severe, may be mistaken for childhood schizophrenia, mental retardation, or both if the child is having seizures frequently and cannot pay attention in school or to parents. Absence seizures may appear as if the person is not paying attention or may be accompanied by chewing or jerking (myoclonic) movements.

9. **Degenerative diseases.** A number of degenerative diseases of the central nervous system, such as Huntington's chorea, idiopathic Parkinson's disease, multiple sclerosis, amyotrophic lateral sclerosis, Gullain-Barré syndrome, Friedreich's ataxia and progressive supranuclear palsy, may present as schizophrenia to the incautious physician. However, the clinician should take into account the low probability of the onset of schizophrenia in older age-groups who are more commonly afflicted by these organic disorders. Although these disorders tend to occur later in life than schizophrenia, some present in the younger age-groups. Because these degenerative diseases carry a worse prognosis than schizophrenia, schizophrenia should be ruled out before making a diagnosis of such diseases as Alzheimer's or Pick's diseases.

10. **Congenital disorders.** Hereditary disorders, such as inborn errors of metabolism, genetic abnormalities, and lipidoses, are probably of little importance in the differential diagnosis of organic mental syndromes presenting as schizophrenia. However, some researchers have made the following discoveries:
    a. A subclinical form of phenylketonuria exists among adolescents and adults, which may be mistaken for schizophrenia.
    b. The smallest child of a pair of twins who has poor motor function and slow development may develop schizophrenia as a result of an intrauterine insult.
    c. Children and adolescents who demonstrate symptoms of minimal brain dysfunction may develop schizophrenia.

11. **Infections.** Infections with bacteria, viruses, fungi, and even parasites can cause organic mental syndromes. Some infectious agents cause cysts or abscesses in the brain with localizing findings on examination. Others may present as a meningitis, encephalitis, or multiple foci.
    a. **Bacteria.** Tuberculosis, syphilis, and organisms, such as *Staphlococcus, Hemophilus,* or *Meningococcus,* are bacterial causes of organic mental syndromes, particularly following or associated with meningitis.
    b. **Fungi.** Fungal causes of organic mental syndromes include histoplasmosis, cryptococcosis, and coccidioidomycosis.
    c. **Viruses.** Viral causes of organic mental syndromes include human immunodeficiency virus (HIV), herpesvirus, equine encephalitis, rabies, coxsackievirus, cytomegalovirus, Epstein-Barr virus, influenza, measles, enterovirus, and polio.
    d. **Parasites.** Infections with parasites that cause organic mental syndromes, while rare, may be dramatic. Causes may include a variety of helminth and protozoan organisms.

12. **Toxicity.** Toxic causes of organic mental syndromes are common and are so varied in form, causative agent, and age of onset that they may be very difficult to diagnose accurately.
    a. **Adolescence and early adulthood**
       (1) Drug abuse must be suspected, and use of amphetamines, cocaine, marijuana, phencyclidine, and other hallucinogens must always be part of the differential diagnosis of schizophrenia.
       (2) Intentional abuse of gasoline and toluene-based inhalants are common causes of organic mental syndromes in the adolescent age-group.
    b. **Older patients.** Digitalis toxicity and toxicity from prescribed medications are frequent causes of organic mental syndromes, especially the long- and intermediate-acting benzodiazepines, which accumulate because of reduced metabolism in the elderly. These elderly patients are sometimes believed to be either schizophrenic or "senile."
    c. **All age-groups**
       (1) Other toxic causes of organic mental syndromes include carbon monoxide toxicity from inadequately ventilated wood stoves, lead poisoning, and organic chemicals used in agriculture and industry.
       (2) Common iatrogenic offenders include:
          (a) Anticholinergic toxicity, often from the concurrent prescription of multiple drugs with anticholinergic properties, such as the combination of a low-potency neuroleptic, an anticholinergic agent for parkinsonian symptoms, and a tertiary amine antidepressant
          (b) Antihypertensive medications, which often lead to organic mood syndromes with depression
          (c) Central nervous system depressants, such as benzodiazepines, barbiturates, or methaqualone, and steroids, which may particularly resemble the negative symptoms of schizophrenia

13. **Traumatic insults** to the brain may result from either acute causes or be chronic sequelae of previous injuries; for example, changes in language after trauma may resemble all of the language changes in schizophrenia, producing neologisms.
    a. Acute subdural hematomas may present with bleeds into areas of the brain that demonstrate localizing neurologic findings or may be in the frontal area that tend to present with psychiatric symptoms first.
    b. Chronic subdural hematomas among older patients may present without a known episode of head trauma, following events as subtle as dehydration, which can tear a small blood vessel in the brain.
    c. Direct trauma to the brain and small bleeds into the brain tissue are not infrequently found among head trauma victims, even though these patients may not admit to the traumatic incident, particularly if it is associated with domestic violence.

    d. Postconcussion syndrome may be found following blows to the head, and the "punch-drunk" syndrome is frequently found among alcoholics and others suffering from head trauma.

  14. Endocrine disorders
    a. Thyroid problems are common causes of organic mood syndromes. In severe hypothyroidism, unusual affects and thinking patterns may be mistaken for schizophrenia.
    b. Parathyroid problems with resulting calcium abnormalities lead to unusual organic mental syndromes.
    c. Pituitary adenomata are notorious for presenting with odd psychiatric pictures as are Cushing's and Addison's diseases.
    d. Pheochromocytoma may resemble panic disorder or may be mistaken by inexperienced clinicians for anxiety accompanying psychotic decompensation.

  15. Neoplasms. Both primary and metastatic tumors of the brain should be kept in mind as causes for both localizing and generalized organic mental syndromes. In addition, tumors in other parts of the body cause organic mental syndromes through paraneoplastic effects that are not completely understood.

B. Mood disorders are often accompanied by symptoms that are confused with those of other psychotic illnesses, including schizophrenia. Depression with severe melancholic features is, for example, a more common cause of the catatonic syndrome in some studies than schizophrenia. Mood congruent delusions and hallucinations are a common feature of severe mood disorders. Manic patients who experience behavioral, hallucinatory, and delusional symptoms may create such diagnostic confusion that it is impossible to determine at the initial interview from which illness the patient is suffering. Studies from others countries have suggested that in the 1950s and 1960s psychiatrists in the United States grossly overdiagnosed schizophrenia, missing other diagnoses, particularly bipolar disorder. The *DSM-III* and *DSM-III-R* are now consistent with the diagnostic criteria used elsewhere in the world. Family history, age of the patient, previous psychiatric history, physical examination, and clinical observations must be used to differentiate mood disorders from schizophrenic disorders.

  1. Manic episodes. Manic patients who present with irritability, suspicions of persecution, delusions, and hallucinations may be indistinguishable from patients with schizophrenia. At the height of a manic episode, the patient may demonstrate bizarre behaviors, incoherence, and other features thought to be pathognomonic of schizophrenia. Careful family histories and longitudinal observations may be required to differentiate these conditions. If organic causes for the manic syndrome and personality disorder have been ruled out, a manic episode by definition implies that the patient suffers from **bipolar disorder**.
    a. Patients with bipolar disorder usually suffer from both manic and depressive episodes at some time in their lives, but in some cases, only mania is present in the lifetime course.
    b. The typical patient with bipolar mood disorder suffers more from manic episodes early in life and from depression in later years.
    c. In many cases, there may be two or more mood cycles a year, including mania and major depression.
    d. In extreme cases, patients may experience over four episodes of illness a year and up to several a day. These patients are called **rapid cycling bipolar disorder** patients.

  2. Major depressive episodes (including those associated with bipolar disorder). Patients with severe depressions may present with paranoid symptoms, social withdrawal, and severely restricted affect, which are suggestive of schizophrenia. Patients who develop melancholic features and delusions concerning cancer, a rotting body, guilt, and other mood congruent delusions particularly resemble schizophrenic individuals. Likewise, indecisiveness, slowing of thoughts, and lack of spontaneity in speech and behavior may resemble the negative symptoms of schizophrenia.

  3. Seasonal mood disorder. Although rare, this disorder represents a treatable diagnostic entity in the differential diagnosis of schizophrenia. Patients with this condition exhibit symptoms most commonly associated with "atypical depression" of hypersomnia, hyperphagia, weight gain, and decreased libido. Usually these symptoms appear in the fall and winter on a yearly basis, although other patterns have been described. Many of these patients report symptoms of mania or hypomania. Although seasonal exacerbation of symptoms in a supposedly schizophrenic patient should suggest the possibility of a seasonal mood disorder, it remains an uncommon finding.

  4. Postpsychotic depression. There is some controversy as to whether postpsychotic depression represents a true depression with the same biologic features as a major depressive episode or if it represents a phase of predominant negative symptoms of schizophrenia. Likewise, oversedation and parkinsonian symptoms, including akathisia, akinesia, and rigidity, may resemble the clinical picture of depression.

5. **Schizoaffective disorder.** The *DSM-III-R* lists this disorder as a "psychotic disorder not elsewhere classified"; that is, it is not classified as a schizophreniform or mood disorder. Patients present with either a manic episode or a major depressive episode with acute psychotic symptoms suggestive of schizophrenia or as an episode of psychotic symptoms without mood symptoms (in an individual in whom a mood disorder has been previously diagnosed). It is still a matter for debate whether this disorder is truly an intermediate condition. Patients with this disorder:
   a. Have a family history more positive for mood disorder than for schizophrenia
   b. Have a prognosis intermediate between mood disorders and schizophrenia
   c. Frequently respond to combinations of medications and treatments used for both schizophrenia and mood disorders.

6. **Schizophreniform disorder.** This diagnostic category was created in the *DSM-III* and *DSM-III-R* to differentiate psychotic patients who are regarded as "good prognosis" schizophrenics from "poor prognosis" schizophrenics as defined under older diagnostic systems. Patients with symptoms suggestive of schizophrenia for whom no organic cause for psychotic symptoms has been found and who meet the diagnostic criteria for schizophrenia, except that their symptoms have lasted less than 6 months, are appropriately diagnosed as having schizophreniform disorder. A few patients with schizophreniform disorder eventually meet the criteria for schizophrenia, although the majority will recover, never having met the diagnostic criteria for schizophrenia.

7. **Brief reactive psychosis.** Like schizophreniform disorder, this diagnostic category describes patients who were previously considered schizophrenic under old diagnostic criteria but whose good prognosis differentiates them from the patients diagnosed as schizophrenic under current criteria. Patients with brief reactive psychoses:
   a. Must have psychotic symptoms
   b. Demonstrate marked emotional turmoil
   c. Experience the onset of psychotic symptoms following a stressful life event
   d. Have no prodromal symptoms of schizophrenia
   e. Have made a full recovery to premorbid levels of functioning within a month at most

8. **Atypical psychosis.** This category is reserved for patients with some diagnostic features of schizophrenia but whose clinical picture does not fit all the criteria for schizophrenia. This diagnostic category is appropriate for patients with nonorganic psychotic presentations, which, after exhaustive examination, do not fit another diagnostic criterion for classification of psychotic symptoms. Atypical psychosis is a diagnosis of exclusion.

9. **Personality disorders.** With the decline of the use of such terms as "process schizophrenia" and "pseudoneurotic schizophrenia," there has been less diagnostic confusion between schizophrenia and personality disorders. However, in the case of several specific personality disorders, features of the clinical presentation may be confused with those of schizophrenia. Personality disorders most likely to be confused with schizophrenia include the following (using *DSM-III-R* nomenclature):
   a. **Paranoid personality disorder.** People suffering from this disorder interpret the actions of others as deliberately demeaning or threatening. Behavior is characterized by questioning the loyalty of others, holding grudges about insults or slights, and lacking trust in others. This disorder can be differentiated from paranoid schizophrenia in that it lacks acute psychotic episodes and extreme deterioration.
   b. **Schizoid personality disorder** is often found among biologic relatives of schizophrenics, suggesting that these disorders share some as yet undetermined genetic commonality. The lack of social interests of these patients results in a very restricted life-style, which may be confused with the social deterioration of schizophrenia. However, the lack of hallucinations and delusions differentiates these patients from schizophrenic patients.
   c. **Schizotypal personality disorder.** Like schizoid personality disorder, schizotypal personality disorder is frequently found among biologic relatives of schizophrenics. Because of the odd beliefs, magical ideation, and eccentric behavior and appearance, this disorder may be confused with schizophrenia; however, it can be differentiated from it because of the lack of a history of an active phase as in schizophrenia.
   d. **Borderline personality disorder.** People with this personality disorder suffer from a lifelong pattern of identity instability and disturbance, such as sexual identity, career choice, self-image, and chaotic social networks. In severe cases, psychotic features may

appear in response to stress but are not of sufficient duration or intensity to warrant a diagnosis of schizophrenia.

    e. Avoidant personality disorder is characterized by limited social and personal contacts because of fear and social discomfort rather than lack of interest. It is unlikely that this disorder would be confused with schizophrenia under modern diagnostic criteria, but under older diagnostic systems, many of these people would have been considered "process" schizophrenics.

    f. Other personality disorders. A variety of other personality disorders exhibit symptoms of sufficient severity that they may sometimes be misdiagnosed by the incautious clinician as schizophrenia.

        (1) Dependent personality disorder may be mistaken for exhibiting schizophrenic ambivalence, lack of drive, fear of being alone and other features.

        (2) Obsessive–compulsive personality disorder may demonstrate such restrictions of affective expression that it is mistaken for the flattened affect of older diagnostic systems for schizophrenia. Additionally, ambivalence, circumstantial speech, and other features may give the impression of schizophrenia without a diagnostic evaluation.

C. Religious and cultural subgroups. Diagnosticians from one culture may confuse culturally based beliefs and behavior patterns with symptoms of schizophrenia. Religious beliefs, if held by a group of people of which the patient is a member, cannot be considered psychotic by members of another group or culture. Likewise, cultural differences in body language and acceptable affective expression may be interpreted as bizarre by clinicians from other cultures. This diagnostic confusion is best avoided by consulting a clinician from the same culture as the patient or a clinician experienced with that culture.

VIII. ETIOLOGIC THEORIES. The search for the etiology of schizophrenia must surely be one of the longest investigations in medicine. Modern diagnostic criteria appear to permit better identification of risk and pathologic mechanisms than in the past.

    A. Genetic theories. With the new restricted criteria for the diagnosis of schizophrenia, evidence for genetic transmission of risk for schizophrenia seems substantial and is widely accepted; however, the nature of this genetic transmission remains elusive.

        1. Possible mechanisms. As early as the 1920s, simple mendelian models for the transmission of a gene for schizophrenia were found to be inapplicable. Since then, several models for the possible genetic transmission of schizophrenia have been developed.

        a. A single gene with variable penetrance. This model proposes that a single gene may transmit the schizophrenic genotype that may or may not be expressed as a result of environmental, social, or psychological factors. Such a monogenetic mechanism was hypothesized to be:

            (1) An inherited biochemical or metabolic disorder

            (2) An immunologic defect that might make the individual prone to infection by as yet unknown viral pathogens

            (3) A defect in a specific protein or enzyme

            (4) A defect in personality organization, which predisposed the individual to the eventual development of schizophrenia

        b. A single gene whose expression is modulated by polygenes. This model proposes that the basic gene for schizophrenia is transmitted in a simple, known pattern and that a combination of other genes regulate the expression of the schizophrenic phenotype. This hypothesis is at least partially supported by the following findings in relatives of schizophrenics:

            (1) Increased saccadic eye movements

            (2) Schizophrenic spectrum personality organization

            (3) High levels of creativity in biologic relatives of schizophrenics

        c. Polygenes. This model supposes that the development of schizophrenia is the result of the expression of multiple genes, which produce the schizophrenic phenotype. Although evidence for this model is good, isolation of these combinations of genes requires sophisticated mapping of human DNA and techniques of frequency analysis. This model appears to account for the differences in severity of the disease, the variable rates of pathology in families, and other puzzling findings.

        2. Evidence. A variety of study designs have been used to gather evidence of genetic transmission of schizophrenia or a risk factor that predisposes to the development of schizophrenia.

   a. Family studies
- **(1)** It has recently been reported (as this chapter goes to press) that a genetic linkage of schizophrenia with two polymorphisms on the long arm of human chromosome 5 was found in several Icelandic and British families. In this study, this dominant schizophrenia susceptibility allele did not lead to schizophrenia in all cases, but predisposed individuals to the schizophrenia spectrum disorders. This study provides the first strong evidence for a single gene as an etiologic agent of schizophrenia.
- **(2)** Another study of selected Swedish families found that the gene on the chromosome 5 is *not* involved in the transmission of schizophrenia in these Swedish families. This finding strongly suggests that several mechanisms, at least one of which is genetic, participate in the etiology of schizophrenia.
- **(3)** The most common research method used in family studies compares the prevalence of schizophrenia in families of schizophrenics with control families, which consist of both normal controls and controls with other psychiatric disorders. In studies completed since the establishment of modern diagnostic criteria, the risk of developing schizophrenia in relatives of schizophrenics appears to range from 3.5%–6.0% in contrast to previous rates of 0.2%–1.7%. These studies do not, however, establish the mode of transmission, that is, whether or not the increased risk in these families is due to environmental or genetic causes.

   b. Twin studies compare the rates of concordance for monozygotic and dizygotic twin pairs in which one member of the pair is diagnosed as schizophrenic. An assumption is made in these studies that the twins all experience an equal environment, which may not be true. Also, these studies have not used raters who are blind to the diagnosis of schizophrenia in one twin. Therefore, these studies cannot claim to answer absolutely the question of genetic transmission of schizophrenia.
- **(1)** Recent twin studies demonstrate concordance rates for monozygotic twins to be between 33% and 60%.
- **(2)** The same studies demonstrate a same-sex dizygotic twin concordance rate of 6%–21%.
- **(3)** Studies that show low rates of concordance for monozygotic twins demonstrate low rates of concordance for dizygotic twin pairs.
- **(4)** Dizygotic twin pairs and nontwin siblings both show a concordance rate of 10%–12% as would be expected.

   c. Adoption studies seek to separate social and environmental factors from genetic factors that might cause schizophrenia. These studies find no role for "vertical cultural transmission" of schizophrenia in families, no increased rate of schizophrenia in nonbiologic relatives of schizophrenics, but an increased rate of schizophrenia and schizophrenia spectrum disorders in biologic relatives of schizophrenic adoptees.
- **(1)** Some studies followed adopted-out children of schizophrenics.
- **(2)** Other studies looked for schizophrenia in the families of origin of adopted-out schizophrenics compared to rates of schizophrenia in the familes of nonschizophrenic controls.
- **(3)** A third type of study looked for rates of schizophrenia in step-siblings of schizophrenics.

B. Biochemical theories. It is clear that neurotransmitters in the brain are involved in the pathophysiology of schizophrenia. However, their specific role is undetermined. Specific neurotransmitters may be directly involved in the cause of schizophrenia. Schizophrenia may be caused by alterations in specific neurochemical systems as a result of some other more fundamental pathophysiologic process in the brain.

   1. Neurotransmitter systems
     a. Dopamine. One of the oldest biochemical theories of the etiology of schizophrenia is that dopamine and dopaminergic receptors are involved in the pathophysiology of this disorder.
      (1) Theories
- **(a)** Current theories suggest that dopamine receptors, particularly the D-2 receptor, are involved in schizophrenia. Areas of the brain suspected to be involved include the mesolimbic, prefrontal, and striatal dopaminergic systems.
- **(b)** Hypo- and hyperdopaminergic schizophrenic conditions that are measured by receptor density and receptor sensitivity may represent different schizophrenic syndromes in which negative or positive symptoms predominate.
- **(c)** Other theories suggest that dopaminergic autoreceptors (i.e., presynaptic receptors that provide feedback regulation to the dopaminergic neurons) may be involved in schizophrenia or, at least, in the treatment of symptoms.

(d) Some theories suggest that dopamine systems reflect only a link in chains of neurons involving multiple neurotransmitters, and problems with other types of neurons are reflected in dopaminergic systems as a secondary effect.

(e) Outdated theories proposed that there were "bad" dopamine molecules, such as isomers of dopamine.

(2) Evidence

(a) The most convincing evidence for the role of dopamine in schizophrenia is pharmacologic. Neuroleptic medications appear to exert their primary effect of alleviating the positive symptoms of schizophrenia through the blockage of dopamine receptors. However, while this evidence appears suggestive, it is indirect evidence that could be accounted for in other ways. The widespread use of neuroleptics, which may alter dopamine receptor density and sensitivity, has confounded more direct evidence.

(b) Postmortem examination of the brains of schizophrenics show increased D-2 receptor density.

(c) Cerebrospinal fluid examination for dopamine-related compounds demonstrate equivocal results.

(d) Discriminating between subtypes in which positive and negative symptoms predominate may clarify two different patterns of dopamine receptor increases and decreases.

b. Neuropeptides. Over 40 neuropeptides with possible central nervous system activity have been identified. Unlike monamines, neuropeptides are synthesized in the soma of the cell, packaged, and transported to the synapse. They are inactivated by peptidases in the synapse and not reabsorbed into the presynaptic neuron. In contrast to the monoamine neurotransmitters, the action of the neuropeptides is long-acting. They have unique anatomic localization in the brain and are correlated with behavioral, pharmacologic, and electrophysiologic findings that make it clear that they play significant roles in behavior.

(1) Theories. Studies of the possible roles of specific neuropeptides in schizophrenia are in their infancy and are plagued by methodologic problems. Nevertheless, the overlapping distribution of neuropeptide systems, such as cholecystokinin with dopaminergic systems in the brain, are typical of the enticing findings.

(2) Evidence. The evidence suggesting roles for specific neuropeptides has been gathered through postmortem examination of brain and cerebrospinal fluid for comparisons of receptor and peptide levels and through the administration of peptides and peptide receptor antagonists.

(a) Although assays for opioid peptides have not provided significant results, administration of destyrosine-γ-endorphin has produced neuroleptic-like activity.

(b) Preliminary findings suggest that cholecystokinin, neurotensin, and δ-sleep-inducing peptide systems may be altered in schizophrenia.

(c) Reports of the ability of naloxone to transiently reverse schizophrenic symptomatology in some patients are inconclusive.

c. Norepinephrine

(1) Theories. Few theories of the role of norepinephrine in schizophrenia suggest that norepinephrine acts alone in the pathogenesis of this illness. Rather, current models of the role of norepinephrine suggest that norepinephrine dysregulaton exposes fundamental defects in the functioning of dopamine or other neurotransmitter systems. Acutely paranoid psychotic states may be accompanied by increased levels of norepinephrine in the brain, while chronic schizophrenic patients appear to show state-dependent fluctuations, depending upon the transient variation in emotional and arousal states. Individual theories concern the increased, decreased, and defective metabolism of norepinephrine.

(2) Evidence. There is a great deal of evidence that norepinephrine is involved in the pathophysiologic process of schizophrenia, but there is little evidence about its precise role.

(a) Low dopamine-β-hydroxylase levels in the cerebrospinal fluid appear to be correlated with better psychosocial functioning in schizophrenics.

(b) In autopsy brain tissue, decreased levels of dopamine-β-hydroxylase and 3-methoxy-4-hydroxyphenylglycol (MHPG) were found in schizophrenics with brain atrophy.

(c) Increased norepinephrine and MHPG have been found in some areas of the brain, and increased norepinephrine has been found in plasma and cerebrospinal fluid of schizophrenics.

d. Serotonin. This neurotransmitter has long been of interest in the pathogenesis of schizophrenia because of findings that hallucinogens with psychotomimetic properties appear to be active in the serotonin systems of the brain.

(1) It may be that serotonin is active in the pathophysiology of schizophrenia as a modulator of other systems, such as dopamine.

(2) Like norepinephrine, abnormalities of the serotonin systems in schizophrenia are manifested by increased levels of serotonin itself and its metabolite, 5-hydroxyindoleacetic acid, in cerebrospinal fluid.

(3) Serotonin and its metabolites appear to be:

  (a) Increased in chronic patients
  (b) Decreased in paranoid and acute patients
  (c) Correlated with agitation
  (d) Affected by antipsychotic medications

(4) When fenfluramine, a serotonin antagonist, was given to several patients and then withdrawn, the negative symptoms of these patients improved. This finding suggests a possible role for this medication in receptor upregulation.

e. γ-Aminobutyric acid (GABA). Interest in GABA has been generated by the hypothesis that GABA may be inversely related to dopamine activity in the brain.

(1) The best studies report that there are no significant differences in GABA levels in the cerebrospinal fluid of medicated and drug-free schizophrenics and normal controls. On the other hand, low levels of GABA are found early in the course of schizophrenia and increase with the duration of the illness.

(2) Baclofen is a $GABA_B$ receptor agonist that produces exacerbations of schizophrenic symptoms.

(3) Benzodiazepines, which work in part as GABA agonists, alleviate both positive and negative psychotic symptoms in some patients.

(4) Low levels of GABA have been found in patients with a number of psychiatric disorders, most significantly depression.

f. Prostaglandins (PGs) have been of interest in schizophrenia, particularly the PGEs, because they are thought to have effects in modulating catecholamine systems in the brain.

(1) In animals, PGE_1 can produce catalepsy in animals, and high levels of PGE_1 are found in endotoxin-induced cataleptic states.

(2) Stimulation of PGE_1 production in platelets results in increased synthesis of PGE_1 in normal individuals but not schizophrenics.

(3) Quantitative measures of PG levels in cerebrospinal fluid demonstrated that PGE_2 and PGFs were absent in schizophrenics in contrast to patients with mood disorders who had demonstrable levels of both compounds.

g. Phospholipids are constituents of membranes of all cells, including neurons. The possibility that phospholipids may have a role in mental illness and in schizophrenia in particular has arisen only recently.

(1) Phosphatidylcholine, phosphatidylserine, and phosphatidylethanolamine have attracted interest for their potential roles in schizophrenia.

  (a) Phosphatidylserine has been found to be significantly increased in the neuronal cell membranes of schizophrenics.
  (b) Phosphatidylserine is found in high concentrations in neuronal tissue and may have a role in catecholamine neurotransmission and a possible role as a second messenger across cell membranes.

(2) Recent studies have focused on the positive lithium response in some schizophrenics as predicted by the theories concerning the methylation of phospholipids and phosphatidylserine.

h. Other neurotransmitters. A variety of other neurotransmitters and possible neurotransmitters have been investigated for roles in the pathogenesis or pathophysiology of schizophrenia.

(1) Phenylethylamines are endogenous amines, which appear to have amphetamine-like properties though interest in these substances has waned in recent years.

(2) In addition to GABA, dopaminergic systems also interact with acetylcholine and glutamate.

(3) There has long been interest in possible endogenous hallucinogens in the brain that might act to produce schizophrenia either as a result of increases from a normal level of a particular neurotransmitter or as a result of alterations of a normal neurotransmitter molecule. Interest in possible endogenous hallucinogens has increased following the discovery of what appears to be a phencyclidine (PCP) receptor in the brain.

2. Role of enzymes. Enzymes, as part of the neuronal systems that may have a role in schizophrenia, are involved in the synthesis, transportation, inactivation, and degradation of neurotransmitters.

a. Monoamine oxidase (MAO)

    (1) Theory. MAO has a role in the catabolism of amine neurotransmitters, including norepinephrine, dopamine, and serotonin. Decreased levels of MAO could make more of these neurotransmitters available within the synapse, potentially causing or exacerbating schizophrenia.

    (2) Evidence. Platelet MAO activity has been found to be lower in schizophrenics than normal controls in some studies. However, reduced platelet MAO has also been found in association with other psychiatric illnesses. Recently, MAO-B plasma levels have been found to vary with ventricular enlargement in schizophrenia, suggesting cerebral atrophy.

b. Catechol-O-methyltransferase (COMT)

    (1) Theory. When *l*-methionine was given to chronic schizophrenic patients in one series of experiments, some of these patients developed an exacerbation of schizophrenic symptoms. Because COMT is a major extracellular route for catecholamine metabolism, interest in methylation possibly producing aberrant neurotransmitters focused attention on COMT.

    (2) Evidence. No consistent decreases or increases in levels of COMT have been found in schizophrenia. Other amino acids have been found to exacerbate symptoms of schizophrenia, possibly as a result of nonspecific amino acid toxicity.

c. Creatine phosphokinase (CPK)

    (1) Theory. This enzyme catalyzes the reaction by which creatine phosphate and adenosine diphosphate (ADP) form creatine and adenosine triphosphate (ATP). Three isoenzyme forms of CPK exist in the brain and in cardiac and skeletal muscle. It has been found that levels of the skeletal muscle CPK (not brain) are increased in the sera of acutely psychotic patients. CPK is also increased in nonpsychotic relatives of schizophrenics.

    (2) Evidence. CPK increases are not specific for schizophrenia and may be artifacts of increased motor activity.

d. Dopamine-β-hydroxylase (DBH)

    (1) Theory. This enzyme catalyzes the transformation of dopamine to norepinephrine in noradrenergic neurons. DBH is reduced in schizophrenics with increased ventricular size. Some studies correlate low DBH with "reactive" schizophrenia, and high DBH with "process" schizophrenia.

    (2) Evidence. These findings (atrophy levels and "process" levels) appear to be contradictory, and the significance of DBH in schizophrenia remains unclear.

3. Viral etiologies

    a. Theories. Since the last century, possible viral etiologies for schizophrenia have been suspected.

        (1) Throughout this century, post–viral encephalitic conditions with symptoms resembling those of schizophrenia have been reported after known infections with influenza, mononucleosis, Epstein-Barr virus, and currently, human immunodeficiency virus among others.

        (2) The possibility of a neurotropic slow virus, acting on individuals with specific immune deficiencies, has also been proposed.

    b. Evidence. Evidence for the role of viruses causing schizophrenia remains inconclusive.

        (1) The observation that rates of schizophrenia are higher in individuals born in the late winter and early spring fits the seasonal patterns of certain viruses, suggesting a possible infection at birth or close to birth that results in schizophrenia.

        (2) Increased amounts of interferon in cerebrospinal fluid of schizophrenics have been found in some studies, but other studies and attempts to treat schizophrenia with interferon have not been encouraging.

4. Immunologic models

    a. Theory. Defects in the immune system in schizophrenia have attracted interest on the theory that:

        (1) An autoimmune illness might have a role in the pathogenesis of schizophrenia.

        (2) An immune deficiency might predispose the individual to schizophrenogenic viral infections.

        (3) Schizophrenics might suffer immunologic compromise as a result of neurohumoral effects of schizophrenia upon the immune system.

    b. Evidence

        (1) Studies show elevated levels of IgG, IgM, and IgA in subgroups of schizophrenics.

    (2) For years, there has been a search for an humoral factor (i.e., taraxein) that is responsible for schizophrenia. Interest in taraxein has been engendered by a lipid precipitate of brain extract from schizophrenics, which has focused attention on the possibility that taraxein is an autoantibody.

    (3) Other studies have focused upon delayed hypersensitivity and upon other indicators of autoimmune disease.

C. Neurophysiologic theories. Pathophysiologic studies of schizophrenia focus upon the identification of both **trait-specific** and **state-dependent markers** for schizophrenia and the significance of these physiologic mechanisms once they are identified.

  1. Electrodermal activity. Changes in skin conductance have been used as a measure of emotional arousal in a variety of situations, such as in industrial and criminal polygraphy, and in a variety of psychiatric conditions.

    a. It has been proposed that increased skin conductance recovery in response to a standard stimulus may be a trait marker for high-risk children who later develop schizophrenia.

    b. It has also been reported that poor prognosis schizophrenics do not habituate to repeated stimuli as do normal individuals and good prognosis schizophrenics.

  2. Cardiovascular activity. Both tonic (or resting) levels of heart rate and phasic heart rate responses to stimuli appear to have the most significant relationship to schizophrenia of all the cardiovascular physiologic parameters.

    a. Tonic heart rate appears to be elevated in schizophrenics in comparison to controls and does not appear to be affected by neuroleptic medications. This finding may reflect hyperarousal and increased adrenergic tone; however, it is a nonspecific finding that could be affected by the inactive life-styles of most schizophrenics.

    b. Phasic heart response studies. Findings of increased phasic responses have been less consistent than findings of increased tonic heart rates.

  3. Smooth pursuit eye movements are the slow-tracking lateral eye movements seen when an individual watches a swinging pendulum. Normally, the eyes move in a smooth back and forth sinusoidal pattern, but in some schizophrenics and other psychotic patients, this smooth pursuit is interrupted by multiple arrests in which the eye comes to a complete stop, resulting in an irregular pattern.

    a. Findings

      (1) This eye movement pattern is found in 45% of first-degree relatives of schizophrenics and in 10% of relatives of nonschizophrenic controls.

      (2) The concordance rate of this characteristic is higher in monozygotic than dizygotic twins.

      (3) This characteristic is seen in normal individuals as well as schizophrenics, and it may be related to the darting eye movements seen in some schizophrenics in clinical settings.

    b. Evidence. This finding deserves further investigation as a potential genetic trait associated with a risk for schizophrenia. It may be that the inability of schizophrenics to follow a pendulum represents an inability to separate a specific stimulus from extraneous background stimuli. The finding of this abnormality in nonpsychotic relatives of schizophrenics, at a time when new diagnostic criteria permit identification of a variety of schizophrenia-spectrum disorders in these same families, suggests a possible linkage of these eye movement patterns and a gene or genes causing susceptibility for schizophrenia.

  4. Electroencephalogram (EEG)

    a. Techniques. New EEG technologies, including multiple head recordings, computerized power spectral analysis (which is able to demonstrate the total amount of wave activity within defined frequency ranges), spatial mapping of power spectra, and multivariate analysis, have permitted a number of interesting findings.

    b. Findings. To date, no psychiatric disease can be diagnosed definitively on the basis of an EEG alone. The EEG findings in schizophrenia may be more specific to states of emotional arousal, cerebral insufficiency, diffuse neuronal impairment, and other nonspecific states than to schizophrenia. On the other hand, seizure-like phenomena in schizophrenia might represent a new insight into the pathophysiology of schizophrenia. A number of EEG findings in schizophrenia are of interest.

      (1) Chronic schizophrenics have less power in the fast alpha range (11–13 Hz), more power in the fast beta range (20–40 Hz), and more power in the slow theta and delta bands (0.5–8 Hz) than normal individuals. These nonspecific findings are also found in users of LSD, demented patients, and alcoholics.

    (2) Brain electrical activity mapping (BEAM), which generates color maps of EEGs and evoked potential data, has demonstrated bilateral increases in delta activity in schizophrenics, particularly in frontal areas, and increased fast beta activity, especially in the left temporal–parietal area. However, these studies are still plagued with artifacts from eyeblinks and muscle activity, so these data must be interpreted with caution.

    (3) Multivariate analysis techniques are able to solve some of the artifact problems, and it may be possible for these techniques to separate different psychiatric disorders, including schizophrenic subtypes, from each other and from normals.

    (4) Some investigators have reported spike phenomena reminiscent of partial complex seizures from depth electrodes in certain patients with psychiatric symptoms, such as auditory hallucinations.

5. Evoked potentials. While power spectral analysis deals with the spatial distribution of electrical activity in the brain, evoked potentials deal with the temporal dimension of specific electrical events.

    a. Technique. In this technique, a specific stimulus (either internal or external) is delivered at a specific time, and electrical activity in the brain is measured by monitoring specific EEG leads. If the stimulus is delivered repeatedly, using a computer, the results can be averaged with each successive stimulus. As the averaging takes place, all electrical events except those directly related to the stimulus disappear, leaving a temporal tracing of the electrical events following the stimulus. Various amplifiers and filters are used to select specific wave characteristics for examination. Components of this evoked potential are defined as positive (P) or negative (N) and by the time in milliseconds following the stimulus. Thus, a positive peak at 200 msec would be called a P200 wave.

        (1) Waves at less than 50 msec from the stimulus are designated as **early**.

        (2) Waves between 50 and 300 msec are designated as **middle**.

        (3) Waves at greater than 300 msec are designated as **late**.

        (4) Waves vary in shape, latency, and amplitude, depending upon sensory modality and location.

    b. Findings. Although there has been a wide range of findings in evoked potential research on schizophrenia, most of these findings are not specific to schizophrenia and can occur in alcoholics, demented patients, and other conditions.

        (1) **Early evoked potentials** are reported to have shortened latencies in chronic schizophrenics as compared to normal controls. The persistent nonsuppression of an early auditory P50 wave in chronic schizophrenics, despite clinical status or medication level, is reported to be a stable trait as compared to normal controls.

        (2) **Middle evoked potentials** are reported to be reduced in amplitude between 75 msec and 250 msec in schizophrenics. Painful electrical shocks were recorded as producing less absolute amplitude in the N120 wave, accompanied by reduced reports of pain in schizophrenics. These effects are reversed by naloxone, suggesting possible endorphin mediation of this phenomenon.

        (3) **Late evoked potentials.** Of all the findings of the evoked potential research in schizophrenia, the reduction of the P300 wave in schizophrenics is perhaps the most widely replicated. This wave form appears to be related to the presentation of stimuli that are task-related and surprising. It can be evoked by loud noises but has been studied in relation to reaction time to complex task-oriented stimuli. A number of interesting findings are discussed below.

        (4) **Adaptation.** With repeated auditory stimuli, schizophrenics fail to suppress a P50 wave, and this suppression failure has been reported commonly among biologic relatives of schizophrenics, suggesting that this is a possible genetic trait associated with schizophrenia.

           (a) With increasing levels of stimulus intensity, schizophrenics are reported to show an **augmenting (increasing) response** as opposed to the **reducing response** of normal individuals. These findings have prompted speculation about the failure of the evoked potentials of schizophrenics to return to normal and the possible inability of schizophrenics to suppress extraneous perceptual and cognitive stimuli.

           (b) An inverse relationship has been found between augmenting and reducing responses in schizophrenia and levels of MAO in platelets. Patients with chronic schizophrenia appear to have low levels of MAO activity as well as an augmenting evoked potential response.

6. Cerebral blood flow and brain metabolism. Cerebral blood flow and brain metabolism as measured by oxygen and glucose consumption have become a focus of investigation in schizophrenia in recent years as a result of advances in measurement techniques. Older studies measuring overall brain metabolism, using nitrous oxide, have been unable to differentiate schizophrenics from normal controls.

    a. Techniques. New techniques, using xenon-133 gas inhalation and scanning techniques, have provided new insights into cerebral blood flow and brain metabolism in schizophrenia.

        (1) Xenon-133 is a low-energy gamma radiation emitter that exchanges rapidly between blood and tissue. Because of this easy exchange, xenon-133 saturates brain tissue easily. External gamma detectors measure areas of high blood flow in the brain by following desaturation of areas with highest blood flow.

        (2) PET techniques use small atomic weight isotopes with short half-lives as gamma emitters. In addition to the PET equipment, research currently requires a cyclotron to produce these isotopes and a convenient radiochemistry laboratory, which has so far limited the number of facilities that use PET imaging.

            (a) One type of PET study uses 2-deoxyglucose, which is not metabolized completely in the brain, labeled with positron emitting isotopes, such as ^{11}C. By assigning the patient a particular cognitive task, activity associated with the specific task can be assessed.

            (b) Other PET techniques use other compounds, such as [^{11}C] chlorpromazine, which bind to specific receptor groups, giving an estimation of receptor density in illness. Other compounds labeled for the study of receptor distribution included haloperidol, bromspiperone, sulpiride, and raclopride.

    b. Findings. Because of the small numbers of patients in xenon and PET studies of schizophrenia and because of general diagnostic criteria used to identify schizophrenics for these studies, questions exist about which groups of schizophrenics demonstrate these abnormalities.

        (1) Xenon-133 studies of schizophrenics demonstrated reduced blood flow in frontal as compared with posterior brain regions in the resting state as compared with normal controls.

        (2) There are also reports of increased blood flow in the left hemisphere in schizophrenics in comparison with normal individuals who show relatively even distribution in the resting state.

        (3) Schizophrenics showed increased left hemispheric blood flow while engaged in spatial cognitive tasks in comparison with normal individuals who demonstrated increased blood flow to the right hemisphere. Neuroleptics were found to increase right cerebral blood flow in these schizophrenic patients.

        (4) Other studies demonstrated that with a standard attention-holding task (the Wisconsin Card Sort Test), schizophrenics failed to demonstrate the increased blood flow to the dorsolateral prefrontal cortex as demonstrated by normal controls.

        (5) Several PET studies demonstrated low metabolic rates in the basal ganglia of schizophrenics, which appear to be increased by neuroleptics, although this finding has also been replicated in patients with mood disorders.

        (6) Tests of attention administered to schizophrenics and normal controls during PET measurements demonstrated that the right superior frontal gyrus may be involved in attention and that schizophrenics who have difficulty in attention show relative hypometabolism in this area. This finding appears to be normalized by the administration of neuroleptics.

D. Neurologic and neuropathologic theories

    1. Neurologic findings. Minor nonlocalizing neurologic abnormalities have been detected in 60%–70% of schizophrenic patients. These neurologic "soft signs" include defects in stereognosis, graphesthesia, coordination, balance, gait, and tremor. Some examiners maintain that, particularly in chronic patients, soft frontal signs, such as snout, suck, and grasp reflexes, are found with increased frequency. Attenuation of glabellar tap–induced blinking is also reported to be reduced in some unmedicated schizophrenic patients, as well as being a parkinsonian symptom in patients on neuroleptics.

    2. Neuroradiologic findings

        a. Increased ventricular size. The most frequently reported finding in CT scans of the brains of schizophrenics is an increase in the size of the lateral ventricles. This finding implies a decrease in the volume of brain tissue and is reported as ventricle–brain ratio (VBR).

            (1) Methodologic problems, such as patient selection, age adjustment of samples, and technical problems in imaging, continue to obscure findings of increased lateral ventricle size, and several studies have failed to replicate this otherwise frequently positive finding.

(2) Preliminary studies of third ventricle size suggest that it may also be enlarged. Despite the methodologic problems, increases in lateral ventricle size have been correlated with such factors as poor neuroleptic response, poor premorbid adjustment, a predominance of negative symptoms over positive, and a possible pattern of familial transmission identified in monozygotic twins.

(3) A number of studies correlate ventricular enlargement with various neurotransmitter abnormalities, particularly dopamine system abnormalities.

b. Cortical surface abnormalities. Dilation of fissures and sulci on the cortical surface demonstrates loss of brain tissue, and like the enlargement of the lateral ventricles, is increased with age and a variety of neurologic conditions. CT scans demonstrate a range of findings, but the most reliable currently available data suggest that increases in the sylvian fissures, prefrontal cortex, and frontal areas may be the most characteristic patterns of atrophy in schizophrenia, suggesting possible temporal and frontal pathology. The degree of severity of symptomatology has yet to be correlated definitively with cortical abnormalities in schizophrenia.

c. Cerebellar abnormalities. Although cerebellar atrophy, and particularly atrophy of the vermis, have been associated with schizophrenia, their presence in schizophrenia is obscured by the same findings in a number of other psychiatric and neurologic conditions.

d. Magnetic resonance imaging (MRI) uses a radiofrequency energy pulse to unalign atoms briefly with particular nuclear configurations in a high-strength magnetic field and measures the resulting radiofrequency pulse from the realigning atoms. The realignment time measurement is specific to particular atoms, and these "signatures" are used to assemble a computer image of the brain. To date, the signature of hydrogen has been used most commonly in brain imaging. MRI studies of schizophrenia are in a very early stage and are highly inconclusive, although one study supports findings of frontal atrophy in schizophrenics. Because of the radiologic safety and very high resolution of MRI, it is expected to become a critical tool for research in schizophrenia in the near future.

3. **Postmortem findings.** Early studies from decades ago concluded, apparently erroneously, that neuroanatomic studies of the brains of schizophrenics had little to offer. Recent controlled postmortem studies appear to confirm data from CT scans concerning schizophrenia. Evidence has been found of decreased brain volume, increased ventricular size, decreased width, and more histopathologic changes consistent with cell loss and deterioration. In addition, studies of brains of unmedicated schizophrenic patients demonstrate reductions of size of parahippocampal gyri, substantia nigra, amygdala, hippocampal formation, and the medial pallidum. Cell studies demonstrate loss of cells in prefrontal associative areas and a general loss of neurons in relation to glial cells.

E. Psychological theories

1. **Overview.** A number of psychological functions have been studied and abnormalities characteristic of schizophrenia reported. Testing of schizophrenics currently includes both routine diagnostic testing, and tests designed to elicit features of schizophrenia in the experimental setting. Integrating psychological theories of deficits in schizophrenia stem from patterns of deficits seen in some, although not all, schizophrenics.

2. **Routine psychological testing** (see Chapter 1) is used in combination with clinical interviews and historical data to establish the diagnosis of schizophrenia. Projective testing is claimed by some to be highly subjective and unreliable and by others to demonstrate the most distinctive psychological picture in schizophrenia.

   a. The Rorschach Test. Schizophrenics demonstrate abnormal responses to the overall form of the ink blot, which normal individuals tend to see in consistent ways. In contrast to normal individuals, schizophrenics tend to see few people and little movement in the ink blot, and responses tend to be crudely formed. Contrary to popular belief, chronic schizophrenics tend to show primarily a lack of imagination and creativity on these tests, although there may be a tendency toward confabulatory answers and mixing of form perception in "contamination responses."

   b. The Thematic Apperception Test (TAT) is used less for diagnostic purposes than to clarify themes specific to the patient. Interpretation of drawings by schizophrenics tend to be distorted and demonstrate a lack of creativity.

   c. The Minnesota Multiphasic Personality Inventory (MMPI). Valid interpretations require specific training, and a diagnosis of schizophrenia on the basis of an MMPI alone cannot be made.

d. The Wechsler Adult Intelligence Scale (WAIS) measures intellectual performance. In schizophrenia, it is typical to see the verbal IQ preserved, while performance IQ scores are low. Specific subtests demonstrate characteristic "scatter" of unusually low and normal scores.

3. Attention. One of the most consistent psychological findings in schizophrenia is the difficulty of the schizophrenic patient in focusing attention on tasks. This is true for tasks that require sustained attention, focused attention (e.g., to separate a specific pattern or stimulus from background stimuli), or quick reaction times. Some of these findings may persist in schizophrenics after the resolution of positive symptoms; they are also found in relatives of schizophrenics. Possible explanations for these findings are discussed below.

a. These patients may lack an adequate filtering mechanism to attend selectively; that is, the signal-to-noise ratio is low, and there is too much "noise" in the system from irrelevant stimuli. Schizophrenics may be unable to maintain a major response set toward a particular goal in the presence of distracting stimuli and alternative mental sets. Schizophrenics tend to perform better on tasks with more external control and fewer opportunities for autonomous decisions.

b. Another theory proposes a sensory input dysfunction, causing a stimulus overload and hyperarousal states.

4. Cognition and information processing. In addition to attentional deficits, problems with registration, integration, and retrieval of information have been noted in many schizophrenic patients. It may be that the mechanisms for memory storage are overwhelmed by a flood of information or, alternatively, that there is an inability to form integrating constructs that would help to organize data. Conceptual overinclusiveness diminishes with clinical improvement, while idiosyncratic and bizarre thinking persists, suggesting that the latter reflects a more primary defect.

F. Family theories

1. Overview. Theories of family interactions in schizophrenia are presented for historical completeness, realizing that misapplication of these theories may harm patients and their families. It must be noted that some of the older work on families was based upon case data rather than experimentally derived data. Also, the existence of a "prepsychotic" personality has largely been replaced by a risk factor model except as a retrospective finding of the prodromal state prior to the development of a frank psychotic episode. In studies of high-risk children and their families, it is unclear whether unusual and possibly harmful interactional patterns derive from atypical behaviors of the high-risk child, mother, or both.

a. Current studies suggest that family communication styles influence the course and possibly the development of schizophrenia but can be modified through education to reduce the exacerbatory effects of harmful communication patterns on relapse in schizophrenics.

b. Older studies that affix blame for the development of schizophrenia upon family members, particularly "schizophrenogenic mothers," have caused more harm than good in the treatment of schizophrenia.

c. Expressed emotionality, one of the topics in family research receiving a lot of attention, suggests that attributing negative characteristics to the patient by family members is detrimental to the course of schizophrenia. Current findings suggest that noncritical attitudes of family members toward the patient may even improve the outcome in schizophrenia.

d. Political groups, such as the Alliance for the Mentally Ill, have attempted to destigmatize schizophrenics and their families and to promote biologic and social research on schizophrenia rather than affixing blame for schizophrenia upon the family of the patient.

2. Bateson and associates hypothesized that constant exposure to **double-bind communications** in the family are etiologic in schizophrenia. Double-bind communications have the following characteristics:

a. The communication takes place in an important and intense relationship from which the child cannot flee and in which a response is required.

b. The two messages, which are expressed on different levels, such as verbal and nonverbal, conflict with or deny each other.

c. The child is forbidden from commenting on the conflicting messages, which would clarify his or her response; thus, no matter what the child says or does, he or she is wrong on one level or another. According to this theory, psychosis develops as an attempt to deal with such situations. Double-bind communications occur frequently in daily life, but according to this model, vulnerable individuals in schizophrenic families are at a particular risk from this style of communication.

3. **Jackson** elaborated a concept of **familial homeostasis** in which the identified patient's illness is necessary for the maintenance of family equilibrium. Change or improvement in one individual results in pathologic consequences for other family members as the family attempts to reestablish a new equilbrium.

4. **Wynne and Singer**
   a. Wynne originally described **pseudomutuality** in family relationships of schizophrenics. Rigid roles are assigned to members at the expense of individuality, and superficial relatedness is maintained at the expense of genuine intimacy, which naturally requires the acknowledgment of individual differences.
   b. Later, Singer and Wynne identified a **transactional thought disorder**, which is predominantly amorphous or fragmented in any given family and which is present in both parents and offspring. The thought disorder can be documented by psychological tests.

5. **Leff and Vaughan** as well as other investigators studied relapse rates for patients in families that are rated for **expressed emotion**, which is defined in terms of criticism and emotional overinvolvement. Patients returning to families with high expressed emotion had a relapse rate four times higher than that of patients returning to families with low expressed emotion. Maintenance neuroleptic treatment and reduction in total weekly face-to-face contact had a protective value for patients returning to families with high expressed emotion. The relapse rate was 92% for patients coming from families with high expressed emotion who were not on neuroleptics and who did not reduce time spent with these relatives.

6. **Current family interaction research.** Several of the findings noted above have stimulated a wave of research on family interactional patterns and schizophrenia as well as other psychiatric disorders. In contrast to the earliest models of familial pathology in schizophrenia, current models are based upon well-designed studies of families.
   a. **Goldstein and colleagues** conducted a prospective longitudinal study of family interactive patterns and risks for the development of schizophrenia spectrum disorders. Factors studied for possible effects upon the development of schizophrenia spectrum disorders include the following:
      (1) **Communication deviance** was derived from transcripts of parents' responses to seven TAT cards and reflected a communications style with difficulties in maintaining a clear focus of attention and meaning. In the study, communication deviance was a marker that predicted the development of schizophrenia spectrum disorders in some family members, although it was not clear whether this was an effect of communication deviance or whether communication deviance and schizophrenia spectrum disorders were parts of a larger phenomenon.
      (2) **Affective style** was measured from the transcripts of parents' speech in interactions with the child while focused on a family problem and reflected personal criticism, guilt induction, or intrusiveness. Negative affective style was a better predictor of the development of schizophrenia spectrum disorders than high expressed emotion when considered along with communication deviance.
      (3) **Expressed emotion** was coded by raters from audiotypes of interviews with family members and reflected negative parental attitudes or criticism of a specific family member.
   b. **The Finnish Adoptive Study** is a prospective longitudinal study of children of schizophrenic mothers adopted away into families without a history of schizophrenia. Preliminary data appear to support the contention that children of schizophrenic mothers bear a genetic vulnerability to disordered interactions in the rearing environment.
   c. **Family attitudes** are thought by many current family interaction researchers to be the driving force behind expressed emotionality and as such should be amenable to change. Current research demonstrates that participation of the family in a **psychoeducational intervention program** is able to reverse the negative effect of high expressed emotionality on the course of the patient's illness. Other research interventions stress helping families to understand schizophrenia as a chronic illness rather than as a matter of the patient's choice or weakness, thereby reducing blame in these situations.

IX. TREATMENT

A. Overview. Because of the heterogeneity of presentations, courses, and possible etiologic contributions to schizophrenia, treatment programs for schizophrenics must be individualized and comprehensive, taking into account the biologic, psychological, and social needs of the patient. Attention must also be paid to the continuity of care, which involves integrating various types of service, treatment, and rehabilitation into a comprehensive whole in spite of a diverse service delivery network and changing providers over time. For over twenty years, the cornerstone of treatment for schizophrenics and other chronically mentally ill individuals has been to provide care in the least restrictive setting possible, making every attempt to reintegrate the person into the community. Modern approaches to the treatment of schizophrenia include control of the positive symptoms of schizophrenia as well as the reduction of the debilitating negative symptomatology.

B. Hospitalization

   1. Indications. Hospitalization is not indicated because of the appearance of symptoms but rather because of specific problems associated with the person's illness.
   a. Problems requiring short-term hospital care
      (1) Risks of suicidal and homicidal ideation
      (2) Command hallucinations
      (3) Extreme fear
      (4) Significant confusion
      (5) Inability of patients to plan and care for themselves
   b. Problems requiring long-term hospital care
      (1) Lack of appropriate community mental health resources (as in the case of patients from rural areas)
      (2) Provision of rehabilitation services prior to discharge to community programs
      (3) For cases of severely debilitated schizophrenic patients

   2. Goals
   a. Protection. The hospital should be a safe environment where:
      (1) Physical needs are met.
      (2) Stresses are minimized.
      (3) Impulses are controlled.
   b. Diagnosis. Twenty-four hour care allows for extensive observation and evaluation of the patient's problems, strengths, history, supports, and responses to treatment. In addition, access to sophisticated diagnostic laboratory and neuroradiologic tests provides the opportunity to differentiate schizophrenia from organic mental syndromes.
   c. Therapy. Treatments of various types can be started in the hospital, including neuroleptic medication, vocational and psychosocial rehabilitation, and family education, which are designed to return the patient to the community. Treatments can be adjusted to the patient's tolerance and response.

   3. Side effects. There are side effects associated with hospitalization. In spite of the distress experienced before the patient enters the hospital, the patient may experience a loss of self-esteem and social stigmatization as a result of being on a "mental ward." In addition, social supports in the community may be lost. With prolonged hospitalization, the patient risks the loss of social and living skills required to live in the world outside the hospital. This loss of skills is termed institutionalization.

C. Milieu treatment

   1. Definition. The therapeutic environment of the inpatient ward is called the **therapeutic milieu.** Inpatient psychiatric wards frequently use the therapeutic milieu as a major treatment modality for schizophrenic patients. Formal milieu therapy depends upon attention to the social structure of the ward and depends upon adequate numbers of well-trained staff. Interactions between staff and patients and formal social organizations, such as the patient's ward government, are tools regularly used in milieu therapy.

   2. Structure. One aspect of the staff's role in the therapeutic milieu is to support the patient's impaired reality testing, impulse control, and modulation of environmental stimulation. The staff works to reduce the patient's anxiety and controls injurious behavior. The structure of the ward should contain regular, structured activities, time alone, and help with personal hygiene and self-care. Milieu therapy avoids intense probing and anxiety-provoking psychotherapeutic interventions, which can be overwhelming for psychotic patients.

   3. Flexibility. The milieu should be flexible enough to respond to the changing needs of individuals with regard to length of stay, extent of restrictions, contact with family, group involvement, and activity levels. For example, as the patient's positive symptoms resolve, efforts may be initiated to increase the patient's socialization with other patients, structured recreational and vocational activities, and participation in the ward government.

4. **Ward community.** The other patients as individuals and as a group are used as therapeutic agents in the therapeutic milieu. Open, direct communication and individual responsibility is encouraged. The more organized and improved patients can provide hope and act as models for sicker patients. The patients are encouraged as a group to make decisions about daily activities of the ward and to help change maladaptive behavior of patients through open feedback.

5. **Side effects.** Like any treatment, the ward milieu may have significant side effects, which must be monitored. Target symptom–oriented treatment plans and post-hospitalization care plans that involve all of the staff, including staff from programs outside the hospital, may remedy these side effects.
    a. Premature and too harsh confrontation from staff and other patients or too much pressure for recovery may exacerbate psychotic symptoms or delay recovery.
    b. A structured and tolerant atmosphere may promote dependence on the ward, making it difficult to return to the community.
    c. Excessive demands for participation may cause overstimulation and disorganization.
    d. Less ill patients may take advantage of sicker patients, unless the interactions are monitored carefully.
    e. Staff may retain patients in the ward milieu longer than is desirable, creating a tendency for patients to return prematurely to the ward without ever developing a relationship with community services. This appears to be a problem with neophyte therapists who become enmeshed with the patient and his or her social network, believing that only they really understand the patient. This may result in a fragmentation of team efforts, poor communication with outpatient therapists, and other programs. Good supervision can reduce this risk to the continuity of care.

D. **Group therapy.** Group therapy has long been a mainstay of the treatment of schizophrenic patients in both inpatient and outpatient settings. Like other forms of therapy for schizophrenic patients, group therapy is best used in conjunction with other forms of therapy, particularly medications. Although there is a paucity of well-controlled studies of group therapy in schizophrenia, those that exist support the contention that group therapy that focuses on communication, alleviation of symptoms, and social skills produces improvements in social integration and fewer readmissions to the hospital than patients with social skills training alone. There is little evidence that open-ended, insight-oriented group therapy is effective in the treatment of schizophrenics, and some clinicians believe that group techniques that are unstructured and too confrontational may exacerbate psychotic symptomatology.

E. **Individual psychotherapy.** Psychotherapy for schizophrenic patients should be supportive and oriented to helping the patient adapt to the details of daily life. The admittedly sparse research literature on individual psychotherapy of schizophrenia suggests that supportive and adaptive therapeutic techniques are far more effective in the management of schizophrenic patients than insight-oriented techniques that focus on the patient's inner experience.

1. **Therapeutic relationship.** The closeness of the therapeutic relationship must be modified according to the needs of the patient.
    a. Attempts by therapists to establish a close or intense therapeutic relationship may exacerbate symptoms in patients who are highly suspicious or who feel overwhelmed by interpersonal relationships.
    b. Nondirective and affectively restricted therapeutic styles may also cause patients to experience anxiety and exacerbations of symptoms.
    c. Supportive psychotherapy is characterized by a warm, open relationship, which focuses on promoting the patient's self-esteem and helping the patient learn about his or her real strengths and limitations. Effective therapy focuses on practical and concrete issues.

2. **Therapeutic techniques.** The principles of psychotherapy of schizophrenic patients are as follows:
    a. **Education.** One of the main techniques of the therapist of schizophrenic patients is to teach the patient about his or her illness, including techniques of managing stress, understanding symptoms, and the value of compliance with pharmacologic treatments. This approach encourages patients to assume responsibility for treatment.
    b. **Focusing on problem-solving.** The therapist focuses on helping the patient solve concrete problems that arise in daily life. The therapist may offer possible solutions to

problems presented by the patient, including an analysis of possible positive and negative outcomes of each solution. The therapist attempts to develop problem-solving skills for the patient in financial, interpersonal, residential, and other areas of the patient's daily life.

c. **Setting reasonable expectations for change.** The current literature suggests that therapists who have unreasonable expectations for "cure" may convey these expectations to the patient in a counterproductive manner. On the other hand, having generally positive expectations for improving functioning and life satisfaction appear to be correlated with good outcomes.

d. **Expressing emotions effectively.** Therapies that encourage expression of emotion for its own sake or for "cathartic" value may trigger exacerbations in some schizophrenic patients. The therapist should encourage a discussion of private feelings and how to deal with these feelings but not encourage full-blown expressions of anger and hostility.

e. **Crisis intervention.** The therapist may be able to intervene in crises in the patient's life to prevent serious escalations. Unlike the passive roles in other forms of therapy, the therapist may need to become active in working with the patient's family, landlord, or social agencies to reduce the escalation of crises into psychotic episodes.

f. **Concrete limit-setting.** The therapist may need to set concrete limits on the patient, such as avoiding substance abuse and violence. These discussions frequently include discussions of consequences of harmful behaviors.

g. **Managing dependence.** One of the functions of the therapy of the schizophrenic patient is to increase the patient's appropriate socialization with other people in the community. In meeting this goal, the therapist encourages the patient to rely upon a large network of people in the community, rather than upon the therapist alone.

F. **Case management.** Because of the diverse and changing needs of the schizophrenic patient throughout the course of his or her illness, a variety of providers and agencies become involved in the person's care in the hospital and community, creating conflicting treatment expectations and plans among these providers. To facilitate the solution of this problem, the role of the individual therapist is giving way to that of the case manager in many mental health systems. The case manager is not confined to the hospital or clinic and may visit the schizophrenic patient in the community or in the home. Roles of the case manager include:

1. **Evaluation.** The case manager is responsible for collecting other assessments of the patient's medical, psychiatric, social, and financial needs and compiling these into an overall coordinated plan.

2. **Planning.** The overall treatment plan must coordinate diverse service and care providers and attend to the overall continuity of care for the schizophrenic patient. In addition, the case manager must share the overall treatment planning process with other members of the service delivery network.

3. **Linking.** Because of the difficulty that many schizophrenic patients have in gaining access to services required for comprehensive care, the case manager works to link the patient with all elements of the service delivery network. For example, the case manager may help the patient make appointments and even find transportation to these services. The case manager also links different service providers and agencies to solve problems of service delivery.

4. **Advocacy.** The case manager may need to seek resources and services for schizophrenic patients. This may either take the form of **case specific advocacy,** which is aimed at gaining resources for the individual patient, or **class specific advocacy,** which is aimed at gaining services, resources, or access to services for a group of patients.

G. **Family interventions and therapy.** Research on the families of schizophrenics has focused on the role of affective and communications patterns on the development and course of schizophrenia, suggesting that there may be specific interventions for families that may help the course of the patients. Current family research focuses upon reduction of the effects of high expressed emotionality and other forms of intrusive and deviant communication.

1. **Reduction of contact.** In some families with high expressed emotionality, patients limited to less than 35 hours of contact per week by the treatment system experience the same relapse rate as patients with low expressed emotionality families, as long as these patients are maintained on medication. Some studies suggest that this finding is applicable mainly to young male patients living in the parental home.

2. **Psychoeducational interventions.** Promising recent findings suggest that education of

families in conjunction with medications substantially reduces the risks of relapse posed by high expressed emotionality and other environmental stressors. These psychoeducational approaches include a behavioral approach that emphasizes understanding the patient's schizophrenia as an illness and modifying communications skills as a means of reducing high expressed emotionality. In some studies, psychoeducational approaches are significantly more effective in reducing relapses in the course of the illness than individual supportive psychotherapy. Some investigators have suggested that the effect of many of these interventions may be in reducing criticism and blame of the patient for his or her illness.

3. **Change from high expressed emotionality.** Recent investigators suggest that there may be a number of vehicles for changing high to low expressed emotionality families and that no matter which approach is used, the reduction of expressed emotionality accomplishes improvement in the course of schizophrenia.

4. **Crisis intervention.** Families in crisis around the schizophrenic illness of a family member may need concrete assistance in problem-solving, emotional reassurance, and education about the illness. The therapist should try to stabilize the crisis and address the fears or concerns about the illness or its treatment, encouraging the family to take needed legal interventions and other problem-solving steps.

5. **Family organizations.** Some families of chronically mentally ill people have formed organizations to promote education, destigmatization of the mentally ill, and mutual support. These organizations, particularly the National Alliance for the Mentally Ill, have had a substantial impact upon the programs for the mentally ill in the states and on a national level. Preliminary data demonstrate that family membership in such organizations may confer benefits similar to other family interventions in reducing risks from high expressed emotionality.

H. **Psychosocial rehabilitation** has become a significant part of treatment programs for schizophrenia because returning patients to productive lives in the community has become a priority. Goals of these programs are to ameliorate symptoms, remediate disabilities, and overcome handicaps associated with schizophrenia. In the past, patients who left inpatient institutions were found to have no skills necessary for independent living—that is, they lacked the skills in social interactions required for employment and required to form social support networks needed for survival. Preliminary data suggest that patients who participate in psychosocial rehabilitation programs experience recidivism at about half the rates of controls. These programs focus on the following issues:

1. **Social skills training.** Training in this area involves skills required to communicate with strangers and familiar people and to reduce the frequency of symptom-based communication and socially inappropriate behaviors.

2. **Nutrition and food preparation.** Patients who have lived in institutions for much of their lives may be unable to shop, prepare food, and plan a balanced diet. Patients are taught how to shop, cook, and plan meals.

3. **Residential skills.** Many schizophrenic patients have difficulty finding and maintaining housing; thus, training involves finding appropriate housing and being a good tenant. Many community mental health programs offer supervised housing for the transition between inpatient hospitalization and independent community living in addition to skills training.

4. **Managing finances.** Managing money, even if it is received monthly, may pose substantial problems. In extreme cases, patients may spend their monthly checks in a few days or weeks; thus, the patient is often without food for many days and, in extreme cases, may return to the hospital. Financial management skills are part of training for independent living.

5. **Managing the illness.** Patients are taught to manage medication administration, to watch for side effects, and to report potentially dangerous developments to the treatment system in an appropriate and assertive manner.

6. **Recreational activities.** Patients are taught to pursue recreational and physical activities to reduce stress and to promote general health.

I. **Consumer movement.** Self-help groups of schizophrenic and other chronicaly mentally ill people are increasingly prominent on the national scene. Clubs for mentally ill people, such as the nationally known Fountain House, are a source of support and improved self-esteem for people suffering from schizophrenia. Current activities associated with the consumer movement include well-functioning mentally ill patients working in the mental health system with less well-functioning patients, client-operated businesses, and other innovative approaches.

J. Pharmacologic treatment and electroconvulsive therapy (ECT)
   1. Antipsychotic agents
      a. Overview. Neuroleptic medications have revolutionized the treatment of schizophrenia (Table 2-2). In recent years, the risks of neuroleptics, particularly tardive dyskinesia, have prompted conservativism about the use of these medications and have prompted the search for new medications to treat schizophrenia. Although the traditional neuroleptics have differential effects upon D_1 and D_2 receptors, they all exert therapeutic effects through the blockage of the dopamine system.
      b. Efficacy
         (1) Acute psychosis. Neuroleptics are effective in alleviating the positive symptoms of schizophrenia, such as hallucinations, delusions, and agitation. They tend to be less effective in treating negative and social symptoms of schizophrenia, such as blunted affect, apathy, anhedonia, and grandiose and persecutory delusions, especially if they are chronic and well-organized.
         (2) Maintenance. Neuroleptics have well-established roles in preventing relapse in schizophrenia, particularly when used in conjunction with a comprehensive treatment plan.
            (a) Recent research shows that there may be a window of efficacy in risk/benefit of neuroleptics; that is, too low a dose and poor compliance may lead to relapse, whereas too high a dose risks noncompliance and tardive dyskinesia without appreciable benefit.
               (i) Within 6–8 months after discontinuation of neuroleptics, 50% of patients relapse.
               (ii) After 18 months, nearly 75% of medication-free patients relapse.
               (iii) About 25% of patients on medication relapse.
            (b) Two groups of schizophrenic patients may not be effectively treated with maintenance neuroleptics.
               (i) Patients who have had a single acute psychotic episode
               (ii) Very deteriorated chronic schizophrenic patients who may be refractory to treatment.

Table 2-2. Neuroleptic Medications

Generic Name	Trade Name(s)	Approximate Equivalent Oral Dosages (mg)	Usual Inpatient Oral Dosage Range (mg/day)
Phenothiazines			
Aliphatic	Thorazine	100	50–1500
Chlorpromazine			
Piperidine			
Thioridazine	Mellaril	100	50–800
Piperazine			
Fluphenazine	Prolixin, Permitil	2–4	2–60
Trifluoperazine	Stelazine	5	5–80
Perphenazine	Trilafon	10	16–64
Butyrophenones			
Haloperidol	Haldol	2–4	2–60
Thioxanthenes			
Thiothixene	Navane	5	5–80
Dihydroindolones			
Molindone	Moban, Lidone	10	20–225
Dibenzoxazepines			
Loxapine	Loxitane, Daxolin	10	20–225

    c. Choice of agent. The various neuroleptics vary in milligram potency and side effects but are efficacious when given in adequate doses. Although there is no evidence that certain subtypes of patients can be chosen prospectively to respond to certain medications, an individual patient may respond well to a particular drug and not to others. Initially, the choice of drug may depend upon side effect profile (e.g., sedation, α-adrenergic blockage, or parkinsonian effects) and the familiarity of the clinician with the particular medication. After an adequate initial trial, if there is not an adequate therapeutic response, there is justification for trying another neuroleptic from another group that may have different pharmacologic properties.

    d. Dosage

        (1) Acute psychosis. Recent studies demonstrate that a moderate initial dose (400–1200 mg) of chlorpromazine or the equivalent is usually adequate for the control of psychotic symptoms.

            (a) Massive doses used acutely for rapid modification of psychotic behavior in the past have been shown to be no more effective than moderate doses and carry added risks from side effects.

            (b) Whatever the dose, the acute effects of the medication on reducing psychotic symptoms usually occur in 3–10 days.

            (c) In a small number of schizophrenics, a much longer time for neuroleptic response may be needed (up to several months).

            (d) There appears to be a small number of schizophrenics who benefit from very high doses of neuroleptics.

        (2) Stabilization phase. Following initial control of symptoms, the daily dose of neuroleptics should be reduced gradually to a maintenance level. This process may take several weeks. In patients with a first psychotic episode and good prognostic indicators, eventual tapering of the medication to the point of discontinuation may be indicated.

        (3) Maintenance phase. The goal is to maintain the patient relatively symptom-free on the lowest possible dose of neuroleptics. A single daily dose is adequate for maintaining blood levels of the medication.

        (4) Nonresponse. There is a paucity of literature establishing a rational protocol for treating resistant cases. Acutely, agitation that appears to be increasing with increases in medication may be related to akathisia, a parkinsonian side effect of medication.

            (a) There is some evidence that new antipsychotic medications, such as clozapine and the substituted benzamides, may be effective for nonresponsive patients, although these drugs must be regarded as experimental.

            (b) Evidence also suggests that obtaining neuroleptic levels in plasma and adjusting doses accordingly may be another strategy for treating resistant patients.

            (c) In situations where there are adequate levels of neuroleptic but no response to treatment, waiting several months before altering treatment again may be beneficial.

            (d) Shifting medications from one class to another may also be beneficial.

            (e) There is little rationale for adding multiple neuroleptics to a treatment regimen.

            (f) The addition of lithium carbonate or carbamazepine to the neuroleptic may be of benefit in some cases with manic-like features of agitation and increased psychomotor activity.

    e. Route of administration.

        (1) Oral. Neuroleptics are routinely administered as tablets, capsules, or oral elixirs. The main problem with the oral route of administration is patient compliance.

        (2) Intramuscular injection. Most neuroleptics are available in injectable form. This route of administration is used with uncooperative patients in acute treatment settings and in cases in which an adequate plasma level cannot be obtained with the oral route.

        (3) Long-acting injections. Both haloperidol and fluphenazine are available as long-acting injections. Such injections provide neuroleptic medication for one to several weeks and have proven valuable for patients who have difficulty complying with oral medications.

    f. Adverse effects

        (1) Extrapyramidal syndromes result from blockade of DA receptors in the basal ganglia and occur more commonly with the high-potency neuroleptics.

            (a) Acute dystonic reactions, which are more common in young male patients early in treatment, involve sudden tonic contractions of the muscles of the tongue, neck (**torticollis**), back (**opisthotonos**), mouth, and eyes (**oculogyric crises**). As well as being extremely frightening, such reactions can be dangerous if the patient's airway is compromised. They can be effectively treated acutely with benztropine, 1–2 mg intramuscularly, or diphenhydramine, 25–50 mg intramuscularly or intravenously. Prophylaxis is accomplished with regular, orally administered anticholinergic medication.

(b) **Drug-induced parkinsonism** is characterized by cogwheel rigidity, bradykinesia, tremor, loss of postural reflexes, mask-like facies, and drooling. It is more common in elderly patients, and although it usually occurs in the first weeks of treatment, it may appear at varying times with varying doses. It can be effectively treated with any of the antiparkinsonian medications (Table 2-3) and may also respond to a decrease in neuroleptic dosage. Antiparkinsonian agents can generally be tapered and discontinued after 3–4 weeks of treatment in most patients. If the extrapyramidal syndrome remains unresponsive, a change to a different class of neuroleptics, usually one of lower potency, is required.

(c) **Akathisia** is a syndrome of motor restlessness, which may involve the entire body but is often most obvious in the patient's inability to keep his or her legs and feet still. It can be mistaken for anxiety, agitation, or an increase in psychotic symptomatology. The akathisia may respond to antiparkinsonian agents, but if the patient responds poorly, a decrease in dosage or change to another neuroleptic is indicated.

(d) **Neuroleptic-induced catatonia** occurs more commonly with the high-potency agents and is characterized by withdrawal, mutism, and motor abnormalities, including rigidity, immobility, and waxy flexibility. Although it can be mistaken for a worsening of the patient's psychotic symptoms, it is a complication of neuroleptic therapy. It may represent a variant of the neuroleptic malignant syndrome [see section IX J 1 f (2)]. It should be treated by temporarily discontinuing neuroleptic therapy and, upon resolution, changing to a different class of neuroleptic. Amantadine, administered in an oral dose of 100 mg three times daily, may also be helpful.

(e) **Tardive dyskinesia** is a late-onset movement disorder, which is thought to result from a disturbance in the DA-acetylcholine balance in the basal ganglia. In contrast to other neuroleptic side effects of the extrapyramidal system, tardive dyskinesia is associated with relative dopamine overactivity in the DA-acetylcholine balance. Mechanisms theorized to account for this phenomenon include an increase in the numbers or sensitivity of dopamine receptors in certain parts of the brain following chronic blockade with neuroleptics, although these theories do not fit all the data about the physiology of this condition.

   (i) Fasciculations of the tongue may be the earliest symptom, followed by lingual–facial hyperkinesias, which are persistent involuntary chewing, smacking, or grimacing movements.

   (ii) Choreoathetotic movements of the extremities and trunk, including the respiratory muscles, can be extremely disabling in severe cases. The symptoms often appear noticeably when there is a dosage reduction or discontinuation of neuroleptic medication, but they can usually be detected by close examination between neuroleptic doses.

   (iii) The syndrome can usually be reversed if it is detected early, and neuroleptics are discontinued. In severe cases, the movement disorder may be irreversible and can progress with continued neuroleptic treatment. Symptoms are worsened by anticholinergic medication, which should be discontinued if possible. Increased doses of neuroleptics may cause apparent temporary improvement by increasing the DA receptor blockade; however, this ultimately causes further progression of the movement disorder. Patients should be screened every 6 months for early signs and should be maintained

Table 2-3. Antiparkinsonian Medications

Generic Name	Trade Name(s)	Usual Oral Dosage Range (mg/day)
Benztropine	Cogentin	1–8
Trihexyphenidyl	Artane, Tremin	2–10
Biperiden	Akineton	2–6
Amantadine	Symmetrel	100–300
Diphenhydramine	Benadryl	25–200

on the lowest possible dose to minimize this serious complication of long-term neuroleptic use.

    (iv) Patients withdrawn abruptly from neuroleptics sometimes demonstrate a **withdrawal-emergent dyskinesia** with transient features of tardive dyskinesia, lasting for several days. It is not known whether this syndrome is an early form of tardive dyskinesia or has some other pathophysiologic mechanism.

(2) Neuroleptic malignant syndrome is a potentially life-threatening complication of neuroleptic therapy and is characterized by muscular rigidity, fever, autonomic instability, and an altered level of consciousness. Onset of the full-blown syndrome is rapid over 1–2 days after a period of gradual progressive rigidity. Treatment involves immediate discontinuation of the neuroleptic medication and support of respiratory, renal, and cardiovascular functioning and possibly treatment with dantrolene or bromocriptine.

(3) Anticholinergic effects occur with high-potency neuroleptics at a higher rate than with the low-potency neuroleptics. Anticholinergic effects are often seen as a direct result of treatment with a combination of drugs, including neuroleptics, anticholinergic agents used to treat parkinsonian side effects of the neuroleptics, and the inappropriate use of medications for other classes, such as the tricyclic antidepressants. In extreme cases of polypharmacy, combinations (e.g., a low-potency neuroleptic, a tricyclic antidepressant, and one or several anticholinergic agents) may produce a life-threatening anticholinergic delirium. Clinicians must watch for the development of increasing psychotic symptoms with the addition of more or different medications to the patient's treatment plan and should suspect anticholinergic delirium in these circumstances. Levels of anticholinergic side effects include the following:

    (a) Anticholinergic effects of medication at low doses include blurred vision on changing from close to distant objects, dry mouth, urinary retention in men with enlarged prostate glands, and constipation.

    (b) Anticholinergic poisoning includes restless agitation, confusion, disorientation, hallucinations, delusions, skin that is hot, flushed and dry, dilation of the pupils, tachycardia, decreased bowel sounds, and urinary retention. Central anticholinergic poisoning may occur without obvious signs, making iatrogenic anticholinergic poisoning a particularly insidious risk of polypharmacy.

    (c) Anticholinergic abuse. Because of the ability of anticholinergic agents to alter consciousness, patients sometimes abuse prescriptions for anticholinergic agents. Clinicians should treat parkinsonian symptoms with drugs with low-antimuscarinic effects, such as amantadine, in patients at risk for anticholinergic abuse.

(4) Cardiovascular effects of the neuroleptics most commonly include orthostatic hypotension, particularly in elderly patients, resulting from adrenergic blockade. This symptom is most commonly associated with the low-potency neuroleptics. In rare cases, neuroleptics may be associated with serious ventricular arrhythmias with electrocardiographic abnormalities (i.e., T-wave changes, prolonged QT intervals, and others) and with cardiac repolarization abnormalities. Risks of all cardiovascular complications are greatest with the low-potency neuroleptics.

(5) Hypothalamic effects include changes in libido, appetite, and temperature regulation. Because of dopamine's mediation of prolactin secretion in the hypothalamus, hyperprolactinemia may be found, resulting in breast enlargement and galactorrhea.

(6) Jaundice of an allergic cholestatic type occurs most commonly with chlorpromazine and usually resolves following withdrawal of the medication.

(7) Agranulocytosis is a rare unpredictable reaction to the more common neuroleptics and is probably related to interference of DNA synthesis by certain neuroleptics. It is reversible if detected early but may otherwise prove fatal. With the increased use of clozapine in the United States, agranulocytosis may be seen more frequently. In Finland, early use of clozapine produced a number of fatal agranulocytic cases, but the drug offers such promise for treatment of resistant cases of schizophrenia and for the reduction of tardive dyskinesia that it is likely to undergo extensive trials in the United States.

(8) Dermatologic effects include allergic rashes, which respond to discontinuation of the drug, and photosensitivity, which can be treated with sunscreens.

(9) Ophthalmologic effects include a pigmentary retinopathy associated with thioridazine in doses greater than 800 mg/day. Lens and corneal pigmentation has been reported with chlorpromazine, thioridazine, and thiothixene after long-term treatment, but this is rare. More common is blurred vision and worsening of narrow-angle glaucoma secondary to anticholinergic effects.

2. **Benzodiazepines.** There is a growing literature that suggests that benzodiazepines may be of value in reducing anxiety and agitation associated with acute psychotic episodes, particularly in combination with neuroleptics.

3. **Barbiturates.** Amobarbital and pentobarbital have been used in the past for acute sedation of patients resistant to sedation with neuroleptics. Because of the risks of respiratory depression and other side effects, these drugs are not recommended, especially because the benzodiazepines can be used more safely.

4. **Propranolol and other β-blockers.** These medications have been reported to be effective in treating acute psychotic episodes in conjunction with neuroleptics. Propranolol appears to increase neuroleptic levels in the blood and to treat akathisia effectively.

5. **Lithium** may be an effective treatment when there is an affective component to the patient's illness or when there is uncertainty about the diagnosis—that is, whether it is schizophrenia or a schizoaffective disorder. In some cases, lithium may be combined with neuroleptics to improve treatment in resistant cases.

6. **Anticonvulsants.** Recent literature reports that certain anticonvulsants, particularly carbamazepine, may be effective treatment for some schizophrenic as well as bipolar patients. These investigations are in the early stages, and criteria for determining a responsive subgroup have yet to be determined.

7. **ECT** has a secondary role in the treatment of schizophrenia and other acutely psychotic conditions. It is perhaps most effective in patients with affective and catatonic symptoms. Some studies suggest that ECT is acutely more effective than neuroleptics for the treatment of psychotic symptoms, though the risks and public perceptions of this treatment render it clearly a secondary line of treatment. Indications for ECT include:
   a. When life-threatening circumstances, such as severe catatonia or extreme suicidal ideation, are present
   b. When massive doses of neuroleptics are required, and smaller doses can be given following ECT
   c. When the patient is refractory to standard treatment regimens

8. **New antipsychotics.** A number of new antipsychotic agents are in the developmental and testing stages.
   a. Among the most interesting of these is clozapine, a dibenzoxazepine. Although this drug has the capability of producing fatal or serious agranulocytosis, it has been reported to be effective in treatment-resistant schizophrenics. Its effects are very different from the traditional neuroleptics.
      (1) It has very weak effects in animal models of dopamine activity.
      (2) It does not produce parkinsonism.
      (3) It appears to have little potential for producing tardive dyskinesia.
   b. Sulpiride and pimozide are, like haloperidol, more potent in their selective binding to D_2 receptors than traditional antipsychotics, perhaps resulting in effectiveness with different populations of schizophrenics. It is likely that the future of pharmacologic treatment for schizophrenia will see the increased use of receptor-specific pharmacologic agents for the treatment of particular groups of schizophrenics.

SUGGESTED READINGS

American Psychiatric Association: *Diagnostic and Statistical Manual of Mental Disorders*, 3rd ed, revised. American Psychiatric Association, Washington, DC, 1987

Baldessarini RJ: *Chemotherapy in Psychiatry: Principles and Practice.* Cambridge, Harvard University Press, 1985

Hahlweg K, Goldstein MJ (eds): *Understanding Major Mental Disorder: The Contribution of Family Interaction Research.* New York, Family Process Press, 1987

Kennedy JL, Guiffra LA, Moises HW, et al: Evidence against linkage of schizophrenia to markers on chromosome 5 in a northern Swedish pedigree. *Nature* 336:167–170, 1988

Leff JP: Schizophrenia and sensitivity to the family environment. *Schizophr Bull* 2:566–574, 1976

Meltzer HY (ed): *Psychopharmacology: The Third Generation of Progress.* New York, Raven Press, 1987

Sherrington R, Brynjolfsson J, Petursson H, et al: Localization of a susceptibility locus for schizophrenia on chromosome 5. *Nature* 336:164–167, 1988

Strauss JS, Hafez H, Lieberman P, et al: The course of psychiatric disorder: III. Longitudinal principles. *Am J Psychiatry* 142:289–296, 1985

Warner R: *Recovery from Schizophrenia: Psychiatry and Political Economy.* London, Routledge and Kegan Paul, 1985

STUDY QUESTIONS

Directions: Each question below contains five suggested answers. Choose the **one best** response to each question.

1. Negative symptoms of schizophrenia include all of the following EXCEPT

(A) affective blunting and flattening
(B) hallucinations of voices speaking to the patient
(C) lack of motivation and initiative
(D) anhedonia
(E) poverty of thought content

2. Which of the following symptoms of schizophrenia is most likely to be acutely responsive to treatment with medications, milieu therapy, and other inpatient treatment methods?

(A) Auditory hallucinations
(B) Apathy
(C) Poverty of thought content
(D) Anhedonia
(E) Social withdrawal

3. The criteria of Eugen Bleuler for the diagnosis of schizophrenia include all of the following EXCEPT

(A) ambivalence
(B) affective flattening
(C) apathy
(D) autism
(E) loose associations

4. Criteria of Kurt Schneider for the diagnosis of schizophrenia include all of the following EXCEPT

(A) auditory hallucinations
(B) voices heard arguing
(C) thought insertion
(D) ambivalence
(E) somatic passivity experiences

5. Risk factors for the development of schizophrenia include all of the following EXCEPT

(A) poor ego functions as demonstrated by lack of self-object differentiation and an increased vulnerability to narcissistic injury
(B) an environment characterized by high levels of cultural, economic, and psychosocial stressors
(C) a birth in early spring in either hemisphere
(D) a schizophrenic biologic relative
(E) a history of herpes simplex or viral encephalitis

6. Evidence used to support genetic transmission of schizophrenia includes all of the following EXCEPT

(A) risks of developing schizophrenia in relatives of schizophrenics range from 3.5%–6%, in contrast to the rates of 0.02%–1.7% in the general population
(B) monozygotic twins have a concordance rate between 33% and 60% for schizophrenia if one member of the pair has schizophrenia
(C) monozygotic and dizygotic twins of the same sex have roughly the same rates of concordance for schizophrenia
(D) adoption studies find no role for vertical cultural transmission of schizophrenia in families as evidenced by no increased rate of schizophrenia in nonbiologic relatives of schizophrenics
(E) increased rates of schizophrenia spectrum disorders are found in biologic relatives of schizophrenic adoptees

7. A patient who has been diagnosed as schizophrenic asks his psychiatrist about the chances of a younger sister developing the same illness. Leaving aside the question of whether this information should or should not be shared with the patient, the psychiatrist knows that the biologic sister's chances of developing schizophrenia are about

(A) 70%
(B) 40%
(C) 25%
(D) 12%
(E) 1%

8. A 21-year old man is referred to the psychiatrist through a student health service. The psychiatrist notes that the young man seems suspicious, talks vaguely with strange word usage, and seems unable to come to the point or include information in his speech. On further questioning, the man denies hallucinations but does appear to have a number of magical beliefs, which are generally consistent with those of the counterculture but which he has elaborated in an unusual way. His psychosocial functioning seems mildly to moderately impaired, but it seems to have been that way throughout much of junior high school and high school. The most likely diagnosis for the young man at this point is

(A) a personality disorder
(B) undifferentiated schizophrenia
(C) pseudoneurotic schizophrenia
(D) paranoid schizophrenia
(E) organic delusional syndrome

9. Which of the following statements is true of paranoid schizophrenia?

(A) The patient must demonstrate persistent delusions of a persecutory or suspicious nature but need not have other symptoms associated with schizophrenia
(B) Paranoid schizophrenic patients frequently demonstrate marked incoherence and loosening of associations.
(C) Because of interference with social function, paranoid schizophrenics have a worse prognosis than residual or undifferentiated schizophrenics
(D) Paranoid schizophrenics are more likely to have increased numbers of neuropathologic, neuroradiologic, and neurochemical abnormalities than other types of schizophrenics
(E) None of the above

10. A 30-year old American Indian man from one of the plains tribes is brought to the emergency room by relatives. Several days ago he found out that his sister had been killed in an automobile accident. Upon examination, he said he has twice seen his dead sister who appeared to him and asked him to join her in death. The most likely diagnosis is

(A) schizophreniform disorder
(B) brief reactive psychosis
(C) schizophrenia
(D) organic mental syndrome
(E) none of the above

11. Which of the following personality constellations has been found by researchers to predict reliably the development of schizophrenia later in life?

(A) Extreme dependency (e.g., sharing bedrooms with parents until late adolescence and experiencing panic away from home)
(B) Shyness, withdrawal, social awkwardness and inability to form close interpersonal relationships
(C) A pattern of lack of socialization, including cruelty to animals, fire setting, bed wetting and enuresis
(D) overcompliance, overconformity, and high academic achievement
(E) none of the above

12. All of the following neurotransmitters are suspected of being involved in the pathophysiology of schizophrenia EXCEPT

(A) dopamine
(B) prostaglandin E_1
(C) ascorbic acid
(D) norepinephrine
(E) serotonin

13. Common treatment goals for schizophrenic patients include all of the following EXCEPT

(A) continuity of care, such as treatment plans, can be carried through over time and changes in therapists
(B) treatment should be administered in the least restrictive setting
(C) comprehensiveness entails integrating medical, psychological, and social needs of the patient into a coordinated treatment plan
(D) confrontation of the patient's resistance to changes in his or her environment should be systematic, frequent, and assertive
(E) psychosocial rehabilitation should teach the patient social and functional skills, which may have been lost in earlier phases of the illness

14. Case management of the schizophrenic patient involves all of the following EXCEPT

(A) advocacy for the needs of the individual patient
(B) planning the overall treatment program among diverse service and care providers
(C) developing insight to intrapsychic causes of psychotic symptoms
(D) advocacy for groups of schizophrenic and other chronically mentally ill patients
(E) linking different care providers to coordinate treatment

15. A 35-year old man has been hospitalized for a number of years in a state hospital psychiatric unit. As the state hospital treatment team works with the community mental health center to plan his treatment and care and given that the community mental health program contains all of the elements of a comprehensive treatment rehabilitation system for the chronically mentally ill, which of the following elements might reasonably be included in his treatment plan for the immediate period after discharge from the state hospital?

(A) Help in finding an apartment in the community

(B) A psychosocial rehabilitation program beginning while he was still in the hospital and continuing through his community placement

(C) A case manager

(D) Participation in a psychoeducational-oriented group therapy system

(E) A regimen of long-acting injectable neuroleptics monitored by a psychiatrist in the mental health center

16. All of the following statements are true concerning psychosocial rehabilitation programs for schizophrenic patients EXCEPT

(A) a significant component of these programs involves communication skills, reducing symptom-based communications, and socially inappropriate behaviors.

(B) these programs focus on daily living skills, such as nutrition, food preparation, residential skills, and managing personal finances

(C) the major focus of these programs is returning patients to work through vocational training

(D) illness management skills are aimed at helping the patient manage medication administration, side effects, and exacerbations in their illness

(E) recreational activities are taught for their own benefit and for health promotional reasons

Directions: Each question below contains four suggested answers of which **one or more** is correct. Choose the answer

> **A** if **1, 2, and 3** are correct
> **B** if **1 and 3** are correct
> **C** if **2 and 4** are correct
> **D** if **4** is correct
> **E** if **1, 2, 3, and 4** are correct

17. Positive symptoms of schizophrenia include which of the following?

(1) Poverty of thought content
(2) Delusions of thought insertion
(3) Marked affective flattening
(4) Auditory hallucinations of voices speaking about the patient

18. The highest reliability symptoms of schizophrenia in the International Pilot Study of Schizophrenia include

(1) ideas of reference
(2) elated thoughts
(3) hearing thoughts aloud
(4) schizophrenic negativism

19. Psychological tests that *cannot* be used alone to diagnose schizophrenia include which of the following?

(1) Rorschach Test
(2) Minnesota Multiphasic Personality Inventory
(3) Thematic Apperception Test
(4) Wechsler Adult Intelligence Scale

20. Which of the following subtypes of schizophrenia are recognized in the *DSM-III-R* criteria?

(1) Pseudoneurotic
(2) Oneiroid
(3) Hebephrenic
(4) Undifferentiated

21. Correct statements concerning probable trait- as opposed to state-dependent markers of schizophrenia include which of the following?

(1) Resting heart rate in acute psychotic episodes is elevated
(2) Schizophrenics and their relatives appear to show abnormal darting eye movements when following a swinging pendulum with their eyes
(3) On electroencephalogram, schizophrenics have less power in the fast alpha range and more power in the fast beta range and slower alpha and beta bands than normal
(4) Schizophrenics and their biologic relatives consistently fail to suppress a P50 wave on average evoked potentials

22. Which of the following statements could be used to support a diagnosis of a central information processing deficit in schizophrenia?

(1) Poor prognosis schizophrenics do not show habituation of skin conductance to repeated stimuli
(2) When auditory stimulus intensity is increased, schizophrenics are reported to show an augmenting response as opposed to the reducing response of normals
(3) There is a failure in schizophrenics to attenuate to the early auditory averaged evoked potentials P50 and P300 with repeated stimuli
(4) Xenon-133 gas inhalation and positron scanning techniques have demonstrated reduced blood flow to the frontal cortex in schizophrenics in comparison with normal controls

23. Neuroradiologic findings associated with schizophrenia include which of the following?

(1) Gas inhalation studies, using xenon-133, demonstrate reduced blood flow in frontal areas of the brain and possible increased blood flow in the left hemisphere in schizophrenics in comparison with normal controls
(2) Magnetic resonance imaging demonstrates frontal atrophy in schizophrenics
(3) Positron emission tomography shows low metabolic rates for the basal ganglia in schizophrenia, which appear to be normalized with neuroleptic administration
(4) Schizophrenics tend to show a much higher than average rate of calcification of the pineal on skull films, which may be associated with the seasonal onset of schizophrenia and rates of melatonin synthesis

24. Both metabolic studies and anatomic neuroradiologic studies appear to support the contention of a loss of actual brain tissue mass in poorly functioning chronic schizophrenics. These studies and neuropathologic and neuroanatomic studies appear to demonstrate cell and tissue loss in which of the following areas of the brain?

(1) Frontal cortex
(2) Parietal cortex
(3) Temporal cortex
(4) Occipital cortex

25. Neuropathologic abnormalities that have been associated with schizophrenia include

(1) an increase in ventricle size associated with poor neuroleptic response and predominance of negative symptoms
(2) atrophy of auditory cortex associated with persistent auditory hallucinations
(3) dilations of fissures and sulci on the cortical surface, particularly in the area of the sylvian fissure, prefrontal cortex, and frontal areas
(4) atrophy of the ventral medial and ventral lateral nuclei of the hypothalamus associated with appetitive changes in catatonia

26. Correct statements concerning socioeconomic factors that influence schizophrenia include which of the following?

(1) During the Great Depression, the outcome of schizophrenia in the United States and Great Britain was worse than either before or after
(2) In large cities, the incidence of schizophrenia increases with the size of the city
(3) In India, the upper castes experience higher incidences of schizophrenia, partially disproving the drift hypothesis
(4) In the United States, a higher prevalence of schizophrenia is found in lower socioeconomic groups than in other groups, supporting the "drift hypothesis"

Directions: The group of questions below consists of lettered choices followed by several numbered items. For each numbered item select the **one** lettered choice with which it is **most** closely associated. Each lettered choice may be used once, more than once, or not at all.

Questions 27–31

For each enzyme listed below, select the response most likely to be associated with it.

(A) Associated at one time with theories that methyl donors exacerbate schizophrenia
(B) Synthetic enzyme in noradrenergic neuronal systems
(C) No known contribution to schizophrenia
(D) The "muscle" isoenzyme is increased in schizophrenics and relatives of schizophrenics
(E) The "B" isoenzyme of this group is associated with cerebral ventricular enlargement in schizophrenics

27. Creatine phosphokinase

28. Dopamine-β-hydroxylase

29. Monoamine oxidase

30. Catechol-O-methyl transferase

31. Lactate dehydrogenase

ANSWERS AND EXPLANATIONS

1. The answer is B. (*I*) Hallucinations and delusions are positive symptoms of schizophrenia. "Positive" symptoms are those that are additions to the patient's mental state, in contrast to absent, or "negative" symptoms. Negative symptoms are those subtracted from the patient's mental state, such as loss of affect and lack of motivation and initiative.

2. The answer is A. (*I; IX B, C, J*) Generally, the positive symptoms of schizophrenia, including alterations in thinking, perceptions, and behavior, such as hallucinations and delusions, are more responsive to acute treatment than the negative symptoms of schizophrenia. Negative symptoms include affective flattening, social withdrawal, apathy, anhedonia, and poverty of thought and content of speech. Negative symptoms of schizophrenia may be more responsive to rehabilitation programs and other psychosocial interventions than to acute inpatient treatments.

3. The answer is C. (*II B 2*) Eugen Bleuler identified disturbances of ambivalence, autism, loose associations, and affect as characteristics of schizophrenia. These criteria are no longer used in the clinical setting but are of historical importance. Anhedonia, although found in schizophrenia, is not one of the classic "four A's" of Bleuler.

4. The answer is D. (*II C*) Kurt Schneider's diagnostic system for schizophrenia focused on clusters of symptoms that are relatively common and that have a relatively high degree of interrater reliability (i.e., a symptom about whose presence and specific type several raters interviewing the same patient are likely to agree). Ambivalence is the type of symptom about which several raters would likely disagree since it reflects an internal process, evidence of which would be difficult to elicit from the patient.

5. The answer is A. (*III E, F; VI A–C; VII A 11 c*) Although disordered ego functioning is believed by some clinicians to be frequently present in schizophrenia, there is no good evidence that disordered ego functioning in any way predicts the development of schizophrenia. In addition, interrater reliability difficulties in assessing disordered ego functioning would make this criteria very difficult to assess should systematic studies of this factor be undertaken. A birth in early spring, environmental stressors, a schizophrenic biologic relative, and a history of herpes simplex or viral encephalitis are factors that are known to be at least statistically associated with an increased risk for the development of schizophrenia.

6. The answer is C. (*III F*) Monozygotic twins raised together have a concordance rate for schizophrenia of 91%; if raised apart, they are concordant at a rate of 78%, according to one study. Some studies show high rates of mental illness, in relatives of schizophrenics, and adoption studies have shown that there is no increased rate of schizophrenia in nonbiologic relatives of schizophrenics. If there were equal rates of schizophrenia in monozygotic and dizygotic twins, there would be strong evidence for an environmental as opposed to a genetic mode of transmission of schizophrenia, but this has not been found to be true.

7. The answer is D. (*III F 1*) Leaving aside the adjustment of the percentage of risk for the sister's age, the risk of a full sibling developing schizophrenia is 10%–12%, according to an average of most studies of this topic. The risk for the general population is 1%.

8. The answer is A. (*V A 3, 4, B 3; VII A, B 9*) The key feature of the presentation of the 21-year old man described in the question is the lack of a clear episode of psychosis without which he cannot be diagnosed as schizophrenic. Diagnostic systems, which include dated concepts, such as "process schizophrenia" are no longer considered valid. Although organic mental syndrome is possible, there is no evidence that would lead the clinician to suspect this over a personality disorder, such as schizotypal personality disorder.

9. The answer is E. (*V A 3*) According to modern diagnostic criteria, patients with paranoid schizophrenia may not have incoherence, marked loosening of associations, flat or grossly inappropriate affect, catatonic behavior, or grossly disorganized behavior. The prognosis for paranoid schizophrenia is better than that for other types, perhaps because of the late onset that is characteristic. Paranoid schizophrenia tends to be associated with fewer neuropathologic abnormalities and neurochemical findings than other types of schizophrenia. In contrast to other types of schizophrenia, paranoid schizophrenia patients retain good social functioning in spite of frequent interferences with relationships because of delusions.

10. The answer is E. (*VI A; VII A, B 6, 7, C*) The case described in the question of an American Indian who is visited by his recently deceased sister is a normal culture-bound experience for American Indians from Plains cultures. The physician should remember that assessment of psychotic systems by a clinician from one culture in a patient from another culture should not be attempted without specific knowledge of the patient's culture.

11. The answer is E. (*VI A 1–4*) Research has failed to demonstrate the existence of the schizophrenic personality, particularly one that reliably predicts later development of schizophrenia. However, some studies have revealed significant histories in some schizophrenics of extreme dependency, shyness, withdrawal, social awkwardness, inability to form close interpersonal relationships; an asocial premorbid personality, and a pattern of overcompliance and conformity.

12. The answer is C. (*VIII B 1 a, c, d, f*) Dopamine systems are thought to be central in the pathophysiology of schizophrenia. All of the compounds listed in the question—prostaglandin E_1, norepinephrine, and serotonin—except ascorbic acid are currently thought to be neuromodulators of the dopamine systems in schizophrenia. There are no known therapeutic or physiologic influences of ascorbic acid in schizophrenia even though there is massive public lore about its efficacy in a variety of conditions.

13. The answer is D. (*IX A, E, H*) Comprehensiveness and continuity of care are elements of a reasonable care plan not just for schizophrenics but for patients with any chronic illness. Treatment of the patient in the least restrictive treatment setting, which may involve placement in the community as opposed to inpatient hospitalization or voluntary as opposed to civil commitment status, is a common treatment goal. Psychosocial rehabilitation is a central feature in the reintegration of schizophrenic patients into the community, and there is increasing evidence that it may significantly improve the prognosis in long-term patients. Confrontation of schizophrenic patients to overcome their resistances to change is likely to produce exacerbations in psychotic symptomatology, particularly if this intervention is carried out with a high degree of affect on the part of the therapist. Thus, systematic confrontation of schizophrenic patients is not indicated in any reasonable treatment plan.

14. The answer is C. (*IX F 1–4*) The role of a case manager as it is defined in most service systems does not involve sharing the role of the therapist. Furthermore, current therapy of the chronically mentally ill does not involve insight-oriented therapy but rather a supportive, educational, problem-solving approach. Planning, evaluation, linking, and advocacy are all portions of the routinely described duties of case managers. Acting as an advocate of groups of mentally ill patients is included in some definitions of case management, although it is a controversial role; however, class-specific advocacy is a more common and widely accepted role for case managers than insight-oriented therapy.

15. The answer is A. (*IX H 1–6*) After a long period of hospitalization, most schizophrenic patients are lacking in skills required to locate an apartment and to live without supervision in the apartment. Such planning might create crises in the patient's life and would make him or her prone to rehospitalization. If graduated supervised residential care is available in this hypothetical community mental health setting, a supervised residential placement would be much more appropriate in the transition to independent living. Although the use of long-acting neuroleptics may well be indicated because of anticipated medication compliance problems, an ideal treatment program would encourage the patient to assume as much responsibility of self-administration of medications as possible. All the other elements (i.e., a psychosocial rehabilitation program, a case manager, and psychoeducational-oriented group therapy) would be appropriate to good treatment planning after the discharge of the patient.

16. The answer is C. (*IX H 1–6*) This question was presented to emphasize an area of confusion for many clinicians. Vocational rehabilitation focuses largely on job skills and job retraining, while psychosocial rehabilitation, which may include elements of vocational rehabilitation, attempts to teach patients skills required for life in the community outside of institutions, including food preparation, managing finances, residential skills, and social skills. Recreational skills may also be promoted in these programs.

17. The answer is C (2, 4). (*I*) Under most diagnostic systems of schizophrenia, the acutely psychotic symptoms are generally considered positive or present symptoms. These include hallucinations, delusions, ideas of thought insertion, and thought broadcasting. Negative symptoms of schizophrenia are often considered to be long-term residual symptoms. These include affective flattening, poverty of thought content, amotivational states, and anhedonia.

18. The answer is A (1, 2, 3). (*II E 2*) In the International Pilot Study of Schizophrenia, the highest reliability was noted in patient-reported criteria, and the most common symptoms reported by schizophrenic patients included suicidal ideation, elated thoughts, ideas of reference, delusions of grandeur, hearing thoughts aloud, derealization, lack of concentration, hopelessness, and delusions of persecution and reference. Schizophrenic negativism, perseveration, and stereotypic behaviors, which are observed by clinicians rather than reported by patients, rank among the lowest in reliability.

19. The answer is E (all). (*VIII E 2 a–d*) No psychological test, when used alone, can be used to diagnose schizophrenia. Each of the tests listed in the question—Rorschach Test, the Minnesota Multiphasic Personality Inventory, Thematic Apperception Test, and Wechsler Adult Intelligence Scale—demonstrate abnormalities that are frequently found in schizophrenia; however, all of these tests produce these findings in nonspecific ways, which may be precipitated by conditions other than schizophrenia.

20. The answer is D (4). (*V A 4, B 2–4*) Only undifferentiated schizophrenia is recognized in the *DSM-III-R* as a diagnostic type. Pseudoneurotic, oneiroid, and hebephrenic types are not included in the *DSM-III-R* because of a lack of diagnostic reliability.

21. The answer is C (2, 4). (*VIII C 2, 3 a, 4 b (1), 5 b*) Both increased resting heart rate and the nonspecific electroencephalographic abnormalities are likely to represent markers of the acutely psychotic state. Increase in resting heart rate may represent a generally higher level of arousal in schizophrenia. Decreases in alpha and increases in beta, delta, and theta are seen in a number of patients that have various features similar to schizophrenia. In contrast, the nonsuppression of the P50 wave and the abnormal psychotic saccadic eye movements of schizophrenics and their biologic relatives suggest that these traits may be associated with at least some physiologic process that places the individual at risk for developing schizophrenia.

22. The answer is A (1, 2, 3). (*VIII C 1, 5, 6*) Failure of schizophrenics to attenuate to stimuli represents a major fundamental difference in the method in which information is processed in schizophrenia and is supported by their failure to habituate to repeated stimuli, their augmenting (rather than reducing) response to increased auditory stimulus intensity, and their persistent inability to suppress early auditory evoked potentials P50 and P300. In contrast, evidence of diminished cerebral blood flow to anterior areas of the brain, while true, would have only very indirect connections to specific information processing abnormalities.

23. The answer is A (1, 2, 3). (*VIII C 6 b*) Gas inhalation studies, using xenon-133, demonstrate reduced blood flow in frontal areas of the brain and possibly increased blood flow in the left hemisphere of schizophrenics. Magnetic resonance imaging demonstrates frontal atrophy, and positron emission tomography shows low metabolic rates for the basal ganglia in schizophrenia. Although these findings are very preliminary, they point the direction for further investigations in schizophrenia.

24. The answer is B (I, 3). (*VIII D 2 b*) Loss of cells in frontal areas and prefrontal areas appear to be the most widely replicated findings in the neuropathology of schizophrenia. Other studies appear to support a loss of mass in temporal areas of the brain. Neither parietal nor occipital cortical areas are widely found to be abnormal in size or cell count density on most studies.

25. The answer is B (1, 3). (*VIII D 2 a, b*) Although there is some evidence of cerebellar atrophy, particularly atrophy of the vermis in schizophrenia, the only consistent neuropathologic abnormalities appear to be frontal and temporal atrophy reflected by both increased ventricular size and widening of fissures and sulci.

26. The answer is E (all). (*III E*) The course and prognosis of schizophrenia tends to be worse during times of socioeconomic stress in the industrialized world. Data from India, showing a higher incidence of schizophrenia in the upper castes, suggest that the drift hypothesis may not be correct, whereas data from the United States, which show a higher prevalence of schizophrenia in lower rather than higher socioeconomic groups, have been used as evidence for the drift hypothesis. Large cities in the industrialized world show increased incidences of schizophrenia proportionate to their size. This ratio does not apply to cities with populations below 100,000.

27–31. The answers are: 27-D, 28-B, 29-E, 30-A, 31-C. (*VIII B 2 a–d*) The muscle form (not brain as might be expected) of creatine phosphokinase has been found to be increased in schizophrenics and relatives of schizophrenics. This may reflect increased levels of muscle breakdown due to as yet unknown processes or simple increases in muscular activity in this group.

Dopamine-β-hydroxylase (DBH) catalyzes the transformation of dopamine to norepinephrine in noradrenergic neurons. It has been found to be reduced in schizophrenics with increased ventricular size, although its overall significance is yet unclear. Low levels of DBH appear to be correlated with better psychosocial functioning than high levels.

Recent research has focused on the role of monoamine oxidase, subtype B, which is found to be associated with changes in ventricular size in schizophrenia. It is likely to be a nonspecific indicator of pathology rather than being directly associated with schizophrenia.

Catechol-O-methyltransferase (COMT) is a major extracellular route for the metabolism of catecholamines. It was originally found that *l*-methionine exacerbated the symptoms of schizophrenics, and this finding was replicated with betaine. Attention was focused on the possible role of COMT in schizophrenia. However, other amino acids without a likely role in donating methyl groups were found to produce similar symptoms. Interest in this enzyme has waned to some extent.

To date there has been no indication that lactate dehydrogenase is involved in schizophrenia.

3
Mood Disorders
Jon A. Bell

I. DEFINITION. Mood disorders are clinical conditions of which the common and essential feature is a disturbance of mood. The term mood refers to persistent emotional states that affect how an individual acts, thinks, and perceives his or her environment. The *Diagnostic and Statistical Manual of Mental Disorders*, 3rd ed., revised (*DSM-III-R*) classification of mood disorders includes bipolar disorders, which are bipolar disorder, cyclothymia, and bipolar disorder not otherwise specified, and depressive disorders, which are major depression, dysthymia, and depressive disorder not otherwise specified. Disturbance of mood is often accompanied by other signs and symptoms, including psychophysiologic, cognitive, psychomotor, and interpersonal difficulties.

II. HISTORY. Descriptions of depression in scientific and poetic literature date back to antiquity. Vigorous scientific investigation of mood disturbances has taken place primarily in the last century.

A. Jules Falret described patients who became depressed and elated in a cyclic fashion—**la folie circulaire**—in 1854.

B. Karl Ludwig Kahlbaum made similar observations about mania and melancholia in 1882. He felt that these episodes were different stages of the same disease process, which he called "**cyclothymia.**"

C. Emil Kraepelin (1856–1926)

    1. Kraepelin made painstaking observations of patients and described a number of mood disorders, including mania, melancholia, recurrent depression, and mild mood swings. In 1921, he concluded that all of these mood disorders are identical in certain ways. He called the underlying illness "**manic–depressive illness.**" This formulation of a single, underlying disorder with varied clinical manifestations was widely accepted for several decades.

    2. Kraepelin's notion of a single mood disorder with varied clinical manifestations did not withstand the scrutiny of clinicians in the 1930s and 1940s. By the mid-1950s, it was suggested that some individuals suffered only from depression, while others suffered from the cyclic disorder that Kraepelin had described—manic–depressive illness.

D. Karl Abraham (1877–1925) accepted Kraepelin's notion of a single mood illness. In his description of 6 patients, he presented a psychodynamic picture of mood illness, which emphasizes the role of loss in precipitating a mood episode and the element of regression in the clinical presentation.

E. Sigmund Freud (1856–1939)

    1. Freud emphasized the importance of loss in depression. Instead of remaining angry with the lost individual, the anger is turned inward by the depressed person. Freud felt that this phenomenon accounted for the typical findings of guilt, lowered self-esteem, self-reproach, and suicidal ideation. He did not explain all depression in this manner, however. He clearly stated that some depression is psychogenic in origin (i.e., precipitated by loss) and, in other cases, biologically determined.

    2. Freud's conceptualization of two different types of depression gained favor. Depression was classified as either **endogenous** (i.e., biologically determined) or **exogenous** (i.e., precipitated by loss). It was felt that those patients who develop severe depression in the face of some acute precipitant suffer from a different disorder than those without recent loss in their histories. Many advocated different treatments for the two groups. Psychotherapy with a focus on reactions to the acute precipitant was advocated for exogenous or reactive depression.

Medication, electroconvulsive therapy (ECT), or both were prescribed for endogenous depression. This interpretation of depression was accepted well into the 1970s.

F. Biologic features of mood disorders

1. Research, which began in earnest in the 1950s, was triggered by a serendipitous observation made in hypertensive patients treated with the then new drug, **reserpine**. Many of these patients developed severe depression. It was soon realized that alterations in central nervous system biogenic amine functioning (which reserpine caused) altered mood. Since that discovery, much of the research on mood disorders, especially depression, has focused on neurotransmitters and brain pathways.

2. As research proceeded, controversy about the endogenous and exogenous classification of depression grew. Recognition of the clinical similarities between the two groups of depressed patients and laboratory studies, which did not distinguish between the groups, led to the current categorization. It is now felt that the presence or absence of a precipitant is less important diagnostically and therapeutically than the signs and symptoms of depression and their severity.

III. EPIDEMIOLOGY. Interpretation of the data on the epidemiology of mood disorders is complicated by variations in the type of classification used, in the parameters measured, and in the reliability of diagnostic categories. This is particularly true of dysthymia and cyclothymia, which are both relatively new categories.

A. Major depression and bipolar disorder. Major depression is more prevalent than bipolar disorder.

1. **Lifetime risk.** Studies in Great Britain, the United States, and the Scandinavian countries indicate that the risk of developing one of these severe disorders ranges from 0.6%–25.0% over the course of a lifetime.
   a. Lifetime risk for bipolar disorder ranges from 0.6%–2.0%.
   b. Lifetime risk for major depression ranges from 2%–25%. Most authorities agree that an accurate figure is in the range of 10%–15%.

2. **Incidence.** The incidence of bipolar disorder is similar in men and women. Major depression is diagnosed about two times as often in women as in men. Some investigators have speculated that this difference reflects a bias on the part of clinicians in diagnosing depression more readily in women. In our society, women tend to be more emotionally expressive than men, and, therefore, they display sadness or unhappiness more easily than men. Recognition of depression in men is often more difficult. Investigators have pointed to the higher incidence of substance abuse among men and have identified it as a **"depressive equivalent"** or **"masked depression."**

3. **Socioeconomic status.** Major depression and bipolar disorder occur in all socioeconomic groups and do not appear to be more prevalent in one group than in another.

4. **Genetics.** Kraepelin first noted that the risk for developing major depression or bipolar disorder is greater for blood relatives of patients with these disorders than it is for the population as a whole. Families of patients with bipolar disorder are much more likely to develop bipolar disorder than major depression. Families of patients with major depression are much more likely to develop major depression than bipolar disorder.

B. Dysthymia and cyclothymia are relatively new diagnostic classifications. Data on the incidence and prevalence of these disorders are limited. However, some recent studies have been completed.

1. **Prevalence**
   a. Over a period of 1 year, investigators found dysthymia to have a prevalence rate of between 4.5% and 10.5%.
   b. Few studies have been done on cyclothymia. Some investigators have estimated that less than 1% of the population is affected, but further inquiry is needed.

2. **Sex ratio**
   a. As in major depression, dysthymia is reported to be more common in women than in men in a ratio of two or three to one.
   b. There are no data regarding the ratio between men and women for cyclothymia.

3. **Socioeconomic status.** No differences in the occurrence of either dysthymia or cyclothymia have been identified among socioeconomic groups.

4. Genetics. No conclusions can be drawn about familial patterns for either dysthymia or cyclothymia.

IV. DIAGNOSIS. The disturbance in mood seen in mood disorders usually involves either depression or elation, with symptoms characteristic of either a manic or depressive syndrome.

A. The diagnostic categories of major depression and bipolar disorder are distinguished from one another on the basis of whether or not there has ever been a manic episode. Bipolar disorder is characterized by the presence or history of a full manic syndrome with or without a depressive episode. Patients who have suffered only from depressive episodes are diagnosed as having a major depression, which is characterized by the presence of a full depressive syndrome.

1. Symptoms of a manic syndrome. The essential feature of a manic episode is a distinct period when the predominant mood is elated, irritable, or expansive. Other associated symptoms include the following:

a. Elevated or intensified mood. In a manic episode, the elevated mood has various manifestations. Some patients are euphoric, extremely cheerful, or happy. An observer may find the individual's high spirits to be infectious, and only those who know the patient may recognize the excessive cheerfulness. Other patients are expansive: They involve themselves in a large number of activities and may have an insatiable craving for social interactions. They are not selective in their involvement and are propelled by seemingly boundless enthusiasm. Although it is common for the manic individual's mood to be elevated, some patients are predominantly irritable. They have little ability to tolerate frustration, and irritability may progress to hostility, belligerence, and assaultiveness.

b. Hyperactivity. Affected individuals make elaborate plans and engage in numerous endeavors. They may have difficulty sitting down and relaxing. They are always doing something or anticipating what they will do next. Many activities are carried to excess. This agitation often makes it stressful for others to be around the manic patient. Under the pressure of an increased desire to be sociable, indiscriminate contacts with distant acquaintances occur. Late-night phone calls and visits are not uncommon. The inappropriate, intrusive, or threatening nature of these contacts is not appreciated by the manic. Expansiveness, grandiosity, impaired judgment, and boundless optimism frequently lead to wild spending sprees, reckless driving, unwise investments, and intense, exaggerated sexual activity. Excessive alcohol use may occur during mania. Behavior is often flamboyant or bizarre. The usual style of dressing may be replaced by more colorful or outlandish apparel. Individuals may appear to be disorganized or out of control. Some manic individuals accost strangers and attempt to engage them in conversation or in unrealistic schemes.

c. Rapid or pressured speech. Manic individuals speak loudly and are difficult to interrupt. Telling jokes, making puns or plays on words, and a preoccupation with unimportant but amusing details are common. Dramatic or exaggerated forms of expression, such as singing or gesturing, may occur. The sounds of words may enchant the patient, leading to **clanging**, a phenomenon characterized by word selection based on sounds rather than meanings. Irritable individuals are prone to hostile tirades when frustrated.

d. Compromised coherence of thought. Flight of ideas is a pattern of thought characterized by a rapid and continuous flow of speech with sudden changes in topic. These changes are usually based on comprehensible associations, distractions (e.g., noises), and plays on words. In its severe form, flight of ideas is difficult to follow, and the manic individual becomes incoherent and disorganized. Loosening of associations, a phenomenon characterized by rapid changes in topic that are not understandable, also occurs in disorganized manic patients.

e. Distractibility. Typically, manic individuals are very distractible. This is evident in the shortened attention span of these individuals. Flight of ideas reflects distractibility. An inability to begin and complete a task because of distractions due to inadvertent and irrelevant stimuli is common. Signs, colors, lights, and sounds may be sufficient to disrupt concentration and attention.

f. Elevated opinions of self. Just as the mood is elevated and exuberant, the manic individual's opinion of him- or herself is elevated. Some patients are uncritical of themselves; others have grandiose and delusional notions of their own worth and accomplishments. It is not uncommon for manics to believe that they are experts on topics of which they are not; for example, manic individuals tell physicians how to practice medicine. Books are written. Jobs for which qualifications are lacking are actively pursued. In extreme forms, manic patients are delusional. They believe that unique relationships with a deity or powerful political, religious, and entertainment figures exist.

g. Limited need for sleep. Manics go to bed late and are up early, often sleeping just 2–4 hours a day. Even with so little sleep, they are full of energy. Sleeplessness for several days is not uncommon.

    h. Rapid shifts in mood (lability). This phenomenon is characterized by an abrupt change from exuberance and elation to anger or depression. The anger or depression may last a few minutes or a few hours. When angry, manic patients pose a significant danger to others. When depressed, they may act on sudden suicidal impulses. This mingling of manic and depressive syndromes is referred to as **bipolar disorder, mixed**, in which aspects of each syndrome become part of an ongoing clinical picture.

    i. Delusions and hallucinations. Psychotically disturbed manic patients experience delusions and hallucinations. Usually, these phenomena are **mood-congruent** (i.e., consistent with the predominant mood). For example, an exuberant, euphoric patient believes that he or she has a special relationship with God, which is a delusion, and hears God's voice, which is an hallucination. Delusions of persecution may arise for manic individuals who imagine that others are jealous of their powers and relationships. Delusions and hallucinations that have no apparent connection with the predominant mood are **mood-incongruent**. The utility of the concepts of mood-congruence and mood-incongruence is open to question at this time.

2. Symptoms of a depressive syndrome. The essential feature of a depressive syndrome is either a dysphoric mood or a loss of pleasure or interest in usual activities. This mood disturbance is prominent and persistent. It is accompanied by a number of typical symptoms and signs of a depressive syndrome. In making a diagnosis of major depression, weight is given to the severity and duration of symptoms. Two weeks of severe symptomatology is suggested as a guideline. A major depression may occur one time only or may be recurrent.

    a. A dysphoric mood. Patients may complain of feeling "blue," sad, irritable, discouraged, hopeless, or depressed. Alternatively, patients may express a loss of interest in and enthusiasm for everyday activities, saying such things as, "I just don't care about anything" or "Nothing makes any difference to me anymore." These symptoms are prominent and unaltering during the depression.

    b. Changes in appetite or weight. Typically, patients lose their appetites. Interest in food is lost, or food no longer tastes good. Food is consumed only when the depressed individual can force it down. In this situation, weight is lost quickly, often 5–10 pounds in 1 week. Less commonly, individuals increase their food intake during a depressive episode. Frequent and large meals satisfy a craving for food, although there may be little gustatory pleasure. Weight may be gained quickly, up to 20 pounds in 2 or 3 weeks.

    c. Disruption of normal sleep patterns. Some patients report difficulty in sleeping, which may take several forms. Difficulty in getting to sleep plagues many; they lie in bed for 1, 2, even 3 hours and cannot get to sleep (**initial insomnia**). Once sleep is achieved, it may be short-lived. Awakening in the middle of the night (**middle insomnia**) or in the early morning (**early morning awakening**) limits the hours of sleep. Overall, most depressed patients suffer from a lack of sleep. However, some sleep excessively, often 12 hours and more a day (**hypersomnia**).

    d. Altered level of activity. Most patients are less active than usual. The patient tells the examiner such things as, "I just can't get my work done" or "I spend my day sitting and can't get going." Observations of these patients reveal a lack of spontaneous movement and activity. They are motionless. They sit with hunched shoulders. They speak slowly and softly, sometimes so softly as to be inaudible. They are said to be **psychomotorically retarded**. Some individuals are strikingly more active than usual. They are restless and may not be able to sit still in a chair. Pacing, constant use of the hands, doing such things as pulling at clothing and hair, or incessantly smoking cigarettes may be prominent. Patients say that they "cannot sit still." They can be described as agitated.

    e. Lack of interest in sexual activity. Typically, both the frequency and the enjoyment of sex are diminished. Men may become impotent. Women report an inability to feel aroused or excited.

    f. Lack of pleasure and interest in normal activities. Individuals who previously enjoyed their work and hobbies no longer find them satisfying. Little effort is made to participate or engage in activities. This loss of all pleasure is called **anhedonia**.

    g. Fatigue. Individuals complain of low levels of energy, saying such things as, "I just get tired so easily" or "I don't have any energy."

    h. Feelings and thoughts of worthlessness, self-reproach, and excessive guilt. Patients may express an intense sense of responsibility for their thoughts and feelings or for events in their environment. They readily find fault with themselves. Such ruminations may attain irrational proportions, and patients may become psychotic (out of touch with reality). Delusions arise from the individual's preoccupations with self-worth, guilt, disease, death, and decay.

    i. Cognitive impairment. Patients find that they cannot think clearly. They are unable to concentrate. Tasks, such as reading and calculating, may become very difficult, if not impossible, to complete. A lack of attention during everyday activities, such as cooking and

watching television, may leave the patient feeling frustrated and inept. Indecisiveness interferes with daily functioning when even minor decisions cannot be made. These cognitive disruptions are frequently apparent in the diagnostic interview. The patient seems demented when cognitive impairment is severe, a phenomenon referred to as "pseudodementia."
  j. Thoughts of death. This phenomenon may take various forms. Some individuals wish for death or long to be reunited with a deceased loved one. Danger is more imminent for others. Plans for death are formulated. Some make wills and get their affairs in order. Others plan suicide. Reckless driving and excessive alcohol or drug use are examples of covert suicidal behavior that warrant attention.

B. The diagnostic categories of dysthymia and cyclothymia are comprised of long-standing conditions with minimal durations of 2 years. A sustained or intermittent disturbance of mood is associated with signs and symptoms of a mood disorder. Unlike major depression and bipolar disorder, only a partial mood disorder is present. There are never any psychotic features.
  1. Signs and symptoms of cyclothymia. The essential feature of cyclothymia is a chronic mood disturbance of at least 2 years' duration. Numerous episodes of depression and hypomania occur in the course of the illness. Depressive and manic syndromes are not of such severity or intensity to warrant a diagnosis of a full mood disorder.
    a. Periods of normal mood may occur between episodes of depression and hypomania. Individuals are never without hypomanic or depressive symptoms for more than 2 months. Others may have limited or no periods of normal moods.
    b. Dysphoria and hypomania. When affected individuals are depressed, they suffer from a dysphoric mood most of the day on more days than not. At other times, they are hypomanic, a condition in which a muted form of a manic syndrome is present.
      (1) Signs and symptoms of the depressive periods during the first 2 years of mood disturbance do not constitute major depression; that is, the symptoms are less severe and do not cause as pervasive a dysfunction as major depression. Signs and symptoms might include the following:
        (a) Insomnia or hypersomnia
        (b) Low energy or chronic fatigue
        (c) Feelings of inadequacy
        (d) Decreased effectiveness or productivity at school, work, or home
        (e) Decreased attention, concentration, or ability to think clearly
        (f) Social withdrawal
        (g) Loss of interest in or enjoyment of sex
        (h) Restriction of involvement in pleasurable activities or guilt over past activities
        (i) Feelings of being slowed down
        (j) Less talkativeness than usual
        (k) Pessimistic attitude towards the future or brooding about past events
      (2) Signs and symptoms of hypomanic periods are similar to those observed in manic periods except that the individual does not suffer marked impairment of functioning, which always occurs in mania. Signs and symptoms might include any of the following:
        (a) Decreased need for sleep
        (b) More energy than usual
        (c) Inflated self-esteem
        (d) Increased productivity, often associated with unusual and self-imposed working hours
        (e) Sharpened and unusually creative thinking
        (f) Uninhibited people-seeking (extreme gregariousness)
        (g) Hypersexuality without recognition of the possibility of painful consequences
        (h) Excessive involvement in pleasurable activities with a lack of concern for the high potential for painful consequences (e.g., heavy drug or alcohol use, spending sprees, and careless driving)
        (i) Physical restlessness
        (j) More talkativeness than usual
        (k) Optimism and an exaggerated sense of accomplishment
        (l) Inappropriate laughing, joking, or punning
    c. Paired symptoms. A review of these signs and symptoms reveals paired symptoms. An individual is socially withdrawn when depressed and extremely gregarious when hypomanic. Optimism and an exaggerated sense of accomplishment contrast with pessimism and brooding over past events. Paired symptoms indicate that the cyclothymic patient may present a history filled with apparent contradictions. "Sometimes I feel like I'm on top of the world, and other times I feel like I'm at the bottom of the heap" is a typical complaint.

2. Signs and symptoms of dysthymia. Dysthymia features a chronic disturbance of mood involving either a depressed mood or a loss of interest or pleasure in all, or almost all, usual activities. Associated symptoms of a depressive syndrome are not of sufficient severity or duration to warrant a diagnosis of major depression. This chronic condition must be present for at least 2 years in adults and 1 year or more in adolescents and children for the diagnosis to be made.

   a. Periods of normal mood may be present for a few days or weeks. The presence of a normal mood for more than 2 months should lead to further evaluation; a diagnosis of dysthymic disorder is questionable in such a case.

   b. Chronic mood disturbance. During depressive episodes, signs and symptoms include a chronic mood disturbance in addition to two or more of the following, according to the diagnostic criteria of the *DSM-III-R:*

     (1) Poor appetite or overeating

     (2) Insomnia or hypersomnia

     (3) Low energy or fatigue

     (4) Low self-esteem

     (5) Poor concentration or difficulty making decisions

     (6) Feelings of hopelessness

   c. Depression masked behind other complaints. Chronic pain, insomnia, and chronic, unresolved somatic problems are common presenting symptoms to physicians. Hypochondriacal complaints represent the patient's experience of chronic depression.

   d. Alcohol abuse can produce a chronic depression or may represent an attempt to ameliorate dysthymia. The toxic effects of alcohol make it necessary for the patient to abstain before the depression can be fully evaluated.

   e. Double depression occurs in dysthymic individuals. This phenomenon is characterized by the development of a full major depressive syndrome in an individual who already suffers from chronic depression (dysthymia). It should be noted that incomplete recovery from a major depressive episode can lead to chronic depression, also.

   f. Early or late onset. Dysthymia is classified as early or late onset, depending on whether the mood disturbance developed before (early) or after (late) the age of 21.

   g. Primary or secondary dysthymia. Dysthymia is classified as primary or secondary, depending on whether or not the mood disturbance developed in the context of another chronic condition. The presence of a preexisting chronic condition leads to a secondary designation, and the absence of a preexisting chronic condition leads to a primary designation for dysthymia. The chronic condition may be a medical disorder, such as cardiac or renal disease, or a nonmood psychiatric disorder, such as panic disorder or bulimia nervosa.

3. Distinguishing dysthymia and cyclothymia. To distinguish dysthymia from cyclothymia, the evaluator must determine if the patient returns to a normal mood (euthymia) or if the patient becomes hypomanic. The return to euthymia is such a change and relief for some individuals that it may seem to be a period of euphoria or exuberance. The best clues to hypomania are abnormally high levels of activity, poor judgment, and impulsive behavior.

C. Mood disorders classified as not otherwise specified, whether bipolar or depressive, are diagnostic categories, which are used to characterize conditions that do not meet the criteria for major depression, bipolar disorder, dysthymia, or cyclothymia.

1. Bipolar disorder not otherwise specified. Individuals who have manic features but whose symptoms do not meet the diagnostic criteria for bipolar disorder or cyclothymia are classified as having bipolar disorder not otherwise specified. Some individuals have major depressive episodes and hypomanic episodes, a clinical phenomenon also referred to as bipolar II.

2. Depressive disorder not otherwise specified. Similarly, individuals with depressive syndromes whose symptoms do not meet the diagnostic criteria for a major depression or dysthymia are classified as having depressive disorder not otherwise specified. A brief depression of mild or moderate intensity, which does not appear to be a reaction to a recognized stress, is one example of an atypical depression.

V. ETIOLOGIC FACTORS. Numerous studies have been made in an attempt to discover the causes of mood disorders. These studies have examined genetic, biologic, psychological, and sociologic variables. This remains an area of vigorous investigation.

A. Causative factors of major depression and bipolar disorder. Studies of major depression and bipolar disorder suggest that these are genetically influenced disorders. Shifts in an intrinsic activity cycle occur, and characteristic symptoms arise. Abnormalities at the synaptic and cellular levels appear to be part of the usual picture. Psychogenic and psychosocial factors appear to be significant in some cases, but their causation roles have not been determined.

1. **Genetic factors.** There is a greater risk of developing a disorder for the monozygotic twin than for the dizygotic twin of an individual with a major depression or bipolar disorder, suggesting the existence of a significant genetic factor. Families of both bipolar and unipolar (depressed) individuals have been studied.

   a. **An X-linked dominant pattern of inheritance has been found by some investigators in families with histories of bipolar illness**. Others have discovered an inherited abnormality of membrane lithium transport in red blood cells, which suggests an autosomal dominant pattern of transmission with variable expression. Each of these two inheritance patterns has been further delineated. The X-linked dominant pattern features an early onset of bipolar disorder (around 25 years of age) with a positive family history. The autosomal dominant pattern has a later onset (around 40 years of age) with a negative family history. Not all patients fit into these two groups, and more studies are being conducted.

   b. **No markers have been discovered for major depression.** However, groups of depressed patients have been investigated by Winokur in his studies. One group includes women who have experienced a major depression before the age of 40 years. These women have experienced depression more often than the men in their families. There is an increased incidence of alcoholism and sociopathy in their male relatives. Winokur has called the depression experienced by this group **depressive spectrum disease**. The second group studied includes men who experienced their first major depression after the age of 40 years. Men and women in the families of this group experience depression at similar rates. There is little alcoholism or sociopathy among male relatives. The disorder suffered by this group is called **pure depressive disease**. Subsequent studies have questioned Winokur's conclusions. The relationship between depressive disorders and other nonmood psychiatric conditions continues to be an active area of research.

2. **Biologic factors.** In 1921 Kraepelin speculated that mood disorders were due to biologic factors. He considered psychological factors to be coincidental. He hypothesized that some inner control mechanism was accelerated or decelerated in mania and depression, respectively.

   a. **Circadian rhythms** refer to various bodily functions that adhere to 24-hour cycles. Many circadian rhythms have been identified, including diurnal variations in mood, electroencephalogram (EEG) patterns, rest–activity cycles, and the regulation of neuroendocrine functions. Disruption of human circadian rhythms might explain several features of mood disorders, such as difficulty in falling asleep, excessive sleep, early morning awakening, and variations in rest–activity cycles. Patients with major depression have characteristic features in sleep EEG's, including delayed REM-latency and a higher density of REM sleep than normal in the first half of the sleep cycle. The phenomenon of the mood switch in bipolar disorder may be indicative of a malfunctioning circadian rhythm. Animal studies have demonstrated the following:

      (1) Studies of the effects of lithium and alcohol in animals have demonstrated that the intrinsic pacemaker is slowed by these drugs, which lengthens the circadian rhythm cycle.

      (2) Exogenous estrogens accelerate the intrinsic pacemaker, thereby shortening the circadian rhythm cycle.

      (3) Tricyclic antidepressants given to animals with abnormally prolonged circadian rhythm cycles accelerate the establishment of a normal cycle.

   b. **Seasonal mood disorder.** Recently, investigators identified a subgroup of depressed individuals who are afflicted only during the months with fewer hours of sunlight, the so-called seasonal mood disorder. These patients have been successfully treated with increased exposure to light. Animal rhythms change in response to sunlight, and it is speculated that the same is true in humans.

3. **Norepinephrine and serotonin levels** have been implicated in the etiology of depression and mania. These compounds transmit signals in the nervous system when they are released into the synaptic spaces.

   a. Deficiencies in the levels of norepinephrine and serotonin have been discovered in depressed patients. A biochemical profile of patients with these deficiencies has been developed in an attempt to identify subgroups of depression, although this has not significantly influenced clinical practice. Table 3-1 illustrates the two profiles.

   b. Levels of norepinephrine and its metabolites are elevated in mania. In addition, activity in dopaminergic neurons is increased.

   c. Many investigators emphasize the concept of dysregulation of synaptic transmission, rather than a deficiency or excess of neurotransmitter, when discussing disturbances at the

Table 3-1. Biochemical Profile of Depressed Patients

Naturally Occurring Biochemicals	In the Presence of	
	Serotonin Deficiency	Norepinephrine Deficiency
5-Hydroxyindoleacetic acid [5-HIAA] (a serotonin metabolite)	Low levels	Normal or elevated levels
3-Methoxy-4-hydroxyphenylglycol [MHPG] (a norepinephrine metabolite)	Normal levels	Low levels
Growth hormone, in response to insulin	Normal levels	Low levels
Tricyclic antidepressant	Amitriptyline	Imipramine

neuronal level found in mood disorders. The complexities of neurotransmission and receptor chemistry are more adequately accounted for by dysregulation hypotheses. So, too, is the fact that pharmacologic agents, which only rapidly alter the availability of neurotransmitters, are not effective antidepressant agents.

4. Psychological and sociocultural variables. These factors are difficult to measure with precision, thereby making much of this work highly speculative.

    a. Psychogenic theories are based on the notion of loss and speculations about the effect of loss on the individual. The hypotheses of Freud and Abraham have been described in section II D and E.

    b. Studies of families of bipolar patients were conducted by Fromm-Reichmann in 1954 and Gibson in 1959. Each found a similar family profile; however, the significance of these findings is unclear.

    c. Studies of children who lose a parent during childhood through divorce or death suggest that loss by divorce may be more significant in the development of future depressive disorder. It is speculated that this is due to widespread disruption, which occurs in families with divorce.

B. Causative factors of dysthymia and cyclothymia have not been studied as thoroughly as those for major depression and bipolar disorder. These diagnostic categories are relatively new, and no data have accumulated.

    1. Genetics. There is consensus that cyclothymia is a muted form of bipolar disorder. There are similarities in the clinical features. Families of cyclothymic individuals often have other cyclothymic members. Bipolar patients often have cyclothymic individuals in their families. These observations have led to the hypothesis that a lesser but similar disruption of circadian rhythms and cellular mechanisms is present in cyclothymia.

    2. Psychological variables. Dysthymia has been studied more vigorously. Some investigators point to its frequent association with other chronic conditions, such as a personality disorder or chronic medical illness. The significance of this association is not clear, although dysthymia is designated as primary or secondary on the basis of the presence or absence of a preexisting chronic condition. Most investigators have focused on psychological variables in their search for causation. Personality traits of dependency, a tendency to feel guilty or blameworthy, passivity, and a tendency to ruminate have been identified in dysthymic individuals. A difficult adaptation to adulthood is felt to be common in many of these patients. Further study is necessary to evaluate these findings. No biologic data have accumulated.

C. The etiology of disorders not otherwise specified has not been studied. Serious study is hampered because these diagnostic categories are ill-defined.

VI. COURSE AND PROGNOSIS. Data on the age of affected individuals at onset and the rapidity of onset, impairment and complications during acute episodes and long-term, and outcome with and without treatment provide a good picture of the course and prognosis of the mood disorders.

A. Depression and bipolar disorder. The disease course of depression and bipolar disorder has been studied and chronicled since the early part of this century. A group of 208 patients was followed by Rennie from 1913–1916. Relapse (82%) was common among 17 manic individuals as it was (77%) among 121 depressed individuals. Initial manic episodes lasted an average of 3½ months. Initial depressive episodes lasted an average of 6½ months.

    1. Onset of bipolar disorder. Bipolar disorder usually becomes clinically evident before the age of 30 years. Onset is typically sudden with a rapid escalation into the manic state. Manic episodes may last a few days or a few months and tend to be shorter in duration than depressive episodes. A depressive episode occurs at some point during the lifetime of most bipolar individuals, but the first episode of the mood disorder is frequently mania.

   a. **Variable frequency and sequence of episodes.** Some individuals have years of normal functioning between episodes. Others have episodes in clusters. In severe cases, "cycling" occurs, a phenomenon characterized by alternations between mania and depression without periods of euthymia.

   b. **Significant impairment and complications of mania.** Social and occupational functioning typically is severely affected. Impulsive and excessive behavior due to poor judgment and hyperactivity may lead to financial loss or ruin, legal difficulties, family disruption or disintegration, and death from accidents, suicide, or homicide. Substance abuse is common. The facts indicate that manics need protection from the consequences of their actions, which is often best provided in a hospital.

2. **Onset of major depression.** Major depression may occur at any age, even early in childhood. The pattern of onset is variable. Sudden onset may follow a severe stress. Signs and symptoms may develop over days to weeks and include such features as anxiety, phobic reactions, panic attacks, and mild depression.

   a. **Recurrence.** Major depression is recurrent for about 50% of affected individuals. Some investigators point to an increased risk for bipolar disorder in patients with recurrent major depression.

   b. **Variable frequency.** Years of normal functioning may pass between depressive episodes for some individuals. Others have clusters of episodes. A chronic deteriorating course is unusual.

   c. **Impairment in functioning** varies in major depression. Relationships are disrupted. It may be difficult, if not impossible, to work. In severe cases, individuals cannot take care of their own needs. Medical, financial, family, and occupational responsibilities are not fulfilled. The risk of suicide and, less frequently, homicide are the most serious complications.

   d. **Prognosis** is good with proper diagnosis and treatment.

B. **Dysthymia and cyclothymia** are chronic conditions. The clear-cut relapses and remissions observed in major depression and bipolar disorder are not observed in dysthymia and cyclothymia.

1. **Onset of primary dysthymia.** Primary dysthymia often develops before age 21, so-called early onset. Acute, severe depressive episodes do not occur. There may be a family history of mood disorders. Affected individuals have difficulty adjusting to the new tasks and responsibilities of adulthood. Onset of primary dysthymia after age 21 is often gradual and insidious. An early history of good functioning in interpersonal, social, and occupational spheres stands in contrast to new difficulties. Failures at work, problems as a parent, and troubled relationships may be present. Primary dysthymia in the elderly occurs in conjunction with normal aging. Mental deterioration may be hard to distinguish from depression in these individuals. Secondary dysthymia may develop at any time during life in the presence of preexisting, chronic psychiatric or medical conditions.

   a. **Concurrent health problems.** Chronically depressed individuals of all ages tend to experience more health problems than the population as a whole. Some individuals delay seeking timely medical care; others seek health care frequently and become identified as chronic somatic complainers. The chronic patient may not be taken seriously and is more likely to have significant problems overlooked or misdiagnosed by physicians. Finally, some authorities have speculated that depression weakens the body and its normal defenses against illness.

   b. **Chronic impairment** in several spheres of functioning is common in dysthymic individuals. Relationships may be unsatisfying and lack intimacy. Interest in sex and the ability to perform sexually may be limited. Social activities provide little enjoyment or are avoided altogether. Divorce, unemployment, and professional failure occur.

   c. **Self-destructive behavior.** Dysthymic individuals tend to be self-destructive. The most obvious manifestations of this are suicide attempts. Another manifestation is a tendency to have accidents. Careful exploration may reveal ways in which individuals have guaranteed that they will fail at work or in relationships.

   d. **Prognosis.** The most significant variable for prognosis is recognition. Many dysthymic individuals remain undiagnosed. Without diagnosis, chronic impairment, physical illness, and even death by suicide result.

2. **Onset of cyclothymia.** Cyclothymia usually manifests itself in adolescence. It can be recognized as a **change in personality**. An individual becomes moody. The duration and intensity of these periods of elation and depression vary.

   a. **Variable impairment.** Cyclothymic adults may be very successful during hypomanic periods. They are optimistic, energetic, ambitious, creative, and gregarious. However, functioning is very different during depressive periods. Energy for work and interpersonal interactions is low. The contrast between these two periods may be marked, which leads to the perception that the affected individual is erratic and unreliable. Some cyclothymic patients do not even do well when they are hypomanic: Judgment is poor, and social interactions are inappropriate.

    b. Prognosis. The prognosis is unclear at this time.

VII. DIFFERENTIAL DIAGNOSIS. As defined in the *DSM-III-R*, a diagnosis of major depression or bipolar disorder cannot be made if superimposed on schizophrenia, schizophreniform disorder, delusional disorder, or psychotic disorder not otherwise specified or if the syndrome is due to a known organic factor. Diagnosis of dysthymia and cyclothymia cannot be made if superimposed on a chronic psychotic condition or if due to a known organic factor. Therefore, a search for organic causes or another psychiatric illness should be conducted in the diagnostic process.

    A. Major depression and mania may be difficult to distinguish from other psychiatric disorders. Organic syndromes may be clinically difficult to distinguish as well.

        1. Mania-like syndromes can be due to a number of causes.

           a. Drug-related conditions

              (1) Mania can result from the **ingestion of corticosteroids**, which are commonly administered for a number of medical illnesses. Collagen–vascular diseases, such as rheumatoid arthritis and systemic lupus erythematosus, and asthma are two such examples.

              (2) Tricyclic antidepressants may produce a manic state in susceptible individuals.

              (3) Amphetamines and other stimulants produce hyperactivity, pressured speech, and impulsive, excessive behavior, which are all features of mania.

              (4) Manic symptoms are also associated with other drugs, including alcohol, disulfiram, barbiturates, anticholinergics, and benzodiazepines.

           b. Medical conditions

              (1) A neurologic disorder, such as **multiple sclerosis**, may produce a manic-like syndrome.

              (2) Metabolic conditions, such as hyperthyroidism, hyperadrenalism, and hypoadrenalism, have been associated with manic symptoms.

           c. Psychiatric conditions

              (1) A common diagnostic dilemma arises in the evaluation of the acutely psychotic patient. There may be signs and symptoms typical of manic psychosis or signs and symptoms that are not so typical. An acute schizophrenic episode may appear to be mania and vice versa. Because a psychotic individual appears to be schizophrenic acutely does not mean that he or she is not manic. The best allies of the clinician are time and history in making this differentiation. Some patients, however, have persistent features of schizophrenia and mania, a mixed clinical picture called **schizoaffective disorder**.

              (2) Since the intensity and duration of the syndrome differentiate mania from cyclothymia, this distinction can be difficult to make. Once again, history usually resolves the question.

              (3) An individual with a **narcissistic personality disorder** experiences highs and lows. Unlike those occurring in bipolar disorder, these peaks and valleys are short-lived and do not usually include the multitude of symptoms seen in manic and depressive episodes.

        2. Depressive syndromes can result from organic and functional disorders.

           a. Drug-related conditions

              (1) A number of **antihypertensive medications** affect central nervous system amines. It should be kept in mind that the effect of reserpine on patients was an early clue to the role of amines in depression.

              (2) A full depressive syndrome may develop with corticosteroids as well, particularly if they are withdrawn too quickly.

              (3) Chronic use of depressants, such as **alcohol and barbiturates**, makes it very difficult to assess depression. Many authorities feel that a mood disorder cannot be evaluated adequately in this population.

           b. Medical conditions

              (1) Cancer, especially in its advanced stages, may produce a depressive syndrome. Pancreatic cancer presents as depression in 30%–40% of all cases.

              (2) Hypothyroidism also mimics depression.

           c. Psychiatric conditions

              (1) Dementia has many characteristics in common with depression, including lack of concentration, memory lapses, disorientation, and apathy. Both demented patients and depressed patients perform poorly on mental status examinations. Distinguishing between these disorders often requires treatment of the patient for depression. The depressed patient's mental status examination will show improvement, the demented patient's will not. The picture is further complicated by the fact that depression is a common secondary disorder in demented individuals.

(2) Very disturbed, psychotic depressive syndromes can include hallucinations, bizarre delusions, and very regressed behavior. This presentation would raise questions about **schizophrenia** as a diagnostic possibility. Time and history can be helpful in distinguishing one from the other.

(3) The agitation, restlessness, insomnia, and dysphoria suffered in **anxiety disorders** can be similar to signs and symptoms of an agitated depression. For some patients, a period of anxiety precedes a major depression. Follow-up and treatment trials with medication may be necessary to make a diagnosis.

(4) Individuals with **somatization disorders** are often chronically depressed but do not describe themselves as such. Depressed patients who present with somatic complaints have similarities to this group. The severity of symptoms and the presence of other features of the depressive syndrome are helpful in making a diagnosis.

(5) There may be a fine line between major depression and dysthymia. Signs and symptoms differ only in intensity and duration. Patient history is helpful, but follow-up may be necessary to differentiate the two.

B. Dysthymia and cyclothymia. The differential diagnostic considerations for dysthymia and cyclothymia are similar to those for the major mood disorders. Other chronic mental conditions, such as personality disorders and substance abuse disorders, warrant consideration in the diagnostic process.

C. Bereavement is the normal reaction to the death of a loved one. In response to loss, an individual sleeps poorly, eats poorly, loses weight, ruminates about the lost person, has trouble concentrating, is tearful, feels depressed, feels ill at ease, and has thoughts of dying. In short, a full depressive syndrome is a normal reaction to the death of a loved one. This syndrome usually lasts from 2–6 months, depending upon the cultural norms for grieving. Guilt about what was or was not done at the time of death may be prominent. A diagnosis of major depression is not made in this situation. If the syndrome is prolonged, if there is marked functional impairment, if marked psychomotor retardation develops, or if there is a morbid hopelessness and feelings of worthlessness and low self-esteem, a diagnosis of major depression should be entertained.

VIII. TREATMENT. In developing a treatment plan for a patient with a mood disorder, the clinician must consider the patient's lethality (i.e., suicide and homicide potential), resources (both internal, intrapsychic resources as well as external resources), past treatment successes and failures, and the specific diagnosis.

A. Major depression and bipolar disorder are rewarding illnesses to treat because treatment is successful in most cases.

1. Hospitalization. The initial decision in the care of patients with bipolar illness, manic or depressed, and major depression is whether or not hospitalization is needed. Whether the patient in question is manic or depressed, successful treatment depends upon the availability of adequate support to the patient. A loss of support systems or inadequate support may compel the clinician to hospitalize the patient.

a. Suicide or homicide

(1) The risk for suicide or homicide is high for some patients with bipolar disorder. This may be due to an expressed and determined intent to kill themselves or others. Wild, impulsive behavior may create a dangerous situation as well. These patients need to be hospitalized.

(2) Acutely depressed individuals may pose a significant risk for suicide or homicide, and they should be hospitalized. It is estimated that 6% of women and 3% of men are hospitalized for depression during adulthood.

b. Mania

(1) Manic behavior can be ruinous for the patient and others. Financial disaster, loss of career, and family disintegration are just three examples of possible tragic consequences. The hospital can provide a secure, protective environment, which minimizes the destruction that mania can bring to so many lives.

(2) The agitated, driven behavior of acute mania can produce dangerous physiologic changes (e.g., elevated blood pressure, elevated temperature, tachycardia, and dehydration). Unchecked, these changes could lead to significant and life-threatening medical complications. Hospitalization and sedation may be life-saving interventions.

    c. Severe depression may render individuals unable to care for their basic needs, in which case hospitalization may be necessary.

2. Outpatient treatment. Many manic and most depressed patients are treated as outpatients. This can be done even when patients are acutely disturbed. Once the setting for treatment has been determined, decisions about other specific interventions can be made.

    a. Frequent contact is necessary for the acutely ill individual. These illnesses can change suddenly and unpredictably. A turn for the worse can be quickly detected, and appropriate interventions can be made.

    b. Evaluation of lethal behavior. Outpatients should not be significant risks for lethal behavior. Careful assessment for suicide and homicide potential is mandatory and should be an ongoing process.

    c. Support systems of family, friends, clergy, and co-workers should be evaluated for their adequacy relative to the patients' needs. Some individuals need more support than others. If patients cannot bear to be alone, for example, the clinician must determine what their environment can provide.

3. Medication

    a. Mania. Medication provides the clinician with a powerful tool for the treatment of mania. The initial task in the treatment of acute mania is to quiet the agitation that commonly occurs. This is usually accomplished with neuroleptic medications (e.g., phenothiazines and butyrophenones), although in rare cases barbiturates and ECT are used when neuroleptics fail to provide enough sedation.

    (1) Lithium carbonate revolutionized the treatment of mania. Its success is reported to be about 80% in most studies. It is beneficial in both the acute phase of mania and as a prophylactic agent.

        (a) Lithium should not be given until the patient's general medical health is evaluated because of its toxicity and metabolism. Of particular concern are renal, cardiac, and thyroid functioning. Once it has been established that the cardiac rhythm is stable, that renal clearance of lithium will be adequate, and that thyroid functioning is normal, lithium can be administered.

        (b) Lithium carbonate is given in high doses to patients with acute mania. Both the levels (0.8–1.5 mEq/L) of lithium and the side effects (e.g., gastrointestinal upset, diarrhea, tremors, and muscular twitches) govern the dosage. In general, doses ranging from 1–3 g/day are necessary.

        (c) It may be necessary to administer a neuroleptic agent along with lithium carbonate. This has been reported to be a dangerous combination in isolated cases; therefore, the combination should be administered cautiously, keeping the patient well hydrated.

        (d) As the acute phase resolves, the need for lithium diminishes. Therefore, with improvement, the dose is decreased. Once again, levels (0.6–1.2 mEq/L) and side effects govern the dosage.

        (e) Once acute mania has resolved, the question of chronic treatment must be addressed. There is evidence to support the prophylactic efficacy of lithium. Decreasing the frequency and severity of episodes may favorably influence the long-term course of the illness. The risk of administering lithium on a chronic basis must be weighed against the potential disruption of another manic episode. Chronic administration of lithium has been associated with medical complications, which include diffuse goiter, decreased glucose tolerance, an elevated white blood cell count, nephrogenic diabetes insipidus, thyroid deficiency, parathyroid adenomas, and interstitial nephritis.

    (2) Carbamazepine has been a recent addition to the treatment of mania.

        (a) It is used in individuals who either do not respond to or are unable to tolerate treatment with lithium carbonate.

        (b) Usual doses of carbamazepine range from 600–1200 mg/day, resulting in blood levels of 8–12 μg/μl.

        (c) In therapeutic doses, carbamazepine has been shown to be an effective mood-stabilizing drug for both acute mania and prophylactic treatment.

        (d) Patients taking carbamazepine may experience drowsiness or sedation, dysarthria, impaired coordination, or ataxia. If these effects are tolerated initially, they tend to diminish or resolve as the individual continues to take carbamazepine.

        (e) Suppression of production of white blood cells, red blood cells, or platelets may occur during the early stages of treatment with carbamazepine. Neutropenia (low white cell count) exposes the individual to infectious complications. Thrombocytopenia (low platelet count) exposes the individual to bleeding problems. Complete blood counts are recommended on a weekly basis for the first month of treatment, or longer, if the dose is not yet stable. Blood counts are obtained less often thereafter with monthly monitoring for 2 or 3 months followed by quarterly monitoring in the stable patient.

(f) Hyponatremia is another complication in the early stages of treatment. Serum sodium levels should be monitored initially.

(g) Carbamazepine levels may decrease, even though the dose remains unchanged because carbamazepine may induce its own metabolism. Therefore, frequent monitoring of drug levels is necessary in the early stages of treatment followed by quarterly monitoring.

(3) **Clonazepam.** A third drug used for treatment of mania is clonazepam. The use of clonazepam usually follows unsuccessful attempts to treat with lithium carbonate and carbamazepine. The usual dose is 2–6 mg/day.

b. **Severe depression.** Medications have also proven to be very useful in the treatment of severe depression. They shorten the duration of the depressive episode in most cases.

(1) It should be emphasized that **diagnostic precision** aids in choosing the appropriate course of treatment. A bipolar depression is treated differently than a major depression in the patient without bipolar disorder. Lithium should be used in combination with the antidepressant in the bipolar patient.

(2) A history of success with a particular antidepressant should direct the clinician to use that medication for treatment of recurrent depression. Similarly, a history of success with a particular antidepressant in a family member may point to the best choice in medication.

(3) **Tricyclic antidepressants** are usually the first medications tried if the patient's health permits. Patients with cardiac disease should be evaluated before beginning the drugs.

(a) Doses of tricyclic antidepressants vary widely among the different medications and within different patient populations. In general, elderly patients need about one-half of the dose needed by younger adults. The dose should be low at first (e.g., 25 mg of imipramine). These medications have powerful and unpleasant side effects (i.e., dry mouth, blurred vision, dizziness, urinary retention, sedation, and orthostatic hypotension) caused by their potent anticholinergic effects. The dose should be raised slowly, always taking into account the patient's tolerance of side effects. The patient may become very uncomfortable with too rapid a rise in dose, which may affect his or her willingness to comply with treatment.

(b) Tricyclic antidepressants do not provide immediate relief; rather, full therapeutic effectiveness usually is not realized for 4–8 weeks. Some symptoms respond more quickly. For example, insomnia may resolve with the sedating effects of amitriptyline in the first week of medication.

(c) Most clinicians keep patients on antidepressant medication for 4–6 months after they have become symptom-free. At this point, the patient can be tapered off the medication over the course of 1–2 months.

(d) Patients who have recurrent major depressive episodes should continue to take an effective medication beyond 6 months. It appears that ongoing treatment protects against relapse. Some patients may take medication indefinitely.

(e) Some patients do not respond to tricyclic antidepressants. In these cases, the diagnosis should be reevaluated. The patient may have another disorder. A change in medication may be necessary if the physician is certain that the diagnosis is correct. Switching to a different tricyclic antidepressant is common practice. Failure of tricyclic antidepressants to work should lead to psychiatric consultation for the nonpsychiatric physician.

(4) **Monoamine oxidase (MAO) inhibitors** may be prescribed as a second-line drug for depression. These medications are complicated to prescribe. They potentiate sympathomimetic agents, including tyramine and tryptophan, in the diet and interact with numerous other medications.

(5) **Stimulants** can alleviate depression. However, they are not recommended for general use. Although a stimulant may provide rapid and dramatic relief of depressive symptoms, it has not been reliably demonstrated that relief of symptoms endures beyond a week or two. Tolerance usually develops to the stimulant, resulting in loss of relief and an escalation of dose. In medically ill patients who are depressed, stimulants may be useful for short-term, rapid relief of depression. The most commonly used stimulants are methylphenidate (Ritalin) and dextroamphetamine (Dexedrine).

4. **ECT** has been used for several decades. Recently, it has been viewed as inhumane; however, it remains an effective treatment for mood disorders.

a. The precise therapeutic mechanism of ECT is not known. Seizures are induced electrically in a medically cleared patient in a safe environment (often an operating room). The patient is paralyzed so that the seizure will do no harm. In most cases seizures are timed to last around 60 seconds for each treatment. A series of treatments, usually three per week, is given on alternating days. This is terminated when clinical improvement is evident. Memory loss, on a temporary basis, accompanies improvement.

   b. Properly administered, ECT is associated with very low morbidity and mortality. The success rate is greater than 90%.

   c. Patients selected for ECT fall into four groups:

     (1) Patients with a history of good response to ECT

     (2) Severely depressed patients with psychomotor retardation, somatic delusions, delusional guilt, disinterest in the world around them, weight loss, and persistent suicidal intent

     (3) Patients who have not responded to medication or who cannot take antidepressants

     (4) Patients who are manic and who have not responded to other therapy

  5. Laboratory tests can be used in the diagnosis and treatment of depression.

   a. Disrupted neuroendocrine functions may play an etiologic role in mood disturbances. Laboratory tests used to evaluate neuroendocrine function in depressed individuals include the following:

     (1) The dexamethasone suppression test measures the functioning of the hypothalamic–pituitary–adrenal cortical axis. A normal response to a dose of dexamethasone (1 mg at 11 P.M.) is suppression of endogenous cortisol production, which is measured at 8 A.M., 4 P.M., and 11 P.M. The next day about half of depressed patients respond normally, but the other half fail to suppress cortisol production. Other conditions, such as alcohol abuse or chronic medical illness, can produce false-positive results. Nonetheless, the positive result can provide a reliable biologic marker to follow throughout treatment of depression. The response to dexamethasone should return to normal with successful treatment. **This test should not be used to screen for depression**. Some find it useful in sorting out diagnostic questions.

     (2) The thyrotropin-releasing hormone (TRH) stimulation test measures the functioning of the hypothalamic–pituitary–thyroid axis. Serum thyroid-stimulating hormone (TSH) levels are measured after an intravenous dose of TRH. Its utility is limited by the low number of depressed individuals who respond by failing to increase levels of TSH, only about 30%–40%.

   b. Alterations in sleep architecture occur in more than 80% of severely depressed individuals. These changes include decreased REM-latency, increased density of REM sleep in the first half of the sleep cycle, and decreased percentage of deep (stages III and IV) sleep. Due to the time and expense involved with sleep polysomnography, this test is infrequently used clinically.

   c. Serum levels of antidepressant agents can assist in determining the appropriate dose of tricyclic agents, such as imipramine, nortriptyline, and desipramine. Levels for other agents are not clinically useful at this time.

  6. Psychotherapy is a useful and necessary adjunct to all of the previously described therapies. The form and intensity of psychotherapy varies from case to case. Some patients require supportive guidance from a therapist and nothing more; others have more pressing needs for in-depth exploration of problems, relationships, and conflicts.

B. Cyclothymia and dysthymia are not as easily or successfully treated as major depression and bipolar disorder. Substance abuse is a common occurrence among dysthymic individuals. The physician must inquire about this and treat it when necessary.

  1. Hospitalization. Almost all cyclothymic and dysthymic individuals can be treated as outpatients. Suicidal behavior, however, may lead to hospitalization.

  2. Somatic therapies are recommended by some authorities, but this type of treatment is controversial.

   a. Lithium carbonate. Some investigators are optimistic about the response of cyclothymic individuals to lithium carbonate. Stable functioning is envisioned with chronic lithium treatment; however, more data are needed to draw any conclusions.

   b. Antidepressants are reported to be successful for some, but not all, dysthymic patients, and currently it is not possible to distinguish those patients who might benefit and those who will not. Some studies suggest that individuals with secondary dysthymia are more responsive to medication treatment.

  3. Psychotherapy is a common treatment for these patients. Therapeutic techniques reflect theoretical considerations regarding the genesis of a chronic mood disturbance.

   a. Psychoanalytically oriented theories relate the development and maintenance of depression and maladaptive behavior to unresolved early childhood conflict. For example, an individual may have suffered the loss of a parent before the age of 18 years. Depression arises in adult life because the individual experiences a persistent vulnerability to loss, a tendency to feel as overwhelmed and helpless as he or she did when the parent died. Therapy would focus on the patient's vulnerability to loss and related behavior, such as avoiding close relationships.

  b. **Cognitive theories** emphasize the role of how one thinks about oneself and the environment in the genesis of depression. Depression results from a series of "wrong" perceptions, such as "I am a bad person," or "I can't change things." In this school of thought, therapy focuses on these incorrect perceptions and encourages the patient to think "correctly." Cognitive therapy is usually of short duration (a few weeks to months) and is reported to be efficacious.

  c. **Maladaptive behavior theories.** Some authorities argue that depression results from maladaptive personal interactions. Affected individuals have family backgrounds that are characterized by excessive dependency and sibling rivalry. Therapy focuses on interpersonal relationships and attempts to change associated maladaptive behavior.

BIBLIOGRAPHY

American Psychiatric Association: *Diagnostic and Statistical Manual of Mental Disorders*, 3rd ed, revised. Washington, DC, American Psychiatric Association, 1987

Cohen MB, Baker G, Cohen RA, et al: An intensive study of twelve cases of manic-depressive psychosis. *Psychiatry* 17, 2:103–137, 1954

Freud S: Mourning and melancholia. In *Standard Edition of the Complete Psychological Works of Sigmund Freud*, vol 14. London, Hogarth, 1957, pp 243–258

Gibson RN, Cohen MB, Cohen RA: On the dynamics of the manic depressive personality. *Am J Psychiatry* 115(2):1101–1107, 1959

Kaplan HI, Freedman AM, Sadock BJ: *Comprehensive Textbook of Psychiatry*, 3rd ed. Baltimore, Williams and Wilkins, 1980, pp 1035–1072, 1305–1358

Kolb LC: *Modern Clinical Psychiatry*, 9th ed. Philadelphia, Saunders, 1977, pp 438–479

Winokur G, Behar D, van Valkenburg C, et al: Is a familial definition of depression both feasible and valid? *J Nerv Ment Dis* 166(11):764–768, 1978

STUDY QUESTIONS

Directions: Each question below contains five suggested answers. Choose the **one best** response to each question.

1. Most authorities believe that the lifelong risk for major depression is approximately

(A) 5%
(B) 10%
(C) 20%
(D) 40%
(E) 50%

2. All of the following statements about the epidemiology of mood disorders are true EXCEPT

(A) the lifelong risk for bipolar disorder is about 1%
(B) depression may occur at any age
(C) dysthymia is frequently associated with chronic medical and psychiatric illnesses
(D) men are diagnosed as depressed more often than women
(E) the risk for a major mood disorder is greater in family members of those afflicted than in the population as a whole

3. Bipolar disorder is characterized by all of the following statements EXCEPT

(A) some patients have inherited an abnormality of membrane lithium transport in red blood cells
(B) depression follows each manic episode
(C) bipolar disorder is equally common in men and women
(D) bipolar disorder is usually clinically evident before 30 years of age
(E) levels of norepinephrine and its metabolites are often elevated in mania

4. All of the following features are characteristic of mania EXCEPT

(A) hyperthermia
(B) alcohol abuse
(C) thyroid dysfunction
(D) dehydration
(E) suicide attempts

5. All of the following statements about major depression are true EXCEPT

(A) some patients are treated with increased exposure to light
(B) 50% of patients suffer a recurrence
(C) levels of dopamine and its metabolites are decreased
(D) symptoms of dysphoria are unaltering during the episode
(E) medication can shorten the depressive episode in many cases

6. Although data on cyclothymia are not sufficient to draw conclusions, many investigators feel that the disorder is

(A) a muted form of bipolar disorder
(B) more common than dysthymia
(C) best treated with tricyclic antidepressants
(D) more common in women with alcoholic male relatives
(E) none of the above

7. Electroconvulsive therapy is characterized by all of the following statements EXCEPT

(A) the success rate is greater than 90%
(B) it is indicated in manic patients who have not responded to other modes of therapy
(C) temporary memory loss is a common side effect
(D) the therapeutic effect results from seizure activity in the limbic area of the brain
(E) it is associated with low morbidity and mortality when properly administered

Directions: Each question below contains four suggested answers of which **one or more** is correct. Choose the answer

    A if **1, 2, and 3** are correct
    B if **1 and 3** are correct
    C if **2 and 4** are correct
    D if **4** is correct
    E if **1, 2, 3, and 4** are correct

8. Drugs that are known to produce a manic-like syndrome include

(1) amphetamines
(2) tricyclic antidepressants
(3) corticosteroids
(4) reserpine

9. Dysthymia is characterized by

(1) chronic fatigue
(2) social withdrawal
(3) insomnia
(4) hypersomnia

10. Medical diseases that are known to produce a full depressive syndrome include

(1) pancreatic cancer
(2) hypertension
(3) hypothyroidism
(4) peptic ulcer disease

11. Bereavement is characterized by

(1) thoughts of dying
(2) weight loss
(3) sleeping difficulties
(4) a duration of 2–6 months

12. Long-term treatment with lithium carbonate can result in

(1) hypertension
(2) anemia
(3) leukopenia
(4) hyperparathyroidism

13. Side effects of tricyclic antidepressants include

(1) hypertension
(2) dry mouth
(3) diarrhea
(4) blurred vision

Directions: The groups of questions below consist of lettered choices followed by several numbered items. For each numbered item select the **one** lettered choice with which it is **most** closely associated. Each lettered choice may be used once, more than once, or not at all.

Questions 14–17

For each contribution to the study of mood disorders, select the investigator with whom it is most commonly associated.

(A) Kraepelin
(B) Winokur
(C) Falret
(D) Freud
(E) Kahlbaum

14. The role of psychogenic factors, such as loss, in depression

15. The relationship between depression and alcoholism in families

16. Alterations in biologic rhythms

17. Manic–depressive illness

Questions 18–21

For each clinical observation listed below, select the disorder with which it is most likely to be associated.

(A) Bipolar disorder
(B) Major depression
(C) Dysthymia
(D) Cyclothymia
(E) Atypical depression

18. A change in personality in adolescence

19. Uninhibited spending

20. A tendency to experience more health problems than most people

21. Delusions of grandeur

ANSWERS AND EXPLANATIONS

1. The answer is B. (*III A 1 b*) Although the figure is controversial, most authorities agree that 10%–15% of the population will suffer a major depression sometime during their lifetimes. The effects of the disease are widespread, and all physicians must be alert for it, especially since it does not always present in a classic manner (e.g., depression in men may present as substance abuse or be otherwise masked).

2. The answer is D. (*III A 1, 2, 4; IV B 2 g; VI A 2*) Depression is diagnosed in women about two times as often as in men, possibly because women get depressed more frequently than men. The signs of depression (e.g., tearfulness and hopelessness) may be more easily recognized in women because societal norms allow such expressions from women. Examiners may overlook depressive symptoms in men for similar societal reasons.

3. The answer is B. (*III A 2; V A 1 a, 3; VI A 1, 2*) The clinical course of bipolar disorder varies. Many patients have manic episodes without any interceding depressive episodes. Others have many more depressive episodes than manic episodes. Unlike major depression, bipolar disorder is equally common in men and women. Symptoms are usually evident before 30 years of age. Investigators have discovered an inherited abnormality of membrane lithium transport in red blood cells, which suggests an autosomal dominant pattern of transmission. In mania, levels of norepinephrine and its metabolites are often elevated.

4. The answer is C. [*IV A 1 b; VI A 1; VII A 1 b; VIII A 1 a (1)*] Thyroid dysfunction in the form of hyperthyroidism may produce a manic-like syndrome. It is important to remember, however, that a diagnosis of bipolar disorder–manic type can be made only if there is no organic cause (such as hyperthyroidism) of the disturbance. A thyroid deficiency may result from the treatment of bipolar disorder with lithium carbonate. Alcohol abuse and an ongoing risk for suicide are associated symptoms of mania. The agitated state of manic individuals can lead to dangerous physiologic conditions, such as hyperthermia and dehydration.

5. The answer is C. (*IV A 2; V A 2 b, 3; VI A 2 a; VIII A 3 b*) Levels of both norepinephrine and serotonin have been found to be decreased in depressed individuals, although levels may also be normal. To date, dopamine has not been shown to play a role in depression. A group of individuals who are depressed only during months with fewer hours of sunlight have been recently identified. Bodily rhythms change in response to sunlight, and increased exposure to light has proved to be successful treatment in some cases. Symptoms of dysphoria are prominent and unaltering in depressive episodes, which have been shortened in many individuals by medication.

6. The answer is A. (*IV B 1; V B 1*) The signs and symptoms of cyclothymia differ from those of bipolar disorder in that they are less severe. The degree of disturbance is attenuated. There are probably similarities in the biology of the two disorders: Bipolar patients often have cyclothymic individuals in their families. There seems to be disruption of circadian rhythms and cellular mechanisms in cyclothymia but to a lesser degree than in bipolar illness. Treatment with lithium carbonate rather than tricyclic antidepressants is advocated for cyclothymia.

7. The answer is D. (*VIII A 4*) Electroconvulsive therapy (ECT) has been a very effective treatment when judiciously used with patients for whom it is indicated. However, it is not known how it works. The limbic area of the brain is associated with emotional control and expression, but it is not known if ECT affects functioning in this area. Properly administered, ECT is associated with very low morbidity and mortality, and its success rate is higher than 90%.

8. The answer is A (1, 2, 3). (*II F 1; VII A 1*) Reserpine produces a depression by depleting norepinephrine. Amphetamines are potent stimulants, which cause hyperactivity, pressured speech, and erratic, excessive behavior when used chronically. In susceptible individuals (i.e., individuals with bipolar illness), tricyclic antidepressants without lithium carbonate can bring on a manic episode. Corticosteroids produce depression or mania when given in sufficient doses.

9. The answer is E (all). (*IV B 2 b*) Apathy and disinterest in normal activities are typical findings in chronic depression. Affected individuals suffer from low self-esteem, and they shy away from social interactions. These factors contribute to a lack of interest in sex. Sleep disruptions, whether in the form of insomnia or hypersomnia, are characteristic of depression, as are feelings of chronic fatigue.

10. The answer is B (1, 3). (*VII A 2 b*) Hypertension is not known to lead to major depression, although antihypertensive medication, such as reserpine, have been implicated in the illness. Pancreatic cancer presents as depression in as many as 40% of cases, but the mechanism of disturbance is not known. Hypothyroidism leads to fatigue, apathy, and disinterest; affected individuals feel slowed down and become discouraged. Although it is known that thyroid hormone is necessary for normal functioning of the central nervous system, the mechanism by which depression is produced is not known.

11. The answer is E (all). (*VII C*) A full depressive syndrome is a normal reaction to loss. Preoccupation with the loss leads to a decrease in appetite, weight loss, ruminations, troubled sleep, distractibility, thoughts about dying, and impaired concentration. Family and cultural expectations play a role in the duration of bereavement. The typical duration is 2–6 months. Severe, disabling symptoms marked by feelings of hopelessness and worthlessness signal the presence of a major depression.

12. The answer is D (4). [*VIII A 3 a (1) (e)*] Chronic administration of lithium can disrupt calcium metabolism and interfere with the normal actions of calcium. Parathyroid adenomas develop during chronic lithium use, leading to hyperparathyroidism. Blood pressure is not known to increase. Although anemia and leukopenia have not been associated with lithium use, leukocytosis has been.

13. The answer is C (2, 4). [*VIII A 3 b (3)*] Tricyclic antidepressants may produce hypotension. The patient experiences dizziness or lightheadedness. If there are any bowel changes as a result of the medication, constipation is more likely to occur than diarrhea. The powerful anticholinergic effects of tricyclic antidepressants produce a dry mouth (through action on the salivary glands) and blurred vision (through action on muscles that control the eye's ability to focus).

14–17. The answers are: 14-D, 15-B, 16-A, 17-A. (*II C 1, E 1; V A 1 b, 2*) Freud noted that an individual reacts to a loss by becoming angry with the lost individual. However, to remain angry with someone who has died, for example, is not acceptable to most people. Individuals begin to fault themselves for feeling that way, and Freud speculated that the anger is turned on themselves. He found support for this idea in typical symptoms of guilt, low self-esteem, and self-reproach.

Winokur explored the genetics of depression. One pattern that he discovered was what he calls depressive spectrum disease. Women in this group suffer depression before the age of 40 years. Their male relatives have an increased incidence of alcoholism and sociopathy. In another group, men suffer depression after the age of 40 years. There is no increased incidence of alcoholism or sociopathy in male relatives. Winokur has called this pure depressive disease.

Kraepelin emphasized the role of biologic factors in mood disorders. A malfunctioning inner control mechanism could either accelerate or decelerate, leading to mania or depression. However, little that is known of circadian rhythms today was known in 1921.

Based on his observations, Kraepelin felt that a single disorder with varied clinical manifestations must exist. He called this manic–depressive illness, a condition that corresponds to the current bipolar disorder. His ability to find associations between these conditions has promoted both research and improved treatment.

18–21. The answers are: 18-D, 19-A, 20-C, 21-A. (*IV A 1 b; f, B 2 c; VI A 1, B 1 a, 2*) The cyclothymic individual experiences marked shifts in mood, level of energy, enthusiasm, and sociability. These symptoms typically begin in adolescence. An individual who was relatively consistent in interactions with others becomes erratic as these shifts in mood occur. The personality is changed.

The exuberant, enthusiastic manic individual is usually hyperactive. Judgment is often impaired. Money is spent freely, even if money is not there to spend. The financial consequences may be severe.

Chronic depression interferes with health care. An individual may not seek care when indicated because he or she does not have the motivation to do so and may feel unworthy of being helped. Some investigators believe that depression hampers the body's immune system. Symptoms in the chronically depressed may be interpreted as signs of depression instead of signs of physical disease.

Psychotic symptoms occur in both bipolar disorder and major depression. The expansive, exuberant mood of bipolar disorder leads to ideas that reflect that mood. The individual believes that he or she is as important as he or she feels, and delusions of grandeur result. Delusions in depression are usually focused on decay, guilt, and death.

4
Organic
Mental Syndromes
Jon A. Bell

I. INTRODUCTION. Disturbances of thoughts, perceptions, feelings, and behavior may be the result of organic or functional (nonorganic) factors or both. The disturbances in an organic mental syndrome are known or presumed to be due to some organic factor. In a functional disorder, other factors, such as social and psychosocial stress, are considered to be causative or the nature of a suspected organic disorder is unknown, as in schizophrenia.

   An organic mental syndrome is the manifestation of brain tissue dysfunction. Brain tissue dysfunction may be transient or permanent. Psychological and behavioral abnormalities vary due to variability in the area of the brain that is affected, the mode of onset, the progression, the duration, and the nature of the pathophysiologic processes.

II. PATHOPHYSIOLOGY. In all cases of organic mental syndrome, there is a failure of normal metabolic processes, **cerebral insufficiency**. The condition may be reversible or irreversible, depending upon whether or not cellular death has occurred. Derangement of cerebral functioning may result from a number of pathophysiologic or biochemical processes. These include the following:

A. Deficiency of fuels for oxidative metabolism. The brain uses glucose as the major substrate for metabolic processes, although it appears that some use of amino acids and protein may also take place. Oxygen is a second essential fuel. Any lack of fuel can produce cerebral insufficiency, resulting in impaired brain function.

B. Impaired mechanisms of release, conservation, and use of chemical energy. Enzyme systems and metabolic pathways can be disrupted by toxic substances, such as ammonia.

C. Disruption of the process of synaptic transmission. Normally, information passes between neurons via synaptic connections. Pathophysiologic processes may deplete neurons of messengers, such as dopamine and norepinephrine. Neurohumoral functions may also be disrupted.

D. Significant alterations in electrolyte content, hydration, pH, and osmolarity. As with other organs in the body, the brain functions best in a steady, stable environment. Whenever the body's internal environment is changed, optimal functioning is compromised. Changes are reflected at the cellular level as cell pH, electrolyte content, osmolarity, and hydration adjust to the internal environment.

E. Interference with macromolecular synthesis. Macromolecular synthesis is necessary for cellular renewal and continued normal functioning; thus, interference can produce dysfunction, due either to diminished substrate availability or disruption of cellular mechanisms.

F. Disruptions of brain anatomy or disequilibrium in functionally related systems. These disruptions can produce organic mental syndromes because brain function depends upon precise anatomic relationships. For example, a mass lesion compresses the brain and distorts anatomic relationships, leading to deficits in functioning pertinent to the affected locality.

III. CLASSIFICATION. Organic mental syndromes are referred to as organic mental disorders in the *Diagnostic and Statistical Manual of Mental Disorders*, 3rd ed., revised (*DSM-III-R*) and can be divided into the following groups:

A. Disorders with generalized or global cognitive impairment

   1. Delirium. The essential feature of delirium is a clouded state of consciousness, which reduces an individual's awareness of his or her environment. It occurs in all age groups, although the young and the elderly are most susceptible.
   a. Attention deficits. Patients have difficulty attending to both internal and external stimuli.

They are easily distracted and have trouble conversing with others. Patients cannot shift, focus, or maintain attention without considerable effort and concentration. As the delirium advances, patients can no longer overcome attention deficits. They become bewildered and confused.

b. Sensory misperceptions. Early in delirium, perceptions become blurred, hazy, and imprecise. Normal sensory cues, such as sounds and sights, become less reliable and accurate, sensations are not identified readily, and important perceptions cannot be acted upon (such as stopping at a red light or obeying a speed-limit sign). Patients may feel a barrage of sensations and are unable to screen out unimportant sensory information. As the delirium advances, patients may experience hallucinations involving any sensory modality; visual hallucinations are common. They may become convinced of the reality of the misperceptions, illusions, and hallucinations. Emotional and behavioral responses to these sensory disturbances arise. Patients may experience vivid dreams and nightmares as well.

c. Fluctuations in behavior, emotional state, level of consciousness, perceptions, and thinking. One moment patients may be calm, relaxed, and able to think clearly; the next moment, they may be agitated, frightened, and confused. This state of agitation is not constant, however. Patients may become calm again or become lethargic and stuporous within a short period of time.

d. Rapid onset. A delirium may emerge more slowly if the underlying cause is a systemic illness or a metabolic imbalance. Usually the cause produces a more immediate, dramatic change, however. For example, drugs and alcohol have an impact within minutes to hours. A delirium rarely lasts more than a few days. Removal of the offending agent can end a delirious state as can treatment of the underlying cause, such as meningitis.

e. Disordered thought processes. Thoughts are not clear or coherent unless affected individuals exercise great care and effort. Patients are hesitant, vague, and uncertain. Thinking becomes concrete as the delirium advances. Thoughts are fragmented and seemingly without direction or purpose. Switching from topic to topic without apparent transition (**loose associations**) also occurs. Reasoning is impaired. Without an ability to think clearly and without an ability to anticipate the consequences of their actions, patients exercise poor judgment and act in impulsive or dangerous ways. As the delirium progresses, patients may become irrational and may take hold of irrational beliefs (**delusions**). Actions based on these delusions jeopardize the safety of the patients and others, particularly if the delusions are paranoid in quality.

f. Disorientation and memory deficits. Early in delirium, patients lose the ability to keep track of time and may lose track of the date. As the delirium worsens, they become disoriented with respect to place and situation. It is very rare for individuals to forget their identity. Memories of immediate or recent events can be retained only with effort early in delirium. Confusion, bewilderment, and misinterpretation set in as the delirium advances. Memory deficits lead to repetition in speech and behavior.

g. Disturbances in psychomotor activity and the sleep cycle. Patients may be agitated and hyperactive or appear to be quite restless. As the delirium advances, they may become clumsy and awkward. They are unable to perform simple tasks and act sluggishly, groping about in attempts to perform motor tasks. Impairment may be so severe that patients cannot walk or sit. Speech may be pressured or limited early in delirium. Inarticulate, slurred speech is common. Patients may sleep excessively, fitfully, or not at all.

h. Autonomic hyperactivity. A number of causes of delirium produce changes in blood pressure, pulse, temperature, and respiratory rate. The presence of these changes should alert the physician to the possibility of an organic etiology for a behavioral disturbance. Alcohol withdrawal and meningitis are two examples in which vital signs would be abnormal.

i. Variable mood state. The predominant feeling may be fear or anxiety. Some patients are giddy or euphoric. Irritability and anger may be seen. Regardless of the patient's emotional state at any given moment, feelings may change rapidly. Such lability contributes to the unpredictability and impulsiveness of delirious patients. In a fearful frame of mind, they may flee or fight. If patients are depressed, suicide is possible.

2. Dementia. The essential feature of dementia is a loss of intellectual abilities of sufficient severity to interfere with social or occupational functioning or both. This disorder occurs predominantly in the elderly and usually affects both the personality and the cognitive functioning of the patient.

The course varies in dementia. When dementia is the result of trauma, losses appear suddenly and, in most cases, stabilize quickly. In dementia due to degenerative causes, the course is insidious and progressive. The demented patient is more susceptible to delirium. The ability to adapt to new situations is limited and leaves the patient vulnerable to stresses and changes in the environment.

a. Memory loss. Early in the course of dementia, patients are forgetful of details. Such forgetfulness may be minor in scope and is frequently overlooked by others. However, the severity of memory loss increases, and more significant memory lapses occur, such as leaving the stove on. In the advanced stages, patients may have no memory at all. Remote memories tend to be affected later, and recent memories are affected very early in this disorder.

b. **Inability to think abstractly.** Patients experience difficulty with new tasks and may avoid doing anything new. The ability to generalize from past experience or to see the relationships between similar situations may be lost as well.

c. **Impaired judgment.** Behavior may be inappropriate for a given social situation. Coarse and obscene language may be used. Patients may not take care of themselves: They may eat a poor, unbalanced diet and pay no attention to cleanliness and grooming. Patients may live in squalor and filth. Impulsive actions occur; for example, an elderly male patient may become active sexually in an exaggerated or inappropriate way, such as exposing himself to children; bad judgment may be exercised in business deals, and savings may be squandered impulsively.

d. **Personality changes.** Patients who had been orderly and meticulous about cleanliness may become obsessively meticulous or quite slovenly. The active, socially involved individual may withdraw and become isolated and apathetic. Patients may become suspicious, guarded, or paranoid when their failing memory cannot provide information about the events of the day. A misplaced purse leads to the conclusion that someone has stolen it, an open window to the conclusion that someone has broken in. Patients become more dependent on others, and they may become very anxious. Someone who has been congenial and friendly may become irritable and hostile.

e. **Deficits in functioning.** Demented patients may lose some ability to express themselves. Language is used in a vague, imprecise, or stereotypic fashion. Patients may use a few phrases again and again; the vocabulary may become limited, and the ability to name objects may be impaired (**dysnomia**). They may experience difficulty in performing routine, physical tasks, such as shaving and dressing (**apraxia**). In the advanced stages of dementia, patients may be mute and in need of assistance for most tasks, including eating.

f. **Depression.** When dementia is mild, patients are aware of their deficits, which creates both anxiety and depression. Severe depression and suicidal behavior are common. Some patients attempt to compensate for or conceal deficits by excessive orderliness, social withdrawal, or excessive attention to detail. Some patients elaborate and fill in details even when they do not remember (**confabulation**). This usually occurs unconsciously and is not intentional or planned by the demented individual. It does, however, obscure the fact that memory is impaired.

B. **Disorders with selective areas of cognitive impairment**

1. **Amnestic syndrome.** The essential feature in this usually chronic and uncommon disorder is impairment of short- and long-term memory in an individual with a normal state of consciousness. This deficit is attributable to an organic factor, and impairment is moderate to severe. Damage to diencephalic and medial temporal lobe structures leads to this disorder. However, unlike dementia, **there is no loss of intellectual functioning**. Other features include the following:

   a. Affected individuals are unable to learn new material (**anterograde amnesia**) and are unable to recall the past (**retrograde amnesia**).

   b. Immediate memory may be intact.

   c. Individuals may be disoriented and may confabulate.

   d. Amnestic patients may become apathetic and lose initiative.

   e. Patients may have no insight into their deficits and exhibit little concern about them.

   f. Affect may become superficial.

   g. The disorder usually presents suddenly when caused by such factors as anoxia.

   h. Secondary complications arise because of a lack of memory. In severely impaired individuals, dangerous behavior may occur, and supervision may be necessary at all times.

2. **Organic hallucinosis.** The essential feature is the presence of persistent or recurrent hallucinations due to organic factors in an individual with a normal state of consciousness. The course depends on the etiology and may be brief or chronic. Other features include the following:

   a. Hallucinations may involve any sensory modality; they may be as simple as the appearance of colors and as complex as the appearance of talking, moving, odd-looking creatures.

   b. Affected individuals may recognize the hallucinations to be hallucinations or may believe that they are real. If they cannot recognize an irrational basis for the hallucinations, the situation becomes delusional. However, there are no systematized delusions.

   c. Individuals may find the hallucinations pleasant or upsetting.

d. If individuals are distracted by the hallucinations or predicate actions upon them, accidents or dangerous behaviors may occur.

C. Disorders resembling other major disorders

1. Organic mood syndrome. The essential feature of this disorder is a disturbance in mood, resembling either mania or depression, due to a specific organic factor. The patient has a normal state of consciousness. No loss of intellectual functioning is present. The same phenomena that are observed in a mood disorder are present (see Chapter 3, "Mood Disorders").
   a. The intensity of symptoms ranges from mild to severe.
   b. Impairment of functioning may be minimal but can be quite extensive.
   c. Mild cognitive impairment is frequently observed.
   d. The risks of a mood disorder are present in this disorder: Impulsive, poorly considered behavior or self-destructive behavior may occur.
   e. Both toxic and metabolic factors can lead to an organic mood syndrome.

2. Organic delusional syndrome. The essential feature of this disorder is the presence of delusions due to a specific organic factor. The patient has a normal state of consciousness. Other features include the following:
   a. Mild cognitive impairment is commonly seen.
   b. Speech may be rambling and voluminous.
   c. Delusional content is variable and related to the etiologic factors. Persecutory delusions are common.
   d. Although hallucinations may be present, they assume a secondary role in the illness; delusions are the predominant symptom.
   e. The patient can present with any number of symptoms. This condition is subjectively unpleasant in many cases: The patient may be perplexed, unkempt, dysphoric, and anxious. The patient's level of activity may be increased (hyperactivity) or decreased (apathy). Ritualistic behavior, generated by delusional convictions, may be part of this syndrome.
   f. The degree of impairment is usually severe. The patient is not able to discern reality adequately and, therefore, cannot respond appropriately to real situations.
   g. The patient may harm him- or herself or others while responding to delusional ideation.

3. Organic anxiety syndrome. The essential feature of this disorder is severe anxiety caused by a specific organic factor. Recurrent symptoms of generalized anxiety or panic attacks are prominent. The patient has a normal state of consciousness. The same phenomena observed in panic disorder or generalized anxiety disorder are present (see Chapter 6, "Anxiety Disorders").
   a. An inability to sustain attention may be present.
   b. Mild cognitive impairment is often seen.
   c. The degree of impairment, which varies due to individual vulnerability and the etiologic factors, ranges from minimal to severe.
   d. Typical etiologic factors include psychoactive substances (e.g., caffeine or amphetamines, withdrawal from psychoactive substances, such as alcohol or sedative-hypnotics, or endocrine disorders, such as hyperthyroidism or pheochromocytoma).
   e. Symptoms of this disorder are usually relieved when the underlying etiology is removed or treated. In some instances, an unexpectedly prolonged or incomplete recovery may be observed.

D. Organic personality syndrome. The personality is affected in an organic personality syndrome, while impairment in other areas is relatively mild. The essential feature is a marked change in personality due to a specific organic factor, usually structural damage to the brain. The disorder may be transient or persistent; toxic factors generally produce short-lived disturbances, but structural factors (e.g., tumors) generally produce chronic disturbances. The differences in presentation reflect the differences in the nature and location of the pathologic process. The degree of impairment is variable; however, the presence of poor judgment may necessitate supervised care. This disorder may prove to be the first sign of a developing dementia. Observations may include the following:

1. The patient may be paranoid or suspicious.

2. Mild cognitive impairment may be observed.

3. Irritability is common.

4. Frontal lobe dysfunction is associated with:
   a. Emotional lability and unexpected outbursts of anger
   b. Impaired impulse control and poor judgment, such as sexually inappropriate behavior

      c. Apathy, indifference, and loss of interest in one's environment
    5. Temporal lobe dysfunction is associated with:
      a. Verbosity in speech and writing
      b. Religiosity and overly aggressive behavior

E. Substance-induced organic mental syndromes
    1. Intoxication. The essential feature of this disorder is maladaptive behavior and a substance-specific syndrome due to either recent use or the lingering presence of the substance in the body. Other characteristics include the following:
      a. There is no evidence of one of the organic mental syndromes (see section III A–C).
      b. The presenting symptoms depend upon the substance involved.
      c. The patient may suffer from a number of functional disturbances in such areas as:
        (1) Perception
        (2) Sleep (wakefulness)
        (3) Emotional control
        (4) Attention
        (5) Thinking
        (6) Judgment
        (7) Psychomotor behavior
      d. Additional disturbances depend upon:
        (1) The individual's expectations
        (2) Environmental circumstances
        (3) The preintoxication personality
        (4) The individual's biologic state
      e. The course of an intoxication is usually brief. The duration depends upon:
        (1) Amount consumed
        (2) Rate of consumption
        (3) Tolerance of the substance by the individual
        (4) Body size (i.e., the volume of distribution)
        (5) Substance half-life
        (6) Gastric contents (if the substance is ingested)
        (7) Rate of absorption
      f. The degree of impairment is related to the demands of the affected individual's environment. If the intoxicated individual faces little or no responsibility, impairment is minimal; if the intoxicated individual faces significant responsibility, the impairment may be marked.
      g. Coma or seizures may occur in the severely intoxicated patient.
      h. Accidents are a common and, far too often, lethal complication of intoxication.

    2. Withdrawal. The essential feature of this disorder is the development of a substance-specific syndrome that follows the reduction or cessation of intake of a substance used to induce intoxication.
      a. There is no evidence of one of the organic mental syndromes (see section III A–C).
      b. The array of symptoms is contingent upon the substance in use.
      c. The patient may experience a number of physiologic and psychological symptoms, including:
        (1) Malaise
        (2) Lability
        (3) Irritability
        (4) Anxiety
        (5) Restlessness
        (6) A change in sleep patterns
        (7) Impaired attention
        (8) A craving for the substance
      d. This condition may last from a few days to several weeks.
      e. The degree of impairment varies. Factors affecting the impairment include:
        (1) The physical health of the individual in withdrawal
        (2) Environmental elements, such as responsibility
      f. Criminal behavior may develop to acquire the substance.

F. Organic mental syndrome not otherwise specified is a residual category, which includes disorders that are due to a specific organic factor and do not meet the diagnostic criteria for another organic mental syndrome. These disorders feature maladaptive behavior, such as disturbances of consciousness, which occur during seizures.

IV. NEUROLOGIC ETIOLOGIES

A. Epilepsy is a symptom complex characterized by transient, episodic alterations in consciousness, which may be associated with convulsive movements or disturbances in feeling, behavior, or both. Features of epilepsy include:

1. **Disturbances of the electrophysiologic activity of brain cells**, which result in seizures. These physiologic changes are expressed in:
   a. Changes in electrical potential in an electroencephalogram (EEG). Although an EEG can localize the seizure focus in most cases, some disorders are missed due to a lack of abnormal electrical activity at the time of the recording or a seizure focus that is deep in the brain's interior.
   b. Variations in consciousness
   c. Disordered functioning of the autonomic nervous system
   d. Convulsive movements or psychic disturbances

2. **Seizure activity** that is precipitated by the following factors:
   a. Hyperventilation
   b. Sleep deprivation
   c. Sensory stimuli, such as flashing lights, loud noises, and tactile sensations
   d. Trauma
   e. Fever
   f. Emotional stress
   g. Hormonal changes, such as those occurring during puberty and menstruation
   h. Drugs, such as alcohol, phenothiazines, tricyclic antidepressants, and antihistamines

3. **Three major groups of seizures**
   a. **Grand mal seizures**
      (1) An **aura** occurs seconds prior to the generalized seizure. Individuals experience motor (e.g., twitching) or sensory (e.g., smelling, seeing, and tingling) symptoms due to early seizure activity.
      (2) In the **tonic phase**, individuals suffer sudden and complete loss of consciousness. They may fall and be injured. All voluntary muscles contract for 10–20 seconds (the **tonic state**). The pupils are dilated. The corneal reflex is lost. Deep-tendon reflexes are decreased or absent. Inspiration ceases, and the face may take on a cyanotic look. Incontinence may occur. **Babinski's sign** is present.
      (3) In the **clonic phase**, muscles relax and contract intermittently, producing generalized jerking motions. Breathing is restored; saliva may froth up in the mouth. The tongue may be bitten due to the contracting jaw muscles.
      (4) A **postconvulsive coma** follows. The pupils are fixed. Deep-tendon reflexes are absent. The muscular tone is flaccid, and the face is congested. Individuals are bewildered and confused upon awakening. They may perform semiautomatic acts or move about aimlessly. A clouded state of consciousness persists for a few minutes to a few hours, in most cases, but it may last for a few days after several seizures.
      (5) In rare cases, one seizure follows another without intervening consciousness (**status epilepticus**). Unchecked, this condition can lead to exhaustion, hyperthermia, rhabdomyolysis, dehydration, coma, and death.
      (6) **EEG tracings** show a high-frequency, high-voltage pattern.
   b. **Petit mal seizures**
      (1) Individuals experience no aura because the onset is sudden.
      (2) The typical duration is 5–30 seconds.
      (3) Individuals assume a fixed posture. Eyes stare into space. They become inattentive to the task at hand. Muscle tone is lost, and things may be dropped. A rhythmic twitching of muscles may occur. There is an interruption of normal consciousness.
      (4) These seizures may also occur in rapid succession (**petit mal status**).
      (5) The age of onset is usually early in life, from 4–8 years. If the disorder persists beyond the age of 18 years (which occurs in two-thirds of those afflicted), a grand mal seizure disorder may develop.
      (6) EEG tracings reveal alternating fast and slow waves three times per second.
   c. **Psychomotor epilepsy, also known as temporal lobe epilepsy**
      (1) Onset is sudden.
      (2) Duration is usually 30 seconds to 2 minutes.
      (3) Various mood states, such as rage, terror, and alarm, may occur.
      (4) A trance-like appearance is characteristic.
      (5) Seemingly planned outbursts, often aggressive in nature, may occur.

(6) Feelings of bewilderment, excitement, and confusion as well as loneliness, strangeness, and déjà vu can result.

(7) Involvement of the muscles of mastication, speech, and swallowing, producing twitching in the face and garbled speech, is common.

(8) Hallucinations, involving any sensory modality, such as flashing lights, repetitive sounds, and noxious odors, may occur.

(9) Amnesia for the seizure and for the 30 seconds or so preceding the seizure is common.

(10) Psychomotor epilepsy is more common in adults than in children.

(11) An anterior frontal lobe EEG tracing with four to eight spikes per second is characteristic.

(12) Disordered thought formation with delusional ideation may occur in some cases.

(13) There is a resemblance to schizophrenic behavior with psychotic symptoms and erratic actions.

4. **Deterioration in functioning with long-standing seizure disorders.** Patients seem mentally slow and intellectually compromised. Although there may be some organic damage, the psychological effects of low self-esteem and a constricted life-style should not be ignored.

5. **Diagnosis.** In many cases, the diagnosis of a seizure disorder can be made by history and physical examination; in some cases, an EEG tracing provides confirmatory evidence. A few cases elude ready diagnosis. The diagnosis of seizure disorder should be considered when dealing with any acutely confused or delirious patient.

B. **Neoplasms** may be primary tumors of the brain parenchyma or the central nervous system or metastatic tumors from other areas, such as the thyroid or breast. The presence of a neoplasm is underdiagnosed. There is no consistent presentation.

1. **Signs and symptoms** may include:
   a. Signs of increased intracranial pressure, such as:
      (1) Headache
      (2) Impaired consciousness or level of energy
      (3) Papilledema
      (4) Vomiting
   b. Focal neurologic findings, such as weakness
   c. **Psychiatric symptoms** that fall into two groups:
      (1) **Personality changes.** An accentuation of preexisting traits may occur (e.g., the orderly individual becomes obsessed with cleanliness). The personality may be markedly changed with a loss of inhibition, leading to shameless, sexually inappropriate behavior.
      (2) **Cerebral changes.** Any and all functions may be affected. An individual may become absentminded or have frank memory deficits. The ability to reason or calculate may be impaired. Alterations in consciousness are seen; there is especially a tendency towards drowsiness. Interest in sex may be diminished. Perceptual difficulties, including hallucinations, may be present. The patient may be confused and confabulate to cover deficits. Simply paying attention to the task at hand may be difficult.

2. **Tumors in specific locations** tend to present in specific ways.
   a. **Occipital lobe tumors** are associated with simple visual hallucinations.
   b. **Parietal lobe tumors** are associated with sensory deficits and agnosia. Individuals may not recognize or perceive parts of the environment; for example, they may perceive only one-half of a clock face and be unaware of this deficit.
   c. **Frontal lobe tumors** tend to present as gradual, insidious changes in personality. Individuals may become passive and apathetic and have a flattened affect. Another common presentation is irritability and anxiety in individuals who act impulsively and in an uninhibited manner.
   d. **Temporal lobe tumors** usually present a clinical picture similar to that described for temporal lobe epilepsy. Paroxysmal motor, perceptual, and behavioral symptoms are the prominent features.

3. **Symptom intensity** is related to the location and rate of growth of the neoplasm. A rapidly growing tumor can produce a delirious state. A slow-growing tumor can produce insidious personality changes.

4. **Diagnosis** of a neoplasm depends upon history, careful neurologic examination for focal abnormalities, and evidence of increased intracranial pressure. A sudden onset of seizures raises the possibility of a neoplasm. EEG tracings and radiographic techniques, such as computed

tomography (CT) scans, magnetic resonance imaging (MRI) scans, and brain scans are used to confirm the diagnosis.

C. **Head trauma** can cause both acute and chronic disorders, which affect cognition, personality, emotional expression, and physical health.

1. **Acute disorders** commonly present a mixed clinical picture. Of particular concern is the possibility of progression. Close observation is warranted with special attention given to signs of increased intracranial pressure. These disorders include the following:

   a. **Concussion syndrome** refers to a momentary interruption of normal cerebral processes following a severe impact to the head. Features include:
      (1) Rapid and complete recovery
      (2) Amnesia for the event and for the few seconds preceding the event
      (3) Variability in consciousness when the individual wakes up, which ranges from an alert, clear sensorium to a confused, clouded state of awareness
      (4) No neurologic or psychological sequelae, a determination that can be made only after observing for aftereffects

   b. **Traumatic coma** results from a more severe head injury, usually leading to damage to the brain parenchyma. Features include:
      (1) Contusion or laceration of the brain
      (2) A duration ranging from hours to days or, in some cases, weeks
      (3) A period of stupor, restlessness, and confusion following the coma
      (4) Amnesia or delirium possibly following the coma

   c. **Traumatic delirium** begins as an individual emerges from a coma. It is due either to tissue injury or increased intracranial pressure. Features include:
      (1) Bewildered, aggressive, or frightened behavior
      (2) Fluctuations in consciousness
      (3) Hallucinations, most often visual in nature
      (4) Variable duration with a prolonged duration suggesting significant tissue damage
      (5) Gradual improvement for 12–18 months after the injury

   d. **Amnestic–confabulatory syndrome** is characterized by deficits in memory and perception. Features include:
      (1) Confabulation
      (2) Impairment of memory
      (3) Deranged, inaccurate perceptions

   e. **Subdural hematomas** occur in as many as 10% of individuals with head injuries. Venous blood accumulates between the dura and arachnoid membranes. Features include:
      (1) Headache
      (2) Neurologic deficits, reflecting the location of the hematoma
      (3) Variability in the level of consciousness
      (4) Irritability
      (5) Confusion
      (6) A predisposing condition, such as alcoholism, senility, epilepsy, and paresis caused by syphilis, that has spread to the central nervous system

2. **Chronic disorders** develop if recovery of damaged brain tissue is incomplete or if emotional and psychological difficulties linger after head trauma. These disorders include the following:

   a. **Postconcussional syndrome.** Symptoms include:
      (1) Headache
      (2) Anxiety
      (3) Fatigue
      (4) Insomnia
      (5) Dizziness
      (6) Impaired memory
      (7) Impaired concentration
      (8) Narrowing of interests
      (9) Diminished tolerance of alcohol
      (10) Irritability
      (11) Lability
      (12) Decreased sexual potency or drive

   b. **Post-traumatic personality disorder in adults.** Symptoms may include changes in personality. An individual may become:
      (1) Irritable and quarrelsome
      (2) Aggressive
      (3) Impulsive
      (4) Irresponsible and unmotivated

        (5) Paranoid
        (6) Withdrawn
    c. Post-traumatic personality disorder in children. Family relationships, especially between parents and the affected child, may be troubled. Symptoms may include changes in personality. A child may become:
        (1) Impulsive
        (2) Destructive
        (3) Disobedient and disruptive
        (4) Overactive and restless
        (5) Cruel
    d. Post-traumatic defect syndrome. Symptoms include:
        (1) Loss of initiative
        (2) Mental slowing
        (3) Impaired memory
        (4) Impaired concentration
        (5) Confabulation
        (6) Loss of motivation
        (7) Confusion
        (8) Impaired speech
        (9) Motor impairment
      (10) Seizures, especially following penetrating head injuries

D. Presenile and senile dementias. With advancing age, presenile and senile dementias develop in both men and women. These conditions result from a progressive loss of neurons. Changes observed in behavior, cognitive functioning, and personality differ from the normal changes brought on by aging both in degree and in kind. Features of these disorders are listed below.

  1. Signs and symptoms include:
    a. Loss of memory
    b. An impaired capacity to think abstractly
    c. Indifference to social norms
    d. Inappropriate sexual behavior
    e. Carelessness in or indifference about grooming and appearance
    f. Suspicion and distrust of others
    g. Irritability or hostility
    h. Anxiety
    i. Isolation and withdrawal
    j. Depression
    k. Preoccupation with bodily concerns
    l. Progressive loss of cognitive functions
    m. Paranoia or delusional thinking
    n. Impaired judgment
    o. Diminished sensory perception at night
    p. Confusion and agitation
    q. Physical symptoms, including:
        (1) Weight loss
        (2) Unsteady gait
        (3) Slowed speech
        (4) Hand tremors
        (5) Diminished sensory acuity
        (6) Atrophied skin
    r. Hypersomnia
    s. Hoarding of money or worthless objects
    t. Indiscriminate accumulation of animals
    u. Illusions or hallucinations

  2. Common clinical variations include:
    a. Simple deterioration. A **slowly progressive course** is characterized by:
        (1) Progressive memory loss
        (2) Narrowing of interests
        (3) Loss of initiative
        (4) Sluggish thinking
        (5) Apathy
        (6) Irritability
        (7) Nocturnal restlessness
        (8) Eventual loss of contact with the environment

    b. Delirium and confusion. An **acute change** is evidenced by:
      (1) Changes in physical well-being, due to illness, drugs, or toxins
      (2) Perplexity and disorientation
      (3) Insomnia
      (4) Hallucinations
      (5) Restlessness
      (6) Fear and anxiety
      (7) Noisy behavior
    c. Depression, which may be the first recognizable feature of a dementing process. Patients may suffer the following:
      (1) Memory loss
      (2) Intellectual impoverishment
      (3) Agitation or withdrawal
      (4) Hypochondriacal preoccupations or delusions
      (5) Melancholia
    d. Paranoia, the features of which include:
      (1) Irritability or hostility
      (2) Demanding, suspicious, mistrustful relationships with others
      (3) Paranoid delusions
      (4) Illusions or hallucinations, which are common
      (5) An undisturbed consciousness
      (6) An unimpaired orientation, which is usual
    e. Presbyophrenia, the features of which include:
      (1) A defect in retention due to memory loss
      (2) Confabulation to cover memory loss
      (3) Talkativeness and apparent alertness
      (4) Being out of touch with reality
      (5) Restless, nonproductive activity

3. Various neuropathologic lesions have been identified, and different syndromes have been described.
    a. Alzheimer's disease was described by Alois Alzheimer (1864–1915). Primary degenerative dementia of the Alzheimer type, as it is now called, occurs in 4% of people 65 years old, is more common in women than men, and increases in prevalence after age 65. The onset of the disease is usually between the ages of 50 and 65 years. There is an insidious course of 5–10 years with no characteristic symptom complex. Alzheimer and subsequent investigators discovered the following:
      (1) Tangled, thread-like structures, occupying much or all of the cell body of cortical ganglion cells
      (2) Characteristic histopathologic changes called senile plaques, neurofibrillary tangles, and granulovacuolar degeneration of neurons
      (3) Involvement of up to one-quarter of the cells
      (4) Predominance in the frontal and temporal lobes but diffuse cortical involvement
      (5) Changes in the basal ganglia
      (6) Motor disturbances, including weakness, hypertonicity, facial paresis, or contractures in large muscle groups
      (7) Progression to a vegetative state
    b. Pick's disease, which usually afflicts individuals who are between 45 and 60 years old, was first described in 1892 by Arnold Pick in Prague. He discovered the following:
      (1) Atrophy and gliosis in associative areas of the brain
      (2) Little change in motor, sensory, and projective areas of the brain
      (3) Speech and thinking particularly impaired
      (4) Involvement of temporal and frontal lobes
      (5) Degenerative, not inflammatory, lesions
      (6) Severe atrophy with a loss of 25% and more of the brain mass
      (7) Chromatolysis, which is loss of chromatic substance and displacement of the nucleus to the cell periphery
      (8) Changes in the basal ganglia, which are rare
      (9) Women afflicted twice as often as men
      (10) In many cases, the appearance of focal symptoms, such as apraxia, aphasia, anomia, alexia, and agraphia, before generalized dementia
      (11) Motor problems, which are rare
      (12) Hallucinations and illusions, which are rare
    c. Creutzfeldt-Jakob disease is a rare, presenile dementia caused by a slow virus.

    d. **"Senile plaques"** have also been observed in the brains of demented patients. The characteristics are:

      (1) Small areas of tissue degeneration throughout the cortex

      (2) The highest density in the frontal lobes

      (3) Axons with excesses of neurofibrils

      (4) Large dendrites

      (5) Dense, altered mitochondria

      (6) No absolute correlation with the severity of the clinical condition

4. Treatment. Given the progressive nature of these disorders and the grossly compromised capacity of affected individuals to adapt to new situations and to cope with stress, specific interventions are frequently required. Treatment should include:

    a. Provisions for the emotional well-being of the affected individual

    b. A home environment, if possible

    c. Structured care in a nursing home or hospital, if necessary

    d. Assistance to the family in the choice of environment and in understanding the illness

    e. Attention to nutrition and physical health

    f. Sensory stimulation at night, as needed

    g. Psychoactive medications, such as neuroleptics or antidepressants, if indicated

    h. Correction of sensory deficits (e.g., eyeglasses and hearing aids)

E. Compromise of oxygenation and nutrition to the brain from interruptions in intracranial blood flow. Interruptions may be sudden and catastrophic (e.g., a stroke or trauma) or may follow a more insidious course (e.g., progressive arteriosclerosis, which may result in multi-infarct dementia). However, these disorders are not always progressive. The onset of illness usually occurs between 50 and 65 years of age with men afflicted more commonly than women. Dementia, depression, and delirium may present in similar ways. Therefore, careful attention to diagnosis is mandatory. Features of these disorders are listed below.

1. Atheromatous plaques narrow or obliterate vessel lumina, which may cause:

    a. Hypoxia

    b. Disturbed metabolism

    c. Cell death

2. Thrombosis causes 85% of this type of disorder versus the 15% caused by embolic phenomena.

3. Prodromal symptoms include:

    a. Fatigue

    b. Headache

    c. Dizziness

    d. Impaired concentration

    e. Drowsiness

    f. Insidious physical or mental impairment

    g. Alterations in personality

4. Signs and symptoms of compromise include:

    a. Confusion, which is the first obvious symptom in more than one-half of all cases

    b. Incoherence

    c. Restlessness

    d. Clouded consciousness

    e. Other deficits, such as muscular weakness or aphasia

5. Early signs and symptoms of insidious disease include:

    a. Mental fatigue

    b. Loss of initiative

    c. Emotional instability

    d. Irritability

    e. Loss of finer sentiments, such as compassion, sympathy, and altruism

    f. Varying degrees of memory loss

    g. Mistrust of others

6. Signs and symptoms of serious disturbances include:

    a. Nocturnal bewilderment

    b. Anxiety

    c. Violent behavior

    d. Lack of self-care

      e. Diminished judgment
      f. Loss of inhibitions
      g. Disturbances in thinking, including delusions
      h. Evidence of localized strokes
      i. Seizures
      j. Tremors
      k. Periods of delirium

7. Treatment. The distinction between extracranial and arteriolar sources of disease indicates the course of treatment. Early recognition affords an opportunity for treatment with angioplasty or endarterectomy. Decreasing stress and physical exertion may slow the progression of the illness. Sedating medications tend to confuse affected individuals. Neuroleptics are effective in treating nocturnal restlessness.

F. Demyelinating disease. The myelin sheaths that insure proper transmission of neuronal signals are destroyed, and the structural integrity of the nervous system is severely compromised in demyelinating disease. Neurologic and psychologic signs and symptoms result.

1. Acute disseminated encephalomyelitis may involve both the brain and the spinal cord. Its onset is abrupt, usually following either the exanthem of viral illnesses, such as measles, chickenpox, rubella, and smallpox, or vaccination against rabies or smallpox. In some cases, there may be no preceding event.
    a. Signs and symptoms. Initially, the patient experiences headaches, confusion, and a stiff neck. With spinal cord involvement, paralysis and sensory loss are prominent. Stupor, convulsions, and coma reflect brain involvement.
    b. Diagnosis. Significant neurologic findings usually eliminate any question about an organic etiology when psychiatric symptoms, such as confused, erratic behavior, are present.
    c. Course. Mortality rates range from 10%–50%. Morbidity is high. Residual neurologic disturbances are common. Intellectual impairment may be present. Permanent changes in behavior, such as increased aggression or social withdrawal, may be observed.

2. Multiple sclerosis (MS) is a relatively common, chronic demyelinating disease. It features episodes of focal disturbances, which remit and recur. Women are afflicted more often than men. The peak incidence occurs in individuals between 30–35 years of age. It is about eight times more common in relatives of those with MS.
    a. Etiology. The etiology of MS has been intensively investigated. Most researchers believe that a viral agent is causative.
    b. Signs and symptoms include:
      (1) Visual impairment. (About 40% of patients experience visual impairment as an initial symptom. This is due to optic neuritis.)
      (2) Nystagmus
      (3) Dysarthria
      (4) Intention tremor
      (5) Ataxia
      (6) Impaired sense of position
      (7) Impaired vibratory sense
      (8) Bladder dysfunction
      (9) Weakness in limbs
     (10) Paraplegia
     (11) Spatial disorientation
     (12) Altered emotional responses
    c. Diagnosis. Any part of the nervous system may be affected. Therefore, signs and symptoms vary widely. The diagnosis is made when evidence for more than one lesion (i.e., more than one focal disturbance) is present and a remitting and relapsing course exists. Some patients present with psychiatric symptoms. Classically, patients have been described as euphoric or pathologically cheerful. Some patients, however, become irritable or depressed. The presence of fleeting neurologic signs and symptoms may raise the question of somatization. Diagnosis can be very difficult in patients who are somatically preoccupied.
    d. Course. MS typically runs a course of 20 years or more, although some patients suffer a more virulent form of the illness. Over the course of the disease, intellectual impairment may develop. Various psychiatric symptoms develop as well. Personality changes may be evident. Mood swings and depression have been observed frequently. An individual's behavior is altered. He or she may become isolated and withdrawn. Cases of paranoid personality changes are reported.

V. PHARMACOLOGIC ETIOLOGIES

A. Overview. Significant psychiatric disturbances occur in approximately 3% of all patients taking medications. These disturbances may be extensions of the desired effects of the medication or secondary effects. In addition, drugs are used in abusive patterns, which also leads to significant symptomatology. Variables that must be considered when evaluating the role that a drug plays in a behavioral disturbance include:

1. The drug and its actions

2. The amount administered

3. The duration of action

4. The existence of medical illnesses

5. The patient's age

6. The cerebral functioning of the patient

7. The patient's environment (e.g., does it lack stimulation?)

8. Sociocultural factors, such as fears concerning medication

9. Drug interactions

10. The patient's personality

B. Sedative-hypnotics and anxiolytics

1. **Barbiturates** are useful as medications in addition to having high abuse potential. Organic mental disorders may arise acutely, with chronic use, or in withdrawal.
   a. **Acute intoxication** causes generalized central nervous system depression. Signs and symptoms include:
      (1) Dizziness
      (2) Ataxia
      (3) Confusion
      (4) Slurred speech
      (5) A compromised level of consciousness, ranging from stupor to coma
   b. **Severe intoxication** results from a dose of 200–1000 mg of pentobarbital. This may vary, depending upon tolerance or the presence of other sedatives, such as alcohol. A fatal dose is 1000–1500 mg of pentobarbital.
   c. **Chronic intoxication** leads to significant difficulties, although it may go undiscovered until a withdrawal crisis occurs. Symptoms of chronic intoxication include:
      (1) Fluctuations in the level of consciousness
      (2) Somnolence
      (3) Confusion
      (4) Slurred speech
      (5) Ataxia
      (6) Poor judgment
      (7) Hypomania, including irritability, euphoria, emotional lability, and querulousness
      (8) Carelessness about work
      (9) Social withdrawal
   d. **Withdrawal** from barbiturates is hazardous and potentially life-threatening. Withdrawal may occur when the individual is cut off from his or her supply; for example, the patient who is hospitalized for surgery.
      (1) **Signs and symptoms of withdrawal**
          (a) Evidence of increasing central nervous system irritability about 8 hours after the last use of barbiturates
          (b) Muscular twitches
          (c) Tremor
          (d) Weakness
          (e) Dizziness
          (f) Nausea and vomiting
          (g) Sweating
          (h) Hyperactive deep-tendon reflexes
          (i) Headaches
          (j) Postural hypotension
          (k) Onset of grand mal seizures from 30–48 hours after the last use of barbiturates
          (l) Delirium with disorientation and elevated temperature lasting as long as 7 days

      (2) Diagnosis of the magnitude of barbiturate addiction can be made with a pentobarbital tolerance test.

        (a) A liquid dose of 200 mg of pentobarbital is given.

        (b) At 1 hour, the patient should be checked for signs of intoxication.

        (c) If the patient is intoxicated, the level of chronic use is low.

        (d) If the patient is not affected or continues to show signs of withdrawal, a high dose of pentobarbital is needed during the initial stages of withdrawal.

      (3) Withdrawal should be undertaken in a hospital.

        (a) A **maintenance dose** is established, which may be as high as 300 mg of pentobarbital every 6 hours.

        (b) The dose is decreased 10% a day for 10 days.

      (4) Individual psychotherapy, group therapy, or both should follow withdrawal to help the patient deal with stresses without reverting to drug abuse.

2. Tranquilizers. Minor tranquilizers are prescribed for relief of anxiety and for sedation; they are widely used but infrequently abused. Abusers tend to be individuals who abuse other psychoactive drugs. Included in this group are diazepam, alprazolam, oxazepam, meprobamate, chlordiazepoxide, lorazepam, and hydroxyzine hydrochloride. They are neither as toxic nor as potent as barbiturates and the synthetic hypnotics and offer a wider margin of safety. However, acute and chronic intoxication as well as withdrawal may occur.

  a. Acute intoxication results from high doses. The individual may become delirious, hyperactive, and have attacks of rage.

  b. Chronic intoxication leads to tolerance. Difficulties similar to those described for chronic barbiturate intoxication develop (see section V B 1 c).

  c. Withdrawal symptoms may be evident within 24 hours if the agent is short-acting (e.g., oxazepam or alprazolam) or may not be seen for a week with long-acting agents (e.g., diazepam or chlordiazepoxide). The withdrawal syndrome may last 3 weeks or longer. Upon evidence of withdrawal, a withdrawal schedule can be started, using pentobarbital.

3. Hypnotics are given for sleep disturbances. Some drugs, such as chloral hydrate, glutethimide, flurazepam, methyprylon, methaqualone, and ethchlorvynol, produce symptoms similar to those produced by barbiturates and are more potent and toxic than minor tranquilizers.

  a. Side effects. Between 1.0% and 3.5% of hospitalized patients suffer untoward reactions to these drugs.

  b. Serious overdose may occur. Symptoms include convulsions, pulmonary edema, and coma.

  c. Withdrawal syndromes may resemble delirium tremens with an elevated temperature, disorientation, agitation, hallucinations, clouded consciousness, and convulsions.

4. Bromides were once commonly used as hypnotics but have been replaced by other drugs for the most part. However, over-the-counter preparations such as Miles Nervine and Bromo-Seltzer and Neurosine, a prescription drug, still contain bromides. Symptoms may arise from either acute or chronic bromide intoxication.

  a. Acute intoxication is rare because very large doses tend to cause nausea and vomiting. Symptoms may include:

    (1) Confusion

    (2) Weakness

    (3) Ataxia

    (4) Depression

    (5) Delirium with hallucinations

  b. Chronic intoxication results from the ingestion of large doses for an extended period of time or from impaired excretion of bromides due to renal disease. Levels of 150 mg/100 ml are found in the blood. Bromides act by displacing chloride ions. In so doing, the individual's hydration and electrolyte balance may be affected in the intoxicated state. **Chronic brominism may simply produce intoxication**. Signs and symptoms may include:

    (1) Forgetfulness

    (2) Diminished libido

    (3) Irritability

    (4) Slowed speech

    (5) Ataxia

    (6) Tremors

    (7) Sluggish, irregular pupillary reaction

    (8) Vertigo

    (9) Lethargy

   c. Chronic brominism
   (1) Delirium results in about two-thirds of patients with chronic brominism. Signs and symptoms may include:
   (a) Disorientation
   (b) Restlessness
   (c) Anxiety
   (d) Insomnia
   (e) Hallucinations
   (f) Mood disturbances
   (g) Delusions
   (2) Transitory schizophreniform psychosis with paranoid delusions and hallucinations but a clear sensorium may occur in some individuals.
   (3) A bromide hallucinosis, that is, visual hallucinations without delusions or delirium, may also occur.
   d. Treatment for brominism must address both psychiatric symptoms and medical problems. Many bromide abusers also abuse alcohol; thus, brominism may be overlooked in the presence of this more common disorder. Sodium chloride is given to eliminate bromide ions. Fluid intake must be maintained. Significant reduction of bromide levels takes several weeks.

C. Stimulants

1. **Amphetamines** are chemically related to sympathomimetic amines and act primarily on the central nervous system. Included in this group are amphetamine sulfate, methamphetamine, dextroamphetamine sulfate, and methylphenidate. These drugs are widely abused because they produce euphoria and combat fatigue. Overdose, acute and chronic intoxication, and withdrawal all may occur.
   a. Acute intoxication results from the alerting effects that amphetamines have on the central nervous system. Signs and symptoms include:
   (1) Mood elevation
   (2) Tireless, energetic feelings
   (3) Diminished appetite
   (4) Tachycardia
   (5) Elevated blood pressure
   (6) Dilated pupils
   (7) Dry mouth
   (8) Tremors
   (9) Sweating
   b. Overdose of amphetamines may lead to a life-threatening medical crisis. Effects are short-lived, usually lasting 36–48 hours. Signs and symptoms include:
   (1) Restlessness
   (2) Irritability
   (3) Confusion
   (4) Disorientation
   (5) Auditory or visual hallucinations
   (6) Palpitations
   (7) Arrhythmias
   (8) Hyperactive, deep-tendon reflexes
   (9) Circulatory collapse
   (10) Convulsions
   (11) Coma

   c. Chronic intoxication leads to marked tolerance. Cessation of use produces a **withdrawal syndrome** characterized by fatigue, depression, and apathy. In some instances, depression is severe, and the risk of suicide is significant.
   (1) After limited use of amphetamines, an **organic delusional syndrome** may develop, but this is rare. Most commonly, the syndrome develops after prolonged use and chronic intoxication. This condition often resembles paranoid schizophrenia. Signs and symptoms include:
   (a) Disorientation
   (b) Ideas of reference
   (c) Persecutory delusions
   (d) Hallucinations
   (e) Paranoid fears
   (f) Stereotypic actions, such as teeth gnashing and repetitive touching of the face

(2) After chronic use, it may take up to 2 months for the effects of the drug to clear. An organic delusional syndrome may persist during this period, requiring treatment with haloperidol.

2. Drugs related to amphetamines

a. Anorectic agents are used to suppress the appetite. These drugs resemble amphetamines but are less potent. Included in this group are phenmetrazine, diethylpropion, and chlorphentermine. Each can produce any of the conditions noted for amphetamines, including a paranoid psychosis.

b. Analeptic agents are also chemically related to sympathomimetic amines and have an alerting effect on the central nervous system. Two commonly used drugs are aminophylline and caffeine.

(1) Aminophylline is prescribed for many asthmatics and patients with other chronic pulmonary diseases. Both intoxication and overdose can produce delirium with nausea, vomiting, anxiety, agitation, and confusion.

(2) Caffeine is the most commonly used stimulant, found in tea, coffee, and soft drinks. An overdose produces excitement, hyperactivity, flushing, insomnia, tremors, and tinnitus. An overdose may result from as few as 3 or 4 cups of coffee (300 mg of caffeine). Chronic intoxication produces a hypomanic condition with hyperactivity, insomnia, and rambling speech.

D. Psychoactive drugs

1. Antidepressants produce many adverse effects. Drugs in this group include tricyclic antidepressants, including imipramine, amitriptyline, and doxepin, and monoamine oxidase (MAO) inhibitors, including phenelzine.

a. Common adverse effects of tricyclic antidepressants include:
(1) Drowsiness
(2) Fatigue
(3) Tremors
(4) Weakness
(5) Confusion
(6) Agitation
(7) Anxiety

b. Overdoses of tricyclic antidepressants are usually severe, and only 1000–1250 mg of amitriptyline are sufficient for overdose. Initially, the patient becomes agitated, confused, disoriented, and experiences fluctuations in the level of consciousness. Seizures may occur. Stupor and coma eventually ensue. The patient is dangerously ill at this point with an elevated temperature and pulse rate, dilated pupils, and cardiac arrhythmias.

c. Combined use of MAO inhibitors and tricyclic antidepressants can lead to a dangerous syndrome, which is characterized by agitated and delirious behavior, headaches, nausea and vomiting, hyperpyrexia, convulsions, and, possibly, death.

2. Lithium carbonate can produce toxic effects even at therapeutic levels (i.e., 0.6–1.2 mEq/L). However, this is not common.

a. Levels of 2 mEq/L and more lead to a toxic confusional state. Affected patients are agitated, disoriented, and may have a multitude of physical signs and symptoms, including thirst, diarrhea, dizziness, slurred speech, weakness, and tremors. At very high levels (i.e., 4 mEq/L and more), coma and convulsions result.

b. Fluid replacement and administration of sodium chloride cause diuresis of excess lithium and reversal of the toxic condition.

3. Major tranquilizers are used to treat symptoms of psychosis. Drugs in this group include phenothiazines (including thioridazine and chlorpromazine), butyrophenones (haloperidol), thioxanthenes (thiothixene), and others. They are most commonly prescribed for schizophrenic disorders for the reduction of anxiety and the inhibition of delusions, hallucinations, and psychomotor agitation.

a. These drugs tranquilize with minimal narcosis. However, large doses may lead to somnolence, stupor, and coma.

b. Acute delirious reactions have been observed when these drugs are taken with barbiturates or antiparkinsonian agents, probably due to the cumulative anticholinergic effects. Patients become confused, agitated, and disoriented.

c. In less than 1% of patients, seizures may develop. These drugs lower the seizure threshold.

E. Cardiovascular drugs

1. Digitalis levels that are necessary to achieve therapeutic effects are close to the levels that produce toxicity. The toxic effects vary. Nausea and vomiting may occur. Affected individuals

may become restless or apathetic. Some experience nightmares. In severe cases, a delirium develops with features of impaired concentration and cognition, irritability, distractability, delusions, and hallucinations. Effects of digitalis toxicity are greater in the elderly who have poor cardiac reserve and cerebral disease in some cases. The sensory deprivation experienced in the intensive care unit may exacerbate the toxicity of this drug.

2. **Procainamide**, an antiarrhythmic agent, has been noted to produce depression and weakness in moderate doses. Severe depression has been observed at higher doses. In rare cases, a psychosis with hallucinations may occur at high doses.

3. **Propranolol**, used to treat both hypertension and arrhythmias, may produce lethargy and drowsiness at moderate doses. Severe depression or a psychosis with visual hallucinations may occur at high doses.

4. **Reserpine**, an antihypertensive agent, acts in the central nervous system by depleting catecholamines (e.g., norepinephrine), which leads to depression, often of great severity.

5. **Methyldopa**, an antihypertensive drug, has been associated with depression and nightmares, even with usual doses.

6. **Hydralazine**, an antihypertensive agent, may produce headaches, gastrointestinal symptoms, and loss of appetite with moderate doses. At high doses more severe disturbances may occur, including anxiety, confusion, disorientation, depression, and an acute psychosis.

7. **Diuretic agents,** such as hydrochlorothiazide and furosemide, affect fluid and electrolyte metabolism. They may deplete sodium, potassium, and total body fluids with a brisk diuresis. Chloride ions may also suffer depletion, leading to a metabolic alkalosis. Symptoms may be mild, such as fatigue and weakness, or severe, including confusion, disorientation, cognitive impairment, and agitation.

F. Drugs of abuse

1. **Hallucinogenic agents** (i.e., psychedelics and psychotomimetics) are used and abused to obtain alterations of normal perceptual, emotional, and cognitive processes. Drugs in this group include psilocybin, lysergic acid diethylamide (LSD), mescaline, marijuana, tetrahydrocannabinol (THC), and phencyclidine (PCP).
   a. **PCP produces a classic picture of delirium.** Signs and symptoms include:
      (1) Depersonalization
      (2) Confusion
      (3) Disorientation
      (4) Isolation
      (5) Hostility
      (6) Negativism
      (7) Apathy
      (8) Catalepsy
      (9) Agitation
      (10) Violent outbursts
   b. Other hallucinogenic agents do not compromise the level of consciousness but alter the form of consciousness. An organic delusional syndrome may develop with grandiose or paranoid delusions. An organic hallucinosis may develop with one or more sensory modalities involved. Visual hallucinations are commonly vivid.
   c. Treatment of unpleasant or untoward effects ("bad trips") begins with a calm, quiet, reassuring environment. Most patients improve as the drug effects subside within a few hours. Some patients may require tranquilizing with either benzodiazepines or butyrophenones.
   d. Diagnosis of conditions caused by hallucinogenic agents depends upon both a good history and, when available, toxicologic screens. Screens are useful because many of these patients do not know what they have taken.

2. **Alcohol** is the most commonly abused drug. This abuse produces varied clinical conditions, ranging from intoxication to delirious states (see Chapter 5, "Substance Use Disorders").
   a. **Alcohol intoxication** (see Chapter 5, section II A) is characterized by specific neurologic, psychiatric, and behavioral disturbances caused by recent ingestion of alcohol. Blood alcohol levels are greater than 100 mg/dl and may be as high as 400–500 mg/dl. Intoxication may last from 2–3 hours to as many as 12 hours. Duration is related to the amount consumed and the rate of consumption. Chronic heavy drinkers metabolize alcohol at an approximate rate of 30 mg/dl/hr. Those who are not chronic heavy drinkers have a metabolic rate for alcohol of about 20 mg/dl/hr.
      (1) **Neurologic signs of alcohol intoxication** include slurred speech, motor incoordina-

tion, and an unsteady gait. Transient periods of memory loss, so-called blackouts, may occur when drinking.

(2) **Psychiatric signs and symptoms** include impaired concentration, memory, and attention as well as emotional lability, lack of inhibitions, loquaciousness, and irritability.

(3) Maladaptive behavior includes fighting, impaired judgment, impaired social and occupational functioning, and failure to meet responsibilities.

b. **Idiosyncratic alcohol intoxication** is a condition in which marked behavioral changes result from the consumption of a small amount of alcohol. Typically, the disturbance lasts a few hours.

(1) Symptoms include aggressive or assaultive behavior that is atypical for the individual concerned and are usually manifest early in life (i.e., in the late teens or early twenties).

(2) Previous brain injury or current sedative use appear to be predisposing factors.

(3) Temporal lobe seizures may present in this way and should be looked for in any patient with this syndrome.

c. **Alcohol withdrawal syndromes** vary in severity (for specific information, see Chapter 5, section III A).

d. **Alcohol withdrawal delirium (delirium tremens)** is a severe condition that arises within 1 week of cessation of, or significant reduction in, alcohol use. Delirium tremens is most common in individuals between 30 and 40 years of age, although all ages are susceptible. The presence of other illnesses, such as infections or fractures, predisposes an individual to this condition. Cognitive disturbances include impaired attention, memory, and concentration. Behavior is marked by impulsiveness and unpredictability, which is easily understood if it is recognized that cognitive and perceptual disturbances render these patients incapable of responding appropriately to the environment. As in all delirious states, these disturbances fluctuate. The patient may be quiet and calm one moment and wild and combative the next. Fever is common. Dehydration develops because of fluid loss due to urination, fever, and sweating and because of inadequate replenishment of lost fluids by the confused, agitated patient.

e. **Alcohol hallucinosis** (see Chapter 5, section III A 4) is a relatively uncommon condition in which there are persistent hallucinations when an individual, after a long binge, is abstinent from alcohol. This is not a withdrawal state. Typically, the affected individual has not been drinking alcohol for 1–2 weeks when hallucinations begin. They may last for weeks, months, or, rarely, years. No other signs of organic impairment are present. These patients do not have a thought disorder, as is found in schizophrenia.

f. **Alcohol amnestic syndrome** refers to an impairment of memory secondary to prolonged alcohol use. It is rarely seen in individuals who are under 35 years of age. Other evidence of significant alcohol abuse, such as hepatic disease, is typically present in this disorder.

(1) **Wernicke's encephalopathy** develops over a period of a few days to a few weeks. The patient becomes confused and may have difficulty remaining alert. An atactic gait, nystagmus, and ophthalmoplegia (most often involving the sixth cranial nerve) are common findings. Evidence of a peripheral neuropathy includes decreased deep-tendon reflexes, weakness, and diminished sensation. **Thiamine deficiencies** cause pathologic changes in the mamillary body, the walls of the third ventricle, and other areas. A patient may recover from this condition spontaneously within a few days or progress to permanent deficits. These deficits often can be resolved rapidly with the administration of thiamine.

(2) **Korsakoff's psychosis** is the chronic condition that is also known as **alcohol amnestic syndrome**. Short-term memory losses are prominent. Long-term memory may also be affected. With little or no capacity to remember, behavior may be grossly disturbed. **Confabulation is common.** Interpersonal and occupational skills are lost. Depression and social withdrawal may occur. Korsakoff's psychosis does not respond to thiamine, and permanent, often severe, impairment exists.

g. **Dementia** is frequently associated with alcoholism, even though alcohol has never been shown to be a causative agent for dementia. This "diagnosis" is usually made when a patient is alcoholic and no other cause can be found for the dementia.

3. **Cocaine**, an alkaloid derivative of the plant *Erythroxylon coca*, was first used in medicine as a local anesthetic in 1884. Use as a local anesthetic is its only current medical application. Abuse of this substance has increased significantly in the last decade or so. The drug is inhaled (snorted), injected intravenously or subcutaneously, or smoked as "crack," or "freebased." The latter two routes of administration are much more toxic than snorting. Both acute and chronic cocaine use may produce significant psychiatric disturbances.

a. **Euphoria.** Acutely, the drug produces a stimulated, euphoric feeling in the user. This feeling lasts for a brief time, usually no more than 2 hours. Other effects are often present, including:

(1) Severe, acute anxiety with paranoid ideation

    (2) Irritability

    (3) Elevated blood pressure and heart rate

    (4) Dilated pupils, which are reactive to light

    (5) Dry mouth

    (6) Uncharacteristically aggressive behavior

    (7) Hallucinations, usually tactile (e.g., formication—creeping sensations on the skin)

    (8) Cardiac dysrhythmias

    (9) Increased deep-tendon reflexes

    (10) Respiratory arrest and death from high doses via the intravenous or smoking route

    (11) Craving for more cocaine

b. Craving for cocaine leads to chronic abuse. Doses increase, and weekend use progresses to more frequent binging. Chronic cocaine abusers are more likely to inject or smoke the drug because more cocaine can be delivered more quickly by these routes of administration. All of the acute effects listed above may occur as well as those listed below.

    (1) Weight loss due to decreased food intake and poor self-care

    (2) Impaired concentration

    (3) Impaired erectile and ejaculatory function

    (4) Hypersomnia, characterized by daytime sleepiness, frequent napping, difficult arousal from sleep, and the need for 10 or more hours of sleep each day

    (5) Psychotic symptoms, including persecutory delusions, ideas of reference, and perceptual disturbances

    (6) Hostility and aggressive behavior

    (7) Nasal septal perforation from snorting

    (8) Sepsis or bacterial endocarditis from intravenous use

    (9) Seizures with an overdose

c. Psychological dependence. Intense psychological dependence develops in chronic users. Cocaine use governs the lives of cocaine abusers. Unfortunately, tragic financial, occupational, medical, interpersonal, and legal events often occur before the abuser is motivated to seek treatment.

G. Miscellaneous drugs

  1. Anesthetic agents act both locally and systemically with different effects.

    a. General anesthesia is comprised of volatile inert gases, which are rapidly excreted. They do not cause an organic mental syndrome for this reason. The postoperative appearance of an organic mental disorder raises the question of anoxia occurring during surgery instead.

    b. Local anesthesia may produce a toxic reaction when given intravenously. The central nervous system is stimulated by local anesthetic agents, leading to restlessness, tremors, or convulsions. Vital functions may be lost, and death may occur with severe toxicity.

  2. Hormonal agents are given either to augment or to inhibit endogenous activity of the body. Changes in behavior and brain function are felt to be related to the metabolic alterations induced by these agents. Although there is some individual variation, the dose level correlates with the severity of toxicity.

    a. Corticosteroids and adrenocorticotropic hormone (ACTH) produce increased glucocorticoid activity. At moderate doses, the mood may be elevated; the patient may be euphoric. A degree of agitation, restlessness, or insomnia may be present. At high doses (> 40 mg/day of prednisone), a clinical picture consistent with mania or a psychosis with paranoid ideation may be observed. Confusion and disorientation may be seen. Curiously, some patients have an opposite reaction and become severely depressed. Dose reduction is indicated. **Withdrawal of corticosteroids** may deprive the patient of sufficient glucocorticoid activity, which leads to depression, apathy, irritability, or psychosis.

    b. Thyroid hormone (thyroxine) and synthetic preparations, when given in high doses, produce a syndrome that mimics hyperthyroidism. The affected individual experiences weakness, fatigue, tremors, palpitations, anxiety, agitation, insomnia, and heat intolerance. With severe toxicity, a dangerously rapid heart rate, elevated temperature, dehydration, diarrhea, vomiting, and a delirious state develop. The patient is severely agitated, confused, disoriented, and may exhibit psychotic features, such as hallucinations and paranoid thinking.

    c. Iodine 131 (^{131}I) and propylthiouracil may cause either a rapid or a slow, insidious onset of hypothyroidism. If hypothyroidism arises quickly, severe disturbances may be noted, including delusions, hallucinations, and a delirious state.

    d. Insulin and orally administered hypoglycemic agents may produce either acute or chronic hypoglycemia. In mild-to-moderate acute hypoglycemia, the patient may be irritable and difficult to interview; the history may be vague and imprecise. Evidence of impaired cognitive functioning or confusion may be found. The patient may be lethargic and complain of a headache. As blood glucose levels drop, the patient becomes more impaired. A delirious condition may develop with disorientation, agitation, and disturbances in perception and thinking. At low enough glucose levels, coma results. With chronic hypoglycemia, the patient may develop an organic personality disorder with impaired judgment and impulse control, emotional withdrawal, and inappropriate outbursts of emotion. A dementia may develop over time.

3. **Anti-inflammatory drugs**
   a. **Non-narcotic analgesics and antipyretics** are commonly used. Toxic states may arise inadvertently or intentionally with overdoses.
      (1) **Salicylates** (e.g., aspirin) produce agitation, confusion, tinnitus, hallucinations (usually visual), and a delirium at toxic levels.
      (2) At high doses, **phenacetin** produces a depressed mood, lethargy, dizziness, feelings of detachment, and impaired concentration. A toxic delirious state may follow.
   b. **Phenylbutazone** has reportedly caused headaches and psychotic reactions at low doses. At higher doses a delirious condition with hallucinations, convulsions, and coma has been observed.
   c. **Indomethacin** produces headache in as many as 50% of patients. Severe reactions may include depersonalization, confusion, nightmares, depression, hallucinations, ataxia, and delirium.

4. **Drugs used to treat infections**
   a. **Among the antibacterials, sulfonamides, penicillin, and gram-negative agents (e.g., chloramphenicol)** have produced psychiatric symptoms. Confusion, depression, and acute psychosis may occur with sulfonamides. Intravenous administration of penicillin has led to acute psychosis with agitation, anxiety, and hallucinations. Chloramphenicol has caused depression as well as a delirious condition.
   b. **Antituberculosis agents** may produce symptoms due to either acute or chronic use. Acutely, **isoniazid** use may lead to anxiety and restlessness. With prolonged use, irritability, confusion, and paranoid thinking have been observed. A schizophrenic-like syndrome with hallucinations and delusions may arise in severe cases.
      (1) **Cycloserine** use has been associated with confusion, agitation, and delirium.
      (2) **Iproniazid**, a monoamine oxidase (MAO) inhibitor, may elevate the mood as well as produce additional manic symptoms.
      (3) **Ethionamide** use may lead to somnolence and a depressed mood.
   c. **Amantadine**, an antiviral agent, has produced agitation, aggressive behavior, hallucinations, and delirium.
   d. **Chloroquine, quinacrine, and griseofulvin**, which are antifungal and antiparasitic agents, may produce a range of symptoms. Depressed mood, aggressive behavior, and changes in personality have been observed. More severe symptoms include hallucinations, delusions, paranoid ideation, and delirium.

5. **Antineoplastic agents** do not cross the blood–brain barrier. Thus, they rarely have any effect on the central nervous system. *Vinca* **alkaloids** have reportedly produced stupor, hallucinations, and coma, however.

6. **Disulfiram**, in normal doses, may reduce libido and sexual potency as well as levels of energy. The patient experiences weakness, impairment of memory and concentration, somnolence, disorientation, and confusion from acute toxic doses. Chronic ingestion leads to carbon disulfide toxicity. The symptoms of this disorder include parkinsonism, depression, a peripheral neuropathy, and delirium. Of great concern with disulfiram is the acetaldehyde reaction that occurs when alcohol enters the body either by drinking or by absorption through the skin (e.g., when applying cologne or perfume) or mucosa (e.g., when using mouthwash). An acute and severe illness may result with palpitations, chest pain, and possible circulatory collapse.

7. **Anticonvulsants** all have potent effects on the central nervous system. In general, they slow down mental processes and tend to sedate the affected individual. They may produce either an acute or chronic organic mental disorder.
   a. **Hydantoin derivatives** produce a variety of symptoms. Individuals may be irritable or depressed with chronic use. They may experience drowsiness and tremors. Difficulty in walking (ataxia), talking (dysarthria), and seeing (diplopia) are common. Nystagmus may be noted. When very high levels of the drugs are present, full-blown delirium and delusions may occur.
   b. **Oxazolidinedione derivatives** are used for petit mal seizures. At therapeutic levels, ataxia and vertigo (loss of the sense of balance or dizziness) have been observed. More symptoms appear at higher levels. Individuals may become irritable and emotionally labile.

They may be nauseated, may vomit, or both. Drowsiness and diplopia may be present. A common physical finding is nystagmus. With an overdose, individuals are sedated. Incoordination, dysarthria, as well as nystagmus occur.

    c. Succinimide derivatives are also used for petit mal seizures. These drugs have numerous psychiatric effects. Side effects include irritability, drowsiness, dizziness, hyperactivity, euphoria, and headaches. Some patients report nightmares. Concentration may be impaired. An increase in aggressive behavior has been attributed to these drugs. Rarely, some patients develop an organic delusional syndrome with paranoid ideation. Some patients become depressed.

    d. Clonazepam is a benzodiazepine derivative used for the treatment of petit mal, akinetic, and psychomotor seizure disorders. Patients develop tolerance to this drug and, as a result, may experience a withdrawal syndrome. A common effect is drowsiness. Some patients become atactic. At toxic levels, forgetfulness or confusion may be noted. Some patients develop psychotic symptoms, including hallucinations.

    e. Phenacemide is a toxic medication that is rarely used. Individuals may become depressed or very aggressive when taking this medication. Personality changes have been noted as well as psychotic disturbances.

  8. Anticholinergic drugs, including belladonna alkaloids and synthetics, have wide therapeutic application and are sometimes used in abusive patterns. Compounds in the group include atropine, benztropine, scopolamine, propantheline, meclizine, diphenhydramine, and trihexyphenidyl. These drugs act by blocking acetylcholine activity in the peripheral nervous system. Scopolamine is readily available. It is a key ingredient in over-the-counter sleeping preparations. Abuse may be inadvertent or purposeful.

    a. General effects. They include sedation, decrement in bronchial and oropharyngeal secretions, decrement in gastrointestinal and urinary tract motility, mydriasis, and cycloplegia. Sweating is decreased, and heart rate is increased by these compounds. They are used in many medical specialties, including cardiology, ophthalmology, urology, gastroenterology, and psychiatry.

    b. Central nervous system effects. Individuals may become restless and agitated. Emotional lability may be observed. Some individuals are confused and have memory deficits. Outright disorientation and unpredictable, wild behavior occur with toxicity. Convulsions and coma are seen in severe cases.

    c. Gastric lavage and support of vital functions are indicated in an overdose.

  9. L-Dopa. Idiopathic parkinsonism is commonly treated with L-dopa. This drug readily crosses the blood–brain barrier and is broken down to dopamine and norepinephrine, both pharmacologically active biogenic amines.

    a. Side effects. As many as 50% of patients taking L-dopa experience nausea, vomiting, and dyskinesias.

    b. Psychiatric effects. It is estimated that 20%–30% of patients experience psychiatric symptoms. A variety of difficulties have been observed. Some patients suffer mood disorders and become depressed or hypomanic. Others suffer cognitive and perceptual impairment. Individuals may be confused or disoriented. In more severe cases, delirious conditions develop. (Delirious conditions are more common in patients with underlying dementia.) Some individuals become psychotic with paranoid delusions, hallucinations, and psychomotor agitation.

    c. Treatment is straightforward: The dose of L-dopa should be decreased.

VI. ENVIRONMENTAL ETIOLOGIES. Exposure to toxins.

The environment has become a common source of exposure to toxins with pollutants in the air and water. Industrial and occupational pollutants create hazards for workers as well as nonworkers in the area. Some of these toxins, such as toluene or gasoline, have become substances of abuse.

  A. Gases may induce changes in brain function, generally when concentrations rise above tolerated levels.

    1. Oxygen intoxication is the result of the inhalation of pure oxygen at levels of 2 atm or greater. Mood changes are noted. Individuals become irritable and labile. They may complain of dizziness and paresthesias. Loss of consciousness may occur. Treatment is reduction of the oxygen being delivered.

    2. Carbon dioxide intoxication. The effects of carbon dioxide are related to its concentration. Levels between 2% and 10% of carbon dioxide tend to increase the respiratory rate and the depth of respiration. At higher levels, headache, confusion, and delirium result.

    3. Carbon monoxide intoxication. Carbon monoxide forms carboxyhemoglobin in the blood, displacing oxygen and leading to hypoxia. Most individuals experience headache at levels of

20% or less of carboxyhemoglobin. At levels between 20% and 40%, severe headache, nausea, vomiting, dizziness, and dimness of vision result. At levels between 40% and 60%, tachypnea, tachycardia, syncope, and convulsions occur. Above 60%, respiratory failure occurs followed by death. Changes in the globus pallidus and substantia nigra occur with acute, severe carbon monoxide intoxication, leading to parkinsonism and seizures. There is chronic intoxication in smokers and urban dwellers, who experience episodic depressions, withdrawal, apathy, impairment of perception and memory, and disorientation. Slowly, the globus pallidus and substantia nigra are affected. Seizures and movement disorders may develop.

B. **Noxious vapors** are encountered on the job, in the home, and in accidents and are abused for their effects. Exposure may have an excitatory effect. Affected individuals become hyperactive or agitated. Emotional lability may be evident. In others, apathy and disinterest may be prominent. Memory and concentration are impaired acutely. Some individuals become very aggressive. With chronic exposure, personality changes occur. Individuals may be apathetic or exhibit wide shifts in activities and interests. Significant cognitive difficulties and psychotic disturbances, such as paranoid thinking and hallucinations, have been noted in abusers. Many changes become irreversible with chronic exposure.

C. **Exposure to heavy metals** leads to widespread health problems, including psychiatric disturbances. Problems develop when the body's capacity to excrete a heavy metal is exceeded by the amount ingested. Intoxication can be either acute or chronic.

1. **Lead** may enter the body through the respiratory route, the gastrointestinal route, and through the skin. Toxicity is greater if vapors are inhaled than if some lead-containing compound is consumed (e.g., paint and moonshine liquor, which is often distilled in containers with lead solder). Symptomatology is mild with low levels in the blood (i.e., 100–150 μg/dl), and fatigue and anemia may occur. At higher levels (i.e., 150–200 μg/dl), constipation, loss of appetite, and lethargy may accompany abdominal pain. Encephalopathy has been observed when levels are above 200 μg/dl. Individuals experience dizziness and clumsiness and are irritable and restless. An excited delirious state develops, which can proceed to lethargy and coma. As many as 25% of severely intoxicated individuals die, and 40% of those affected who survive suffer severe sequelae.

2. **Mercury** poisons the body through the skin and through respiratory and gastrointestinal routes. In acute syndromes, the mercury usually has been swallowed. A gastrointestinal syndrome with diarrhea, dehydration, and bleeding occurs. Chronic intoxication usually results from inhalation of vapors. Early in the chronic illness, affected individuals may exhibit changes in personality (e.g., irritability, apathy, and lability) as well as tremors, gingivitis, and albuminuria. If the intoxication persists, insomnia, lethargy, depression, timidity, withdrawal from others, despondency, and, in some cases, hallucinations occur. At the same time, physical signs and symptoms worsen. These include anemia, hypertension, colitis, renal disease, loosening of the teeth, and anorexia.

3. **Thallium** is found in rat poisons and in depilatory agents. Initially, intoxication causes pain in the legs, diarrhea, and vomiting. If a chronic condition (or severe acute condition) develops, depression, paranoid thinking, or choreiform movements may result. In severe cases, a delirium develops with possible seizures and blindness. A clue to thallium intoxication can be alopecia.

4. **Manganese** exposure is rare, limited to specific contact with mines or battery casings. Vapors produce intoxication. Headaches, somnolence, and irritability may be seen initially. Later, emotional lability, nightmares, aggressive behavior, confusion, hallucinations, and compulsive and impulsive acts have been observed. Lesions in the basal ganglia and pyramis result, leading to gait impairment, tremors, rigidity of posture, monotonous speech, and micrographia. The recommended treatment is removing the source of exposure. Psychological symptoms resolve in 3–4 months in most cases.

5. **Arsenic** is found in insecticides, disinfectants, and rat poisons. Severe acute intoxication produces a life-threatening condition with fluid loss. Chronic, insidious intoxication produces lethargy, anorexia, and fatigue. Diarrhea and upper respiratory irritation may be present as well. Eventually an encephalopathic condition results, with loss of intellect, apathy, as well as personality changes.

6. **Bismuth** is found in salts used for constipation (this use is uncommon now). The salts may be absorbed, leading to a variety of psychological symptoms, including depression, anxiety, irritability, phobias, and paranoid delusions. Neurologic symptoms also occur, such as incontinence, dysarthria, ataxia, and pseudotremors.

D. Organophosphates are potent acetylcholinesterase inhibitors found in insecticides, such as parathion and malathion. These compounds are introduced into the body via vapors and skin contact. Acetylcholine accumulates at synapses, blocking functioning. Mild acute intoxication produces headache, fatigue, numbness, gastrointestinal upset, dizziness, profuse sweating, excessive salivation, tightness in the chest, and abdominal pain. Severe acute intoxication leads to extreme weakness, difficulty in talking and walking, and muscle fasciculations. A flaccid paralysis may occur. Affected individuals may be delirious. Chronic intoxication may lead to diminished concentration, drowsiness, confusion, memory deficits, psychomotor slowing, slurring of speech, perseveration, depression, lethargy, anxiety, irritability, and unexpected outbursts of aggressive behavior.

VII. NUTRITIONAL ETIOLOGIES.

Nutritional deficiencies can disrupt brain functions. In addition to substrates, such as oxygen, glucose, and amino acids, vitamins and minerals are essential for the proper functioning of enzyme and transport systems, maintenance of membrane integrity, and myelin formation. Vitamin deficiencies result from inadequate intake, impaired absorption, and increased metabolic requirements. These conditions are usually seen in impoverished people, food faddists, and alcoholics.

A. Thiamine is required for the formation of thiamine pyrophosphate, a coenzyme in the carbohydrate degradation cycle. Deficiencies occur in malnourished, starving, or alcoholic individuals.

    1. Beriberi runs a subacute or chronic course. Affected individuals suffer from high-output cardiac failure with cardiac dilation, tachycardia, arrhythmias, edema, and dyspnea on exertion. A peripheral neuropathy results from demyelination of peripheral nerves and dorsal root ganglia. Psychiatric symptoms may include apathy, depression, irritability, impaired concentration, and nervousness. In severe cases, memory and intellect may be permanently compromised.

    2. Wernicke's encephalopathy and Korsakoff's psychosis. For details concerning syndromes associated with chronic alcoholism, see section V F 2.

B. Nicotinic acid is necessary for the formation of coenzymes for tissue respiration. Skin rashes and atrophy of the mucous membranes result from a deficiency. In addition, headache, apathy, confusion, delusions, insomnia, and a clinical picture resembling dementia have been reported. These signs and symptoms respond promptly to the administration of nicotinic acid.

C. Pyridoxine (a form of vitamin B$_6$) deficiency can lead to peripheral neuropathy. It should be noted that isoniazid, the antituberculosis drug, competes with pyridoxine and increases the chance of a neuropathy developing.

D. Cyanocobalamin (vitamin B$_{12}$) is absorbed from the gastrointestinal tract only when the required intrinsic factor has been produced by the gastric mucosa. Important functions of this vitamin include roles in hematopoiesis, nucleoprotein production, myelin production, and gastrointestinal epithelial cell maintenance. With vitamin B$_{12}$ deficiency, megaloblastic anemia and neurologic deficits develop over a period of weeks to months. Myelin is destroyed in the spinal cord, brain, and peripheral nerves. Paresthesias are a common early sign. The gait may become unsteady. Deep-tendon reflexes are diminished. Apathy, depression, irritability, and moodiness are common. Less common are confusion, delusions, paranoid thinking, hallucinations, and a clinical picture resembling dementia. Although neurologic and hematologic symptoms are usually present, some patients present only with psychiatric symptoms. Most patients respond to vitamin B$_{12}$ administration, although the degree of disease progression is a factor to consider. Some patients have enduring deficits.

VIII. METABOLIC ETIOLOGIES

A. Inborn errors of metabolism may produce psychiatric conditions. The list of diseases in which either lipids, carbohydrates, or proteins are mishandled by the body is extensive. Mental changes, including retardation, are common elements of these diseases. These disorders are familial and usually appear early in life. Two disorders, Wilson's disease and acute intermittent porphyria, warrant further description.

    1. Wilson's disease (hepatolenticular degeneration) is inherited as an autosomal recessive defect. Features of the disease are abnormal copper metabolism, degenerative changes in the brain, and cirrhosis of the liver. Copper is deposited in the liver, in the renal tubules, and in the brain (in the corpus callosum and putamen). Signs and symptoms appear in the second and third decades of life. Personality changes may be the first sign. Existing traits may become muted or exaggerated. Irritability and moodiness may be seen. Transient psychotic symptoms, including hallucinations, paranoid thinking, and even manic-like outbursts, have been described. A mild tremor and loss of coordination may be apparent in the handwriting of the affected individual. Speech may become indistinct or frankly dysarthric. Ataxia and chorea may develop. Facial immobility and dysphagia may occur. Cirrhotic changes in the liver and renal tubular damage result from copper deposition in these tissues. Treatment includes administration of D-penicillamine and a copper-restricted diet.

2. **Acute intermittent porphyria** is inherited as an autosomal dominant trait. The lesion is a defect in the regulation of the hepatic enzyme δ-aminolevulinic acid synthetase. An increase in this enzyme produces the episodic characteristic of this disease. Symptoms typically begin after puberty, usually between the ages of 20–40 years and occur more commonly in women than in men. Affected individuals may experience nervousness and emotional instability on a chronic basis. During acute episodes, abdominal pain recurs. Confusion, disorientation, impaired concentration, or frank delirium may appear. Peripheral neuropathies, including cranial nerve palsies, are often seen. Some patients have convulsions and lapse into coma. These episodes can be stimulated by medications, such as estrogens, sulfonamides, and barbiturates. Symptomatic treatment of the pain and psychiatric symptoms is recommended.

B. **Metabolic disorders** are frequently reflected in rapid recent changes in behavior, thinking, and consciousness. The earliest signs of metabolic irregularities are often compromised memory and orientation. Affected individuals may become agitated, anxious, hyperactive, or withdrawn. Failures in perception may occur as hallucinations, or illusions are experienced. Disturbances in thinking (e.g., delusions and paranoid ideation) may develop. Confusion and delirium develop in severe cases as do pronounced neurologic disturbances, such as grand mal seizures. For the most part, EEG changes are nonspecific. The neurologic examination shows nonfocal involvement.

1. **Hepatic encephalopathy** results from severe, acute, or chronic liver disease. Ammonia and other toxins accumulate as a result of hepatic failure. Changes in personality, impairment of memory, intellectual deficits, and disturbances in consciousness ranging from apathy and drowsiness to coma can develop. A flapping tremor (**asterixis**) may appear. Individuals may hyperventilate, reflecting an acid–base disturbance common to hepatic failure. Triphasic wave patterns are seen on EEG. Limiting nitrogenous products in the body is the current treatment of this severe illness.

2. **Uremic encephalopathy** results from either acute or chronic renal failure. Urea and other metabolites, a metabolic acidosis, and alterations in normal electrolyte metabolism due to acidosis produce the signs and symptoms of this disorder. Patients are restless. Memory, orientation, and the ability to maintain consciousness may be compromised. A peripheral neuropathy characterized by diffuse sensory and motor impairment and diminished deep-tendon reflexes may occur. Muscles twitch, and asterixis may appear. In severe cases, seizures have been reported. Dialysis is indicated in most cases. Rapid dialysis can lead to a syndrome called **dialysis disequilibrium**, which is characterized by headache, confusion, changes in consciousness, and convulsions.

3. **Failure to maintain normal serum glucose levels** can lead to an organic mental syndrome. Glucose levels may be too high or too low.
   a. **Hypoglycemic encephalopathy** can result from causes as various as an islet cell adenoma of the pancreas, the administration of too much insulin, adrenocortical failure, hepatic necrosis, and a glycogen storage disease. Hypoglycemic episodes usually occur in the early morning or after exercise. The rate of decline in serum glucose concentration seems to be crucial. Premonitory symptoms include nausea, tachycardia, sweating, hunger, apprehension, and restlessness. As the encephalopathy progresses, disorientation, agitation, confusion, and hallucinations may occur. Diplopia, pallor, increased deep-tendon reflexes, clonus, and seizures may follow. Late in the course, stupor or coma is seen. Many of these symptoms can be confused with an anxiety attack. Treatment with intravenous dextrose is indicated.
   b. **Diabetic ketoacidosis** results from inadequately treated diabetes mellitus. The affected individual has too little insulin available to metabolize glucose properly. This is due either to insufficient doses of insulin or an ongoing condition that increases insulin demands, such as an infection or physical trauma. Early signs and symptoms of diabetic ketoacidosis include weakness, listlessness, fatigue, polyuria, polydipsia, headache, nausea, and vomiting. The patient's condition can worsen over a period of hours to days as ketonuria, ketonemia, dehydration, and acidosis persist. At any point, a more rapid deterioration may occur as the patient becomes confused, stuporous, or comatose. Treatment with intravenous fluids and insulin is indicated. Care must be taken to maintain electrolyte balance as acid–base disturbances are corrected with treatment.

c. Hyperglycemic nonketotic coma is a clinical syndrome seen in association with corticosteroid or diuretic therapy or peritoneal dialysis. It may be the first indication of diabetes mellitus in a patient or a complication arising from inadequately treated diabetes mellitus. It occurs in middle-aged individuals and in the elderly. The condition comes on slowly as the blood glucose level climbs as high as 1000 mg/dl. Unlike diabetic ketoacidosis, there is no significant formation of ketones. As the blood glucose level rises, the kidneys produce increased amounts of urine (polyuria) in an effort to correct the problem. Fluids move from tissues into the vascular space in an effort to lower serum osmolarity, causing intracellular dehydration. Serum sodium levels rise (**hypernatremia**). Patients become lethargic and easily fatigued. Memory difficulties and confusion develop. Coma and seizures may ensue.

4. **Failure to maintain normal serum sodium concentration** may lead to an organic mental syndrome. Levels may be too high or too low. A critical factor is the rate of change in the serum sodium concentration. A rapid change has a more profound effect on the central nervous system.
   a. Hyponatremia is a condition in which there is a relative excess of total body water to total solute (sodium). It results from defects in the urinary dilution system brought about by such conditions as volume depletion, edematous states, adrenal insufficiency, a syndrome of inappropriate antidiuretic hormone (ADH) secretion as occurs with some malignancies (e.g., oat-cell carcinoma of the lung) and central nervous system infections, renal failure, psychogenic polydipsia, and exposure to medications, including oral hypoglycemics, carbamazepine, and amitriptyline. Hyponatremia is usually of little consequence clinically. Symptoms rarely develop if serum sodium concentration is 125 mEq/L or greater. However, with a lower level of serum sodium concentration and rapid onset, marked central nervous system findings are present. Individuals become lethargic and inactive. Confusion develops, leading to erratic behavior and irrational thinking. As the condition progresses, stupor and coma develop. Central nervous system defects result from intracellular fluid accumulation (i.e., brain cells swell up and function inefficiently and erratically); once identified, this situation must be corrected slowly so that affected brain cells may adjust without another rapid change in cellular hydration.
   b. Hypernatremia is a condition in which there is a relative deficit in total body water to total solute (sodium). This condition is the result of losses of hypotonic fluids, which may occur with excessive sweating in the presence of inadequate fluid replacement, in burn victims who lose large volumes of hypotonic fluid through injured skin, and with diabetes insipidus. Brain cells become dehydrated when serum sodium concentrations rise, leading to impaired brain functioning. As with hyponatremia, confusion, lethargy, and alterations in consciousness may develop. This condition should be corrected slowly with hypotonic fluids administered intravenously or orally to avoid further compromise of central nervous system functioning brought on by another rapid shift in cellular hydration.

5. **Hypoxia** has profound effects on brain functioning. Delivery of oxygen to the central nervous system depends upon the respiratory and circulatory systems, the supply of oxygen at the alveolar level, and the capacity of erythrocytes to transport and release oxygen. Numerous conditions can compromise the availability of oxygen to the brain. Cerebral vascular changes occur. Anemia reduces the oxygen–carrying capacity of blood because there are fewer erythrocytes available for transport. In pulmonary diseases, such as emphysema, there is an impaired ability to exchange oxygen at the alveolar level, leading to reduced oxygen partial pressure (PO_2) in the blood and, therefore, to reduced delivery of oxygen to tissues. In congestive heart failure, circulation is impaired. Blood may be poorly oxygenated due to compromised pulmonary arterial circulation, and tissues may receive diminished amounts of blood. Toxins, such as cyanide, and toxin-caused diseases, such as diphtheria, interfere with cellular respiration, producing histotoxic hypoxia. Changes in levels and activity of 2,3-diphosphoglycerate (2,3-DPG), an intracellular enzyme in erythrocytes, affect oxygen transport and release as well. Carbon monoxide poisoning also produces hypoxia. Acute signs and symptoms of hypoxia include impaired judgment, confusion, loss of motor coordination, emotional lability, irrational thinking (e.g., paranoid ideation), and impulsive, erratic behavior. Some individuals are chronically hypoxic. These patients experience fatigue, drowsiness, inattentiveness, a delayed reaction time, diminished work capacity, and confusion. Severe hypoxia can lead to stupor, an obtundent state, and coma.

6. **Elevated and depressed levels of potassium** produce significant neuromuscular effects, especially cardiac arrhythmias, without any significant effect on brain functioning.

IX. **ENDOCRINE ETIOLOGIES.** Endocrine disorders can lead to psychiatric symptoms. In general, changes may be evident in personality, mental functions, memory, and neurologic functions.

A. **Tumors of the pituitary and hypothalamus** can grossly alter neurologic and endocrine functioning. These tumors usually develop quiescently. Headaches are rare because intracranial pressure is not increased. Neurologic signs appear when the tumor is large enough to compress other brain structures. When the optic chiasm is compressed, bitemporal hemianopia develops. Memory and intellect are impaired by pressure to basal frontal and temporal lobe structures. Endocrine disturbances reflect the area of the hypothalamus or pituitary that is affected. Radiographic identification of these tumors is difficult because of their small size.

B. **Tumors of the hypothalamus.** A radical change in appetite leads to obesity or inanition. Sleep may be disturbed. The patient may become emotionally labile and be subject to rage reactions. Excessive water drinking arises in diabetes insipidus, a condition in which ADH is no longer secreted, leading to a failure to reabsorb water in the kidney. Conversely, the inappropriate and excessive secretion of ADH dilutes body fluids, leading to water intoxication and cerebral edema (see section VIII B 4 a).

C. **Elevated or depressed thyroid functions**

1. Individuals with a hyperactive thyroid experience weakness and fatigue. They may suffer insomnia. Weight loss occurs in the face of an increased appetite. Tremulousness and palpitations develop. Patients perspire excessively. Anxiety and restlessness are early signs of **hyperthyroidism.** As the condition progresses, impairment of memory, orientation, and judgment becomes apparent. In severe cases, a manic-like excitement is evident or a schizophreniform picture with delusions and hallucinations arises. Hyperthyroidism may be masked behind a state of apathy, confusion, and depression in the elderly. However, examination usually reveals eye signs (e.g., lid lag and exophthalmos) and other signs of the disorder. Treatment of the hyperthyroidism provides treatment of the associated psychiatric syndrome.

2. **Hypothyroidism (myxedema)** may be caused by overtreatment with ^{131}I, diminished thyroid-stimulating hormone (TSH) or thyrotropin-releasing hormone (TRH) levels, or thyroiditis. The patient is easily fatigued, often sleepy, and experiences weakness. Skin becomes dry and thick. Hair is brittle. Hot or cold temperatures are poorly tolerated. Speech is slowed and may be hoarse. The individual becomes irritable or appears depressed. As the disorder progresses, memory and intellect are impaired, so much so that a person appears demented. In severe cases, the patient becomes obtundent or comatose; if this occurs, the mortality rate is substantial (50%). Early recognition and treatment improves the outcome of hypothyroidism. Early treatment usually reverses all ill effects; left untreated, permanent cognitive deficits may develop.

D. **Elevated or depressed parathyroid functions**

1. **Hyperparathyroidism typically results from parathyroid neoplasms**, which are usually benign adenomas. This disorder leads to elevated serum calcium concentration. (Hypercalcemia may also develop in disease processes affecting bones, such as Paget's disease, multiple myeloma, and metastatic carcinoma). Hypercalcemic patients experience lassitude, anxiety, and irritability. They may become agitated, paranoid, confused, or depressed. Muscular weakness is common.

2. **Hypoparathyroidism** occurs when parathyroid gland functioning is diminished or lost. This condition usually follows neck or thyroid surgery, when the parathyroid glands are excised. Hypoparathyroidism leads to hypocalcemia. Neuromuscular signs and symptoms include increased excitability, transient paresthesias, cramping, twitching, tetany, and seizures. Psychiatric signs and symptoms include confusion, agitation, drowsiness, hallucinations, and depression. Correction of serum calcium concentration eliminates the signs and symptoms.

E. **Abnormalities of adrenal cortical functioning**

1. **Adrenal insufficiency** is a life-threatening condition when its onset is sudden. Vomiting, weakness, dehydration, hypotension, and impairment of consciousness may be present. Without prompt treatment, circulatory collapse and death will follow. Chronic adrenal insufficiency, **Addison's disease**, produces apathy, fatigability, irritability, and depression. Occasionally, a patient becomes confused or psychotic. Treatment with corticosteroids eliminates psychiatric symptoms.

2. **Cushing's disease is a state of adrenal cortical hyperactivity** caused by either excessive ACTH secretion by the pituitary or an adrenal cortical adenoma that produces excessive amounts of corticosteroids. In modern medical practice, Cushing's syndrome is seen to develop in patients taking high doses of corticosteroids long-term for various conditions. Signs and symptoms vary. Some patients are restless, suffer from insomnia, have an elevated mood, and are hyperactive. Others feel anxious or depressed. Psychosis may develop with delusions and

hallucinations. Suicide may occur. Treatment of a tumor or decreasing the dosage of prednisone is indicated and usually remedies the problem.

F. Pheochromocytoma is a catecholamine-secreting tumor of the adrenal medulla. The patient experiences severe anxiety as well as excessive perspiration, palpitations, tremulousness, lightheadedness, headaches, and pallor. These symptoms are very similar to those of panic attacks. Blood pressure is elevated in a sustained or a paroxysmal fashion. These tumors are often very small and difficult to locate. Once found, surgical excision is indicated in most cases.

X. INFECTIOUS ETIOLOGIES. Infections can produce changes in cognition, behavior, and emotional expression. Although these changes may occur with systemic infections, they are much more common with central nervous system infections.

A. High fever. A patient with a systemic infection, such as pneumonia or typhoid, often has an associated high fever. A delirium may be present. The affected individual is confused, agitated, and irritable. The level of consciousness fluctuates. Hallucinations may prove to be very troubling. Erratic, ill-considered behavior may occur. A safe environment with adequate provision for orienting the patient is necessary. As fever diminishes, signs of delirium typically remit.

B. Encephalitides. A viral infection of the central nervous system produces encephalitis. Encephalitides may be acute or chronic.

   1. In acute viral encephalitis, inclusion bodies are formed in the brain. The patient may be excessively sleepy, lethargic, and confused. Other patients are irritable and hyperkinetic. Some experience anxiety, apprehension, and have outbursts of terror or rage. Fever, headache, and photophobia are common physical symptoms.

   2. Chronic viral encephalitides are much less common. Pronounced physical symptoms, such as fever and headache, may be diminished or absent. In adults, chronic encephalitis may present with extrapyramidal symptomatology or with a seizure. In children, alterations in behavior and character may be evident. A well-behaved child may become destructive and inconsiderate of others. There may be no neurologic or intellectual deficits. Viral titers and examination of the cerebrospinal fluid aid in diagnosis. A syndrome characterized by chronic somatic and psychiatric symptoms has been reported in association with chronically elevated titers for the Epstein-Barr virus. The role of this viral infection in the generation of symptoms has not been identified.

C. Tertiary syphilis has devastating effects on the central nervous system. As recently as 1920, 10% of all psychiatric hospitalizations were for general paresis, a form of tertiary syphilis. Currently, general paresis accounts for far less than 1% of admissions. The discovery of penicillin in 1943 provided definitive treatment, although cases are still occasionally seen. A second type of tertiary syphilis, syphilitic meningitis, warrants description also.

   1. General paresis occurs 5–30 years after an episode of primary syphilis, most frequently within 20 years.

      a. Diagnosis is made by examination of the cerebrospinal fluid and serum. Test results of spinal fluid are positive in more than 90% of untreated cases. Protein is elevated two to six times the normal levels. Globulins are disproportionately high. A cell count of more than 100 cells per ml indicates an active infection.

      b. Mortality rates are between 20% and 30%. Untreated individuals have an average life expectancy of 4 years. Active, adequate treatment with penicillin yields good results.

      c. Marked personality changes and neurologic signs may be noted, including:

         (1) Irritability
         (2) Impaired concentration
         (3) Depression
         (4) Periods of confusion
         (5) Sleep disturbances
         (6) Headaches
         (7) Indifference or apathy
         (8) Impaired judgment
         (9) Grandiose delusions
         (10) Impaired memory
         (11) Erratic emotional reactions
         (12) Loss of muscle tone
         (13) Fatigue
         (14) Papilledema

(15) Optic atrophy (in 65% of individuals)
(16) Argyll Robertson pupils
(17) Speech disturbances
(18) Gait disturbances
(19) Spasticity

2. **Syphilitic meningitis** primarily involves the meninges, unlike general paresis, which affects brain parenchyma. It usually arises 1–3 years after a primary syphilitic infection. In general, the personality is less affected when the brain parenchyma is not involved.
   a. **Basilar meningitis.** Inflammation of the meninges around the base of the brain is basilar meningitis. The patient is usually clearly impaired with neurologic signs. Headache, dizziness, sleepiness, confusion, and impaired memory are accompanied by pupillary abnormalities, ptosis, deafness, and a facial palsy.
   b. **Vertical meningitis** results from inflammation involving the brain's convex surfaces (the cerebral hemispheres). Symptoms include severe nocturnal headaches, frequent dizziness, irritability, inability to sustain effort, slowed thinking, amnesia, aphasia, retarded speech, and seizures. Diagnosis by serology and examination of the cerebrospinal fluid should lead to successful treatment with penicillin.

D. **Meningococcal meningitis** may present as a delirium. The patient is confused, mumbles or rambles in his or her speech, and is restless and disoriented. Its course may be fulminant. Acutely, the patient may be noisy or violent. In subacute cases, drowsiness and confusion are prominent. Chronic cases present with impaired concentration, or, in children, impaired intellect. Meningeal irritation (i.e., a stiff neck) and fever are usually present. Examination of the cerebrospinal fluid reveals depressed glucose levels, purulence (i.e., the presence of leukocytes), and diplococci. Prompt diagnosis and treatment typically yield a full recovery.

E. **Tubercular meningitis** is a condition that develops when tuberculosis spreads from the lungs to the central nervous system. Its onset is insidious. Early symptoms include fatigue, irritability, peevishness, and disturbed sleep. If intracranial pressure increases, the patient experiences headaches, confusion, and clouded consciousness. As the disease progresses, meningeal irritation is evident. Examination of the cerebrospinal fluid reveals decreased glucose levels, elevated protein levels, an increased cell count, and the presence of tubercle bacillus upon stain or culture. Early treatment with isoniazid and streptomycin yields the best outcome.

F. **Sydenham's chorea** is a condition that develops following recurrent streptococcal infections (usually tonsillitis). Typically, a rheumatic condition accompanies the recurrent infections. In the brain, the cerebral cortex and basal ganglia are affected. Children are affected more often than adults, and females more often than males. The illness usually runs a 2- or 3-month course, although relapses may occur. Treatment with salicylates and bed rest is indicated. Signs and symptoms include:

1. Emotional instability

2. Impaired memory

3. Impaired concentration

4. Irritability

5. Abnormal movement, including grimacing and jerky movements of the limbs

XI. **AUTOIMMUNE ETIOLOGIES** are those conditions in which the body initiates an immune response against its own tissue (i.e., pathogenesis involves immunologic mechanisms). This process may involve the central nervous system and, therefore, lead to psychiatric signs and symptoms.

A. **Systemic lupus erythematosus (SLE)** is a disease of unknown cause. It is clear that a group of antibodies to substances found in cell nuclei are formed, so-called **antinuclear antibodies**. Antibody–antigen complexes form and are deposited in renal glomeruli and in blood vessels, leading to tissue damage. SLE occurs in women nine times as often as in men. Although it occurs in all age groups, it is more common in individuals between 20 and 50 years of age. Overall, between 2 and 3 of every 100,000 individuals are affected. The 5-year survival rate is about 80%.

1. Some patients present initially with psychiatric complaints, especially mood symptoms. Emotional lability and psychotic symptoms, such as delusions and hallucinations also occur. Signs and symptoms include:
   a. Arthritis and arthralgia
   b. Fever

      c. Malaise
      d. Weight loss
      e. Anorexia
      f. Skin eruptions
      g. Seizures
      h. Cognitive deficits

  2. Patients with severe renal or central nervous system disease experience high morbidity and early mortality. Central nervous system lesions include necrotizing vasculitis of arterioles and capillaries, microinfarcts, and deposition of immunoglobulins and complement in the choroid plexus.

  3. A positive antinuclear antibody titer, evidence of renal disease, anemia, leukopenia, and thrombocytopenia, and biopsy aid in diagnosis, although other autoimmune diseases may be difficult to rule out.

  4. Some patients with SLE recover spontaneously. Some respond to steroids. Some are unresponsive to treatment. High doses of corticosteroids can also produce psychiatric symptoms, further complicating the evaluation of emotional and behavioral changes in these patients.

B. Vasculitides are autoimmune diseases that primarily involve blood vessels, often in the brain. Psychiatric symptoms may occur.

STUDY QUESTIONS

Directions: Each question below contains five suggested answers. Choose the **one best** response to each question.

1. Dementia is characterized by all of the following statements EXCEPT

(A) demented patients are often depressed
(B) the ability to generalize from past experiences and to see the relationships between similar situations is lost
(C) an early feature of dementia is an inability to recall events of the distant past
(D) demented patients may experience hallucinations
(E) Creutzfeldt-Jakob disease is a dementia caused by a slow virus

2. Organic mental conditions due to vascular disease are characterized by all of the following statements EXCEPT

(A) early signs of vascular disease include memory loss, irritability, and mental fatigue
(B) these conditions usually occur in individuals between 50 and 65 years of age
(C) insomnia is treated with sedating medications
(D) men are affected more often than women
(E) signs and symptoms of these disorders result from cellular hypoxia and disrupted metabolism

3. Alcohol abuse is characterized by all of the following statements EXCEPT

(A) chronic, heavy drinkers metabolize alcohol at a rate of 30 mg/dl/hr
(B) rapid consumption of large amounts of alcohol may cause death due to respiratory arrest
(C) subdural hematomas are more common in alcoholics than in the population as a whole
(D) chronic, heavy alcohol use frequently causes dementia
(E) the duration of intoxication is typically 12 hours or less

4. A 32-year-old man is noted to have an unsteady gait, a sixth cranial nerve palsy, and spider angiomas when examined in the emergency room. He is confused and agitated. He should be treated with

(A) haloperidol
(B) pentobarbital
(C) anticoagulants
(D) thiamine
(E) salicylates

5. A 46-year-old woman has been found unconscious in the garage. The car was running, and all the doors to the garage were closed. Upon examination she is confused. The most likely cause of her confusion is

(A) lead poisoning
(B) hypoxia
(C) hypoglycemia
(D) gasoline inhalation
(E) none of the above

6. A 58-year-old man complains of moodiness and disinterest in his normal activities. At times he is confused and forgetful. His gait is unsteady. Deep-tendon reflexes are diminished. He frequently experiences tingling in his legs. What is the most likely diagnosis?

(A) Hypothyroidism
(B) A cerebellar neoplasm
(C) Multiple sclerosis
(D) Vitamin B_{12} deficiency
(E) Manganese intoxication

7. A 26-year-old woman presents with a history of emotional lability and anxiety punctuated by episodes of confusion and abdominal pain. She takes birth control pills but uses no other drugs or medications. Which of the following diagnoses is most likely?

(A) Acute intermittent porphyria
(B) Toxic vapor exposure
(C) Premenstrual syndrome
(D) Petit mal seizures
(E) Presenile dementia

8. A 29-year-old man presents with a history of three discrete episodes of elevated mood and hyperactivity; he has noted a tendency to get "lost" during these episodes. Once he experienced a loss of vision in the right visual field. Which of the following conditions is the most likely diagnosis?

(A) Multiple sclerosis
(B) Vitamin B_{12} deficiency
(C) Herpes encephalitis
(D) Systemic lupus erythematosus
(E) General paresis

Directions: Each question below contains four suggested answers of which **one or more** is correct. Choose the answer

A   if **1, 2, and 3** are correct
B   if **1 and 3** are correct
C   if **2 and 4** are correct
D   if **4** is correct
E   if **1, 2, 3, and 4** are correct

9. Features of delirium include

(1) emotional lability
(2) disorientation
(3) rapid onset
(4) depression

10. A 54-year-old woman has suffered a fractured hip. On the second day following surgical repair, she becomes agitated and uncooperative. On the third day, she appears to hallucinate and calls the nursing staff by the names of her children. She is febrile and tachycardiac. Causes for this behavior include

(1) alcohol withdrawal
(2) intravenous penicillin administration
(3) sepsis
(4) general anesthesia

11. A 16-year-old boy angrily accuses his father of spying on him and then assaults him. This is the first known episode of violent behavior on his part. At the hospital his condition fluctuates between apparent calm and extreme belligerence. Initial evaluation and treatment measures include

(1) a toxicologic screen
(2) a pentobarbital tolerance test
(3) seclusion and restraints
(4) naloxone administration

12. A 67-year-old man is detained by the police after he has been caught exposing himself to schoolchildren. There is no history of such behavior. Likely causes of this behavior include

(1) petit mal seizure disorder
(2) Alzheimer's disease
(3) digitalis toxicity
(4) intracranial neoplasm

13. A 68-year-old woman with chronic obstructive pulmonary disease is brought to the hospital by her husband. Four times in the last month he has found her wandering about their yard at 2 A.M. in her bedclothes. Which of the following etiologic factors should be considered?

(1) Hypoxia
(2) Aminophylline toxicity
(3) Senile dementia
(4) Cerebrovascular disease

14. A 37-year-old man is brought to the emergency room by the police. He was apprehended while driving 100 mph on the highway at night without his headlights on. He is agitated and belligerent. He warns the physician that he has spoken to God and that God will punish those who have incarcerated him. Diagnostic possibilities include

(1) hyperthyroidism
(2) arsenic intoxication
(3) amphetamine intoxication
(4) Addison's disease

15. Cocaine abuse can manifest as

(1) sexual dysfunction in men
(2) an increased need for sleep
(3) severe anxiety and paranoid ideation
(4) hallucinations

16. Shortly after surgery for thyroid carcinoma, a 51-year-old woman becomes depressed. She complains of drowsiness and feels confused. Laboratory tests that should be ordered include measurement of

(1) serum cortisol level
(2) arterial blood gases
(3) hemoglobin level
(4) serum calcium level

Directions: The groups of questions below consist of lettered choices followed by several numbered items. For each numbered item select the **one** lettered choice with which it is **most** closely associated. Each lettered choice may be used once, more than once, or not at all.

Questions 17–20

For each sign or symptom listed below, select the disease process with which it is most apt to be associated.

(A) Frontal lobe neoplasm
(B) Occipital lobe neoplasm
(C) Temporal lobe neoplasm
(D) Parietal lobe neoplasm
(E) Pituitary neoplasm

17. Paroxysms

18. Apathy

19. Uninhibited behavior

20. Visual hallucinations

Questions 21–24

For each sign or symptom listed below, select the alcohol-related syndrome with which it is most commonly associated.

(A) Delirium tremens
(B) Intoxication
(C) Hallucinosis
(D) Korsakoff's psychosis
(E) Wernicke's encephalopathy

21. Visual and tactile hallucincations

22. Blackouts

23. Confabulation

24. Dehydration

ANSWERS AND EXPLANATIONS

1. The answer is C. (*III A 2 a*) Short-term memories, such as one's daily activities, register in the brain each day. Long-term memories, such as recollections from childhood, are already stored in the brain. In the initial stages of dementia, the ability to form enduring new memories is lost. Old memories persist until the later stages of the disease.

2. The answer is C. (*IV E 1–7*) Confusion is one of the more problematic symptoms of cerebral vascular insufficiency, and sedating medications exacerbate confusion. Although nocturnal restlessness often must be treated, a sedative is not indicated. More appropriate treatment is low-dose neuroleptic medication (e.g., 1–2 mg of haloperidol).

3. The answer is D. (*V F 2*) There are many patients who present with dementia and who have a history of alcoholism. Often there is no alternative disease process that can be identified. The dementia is explained by attributing it to alcohol abuse, but no cause-and-effect relationship has been established. Individuals who are severely affected with Korsakoff's psychosis are rare, and thiamine deficiency is implicated in the pathophysiology of that condition.

4. The answer is D. [*V F 2 f (1)*] The psychiatric findings of confusion and agitation are nonspecific. However, when considered in light of a gait disturbance and ophthalmoplegia in an individual with skin lesions that are found in chronic alcoholics, a presumptive diagnosis of Wernicke's encephalopathy can be made. Treatment with thiamine is indicated, which may reverse this patient's condition. Less fortunate patients develop Korsakoff's psychosis.

5. The answer is B. (*VI A 3, C 1*) Automobile exhaust contains carbon monoxide, and carbon monoxide poisoning produces hypoxia. Hypoxia leads to confusion, which may be transient or persistent, depending upon the degree and duration of oxygen insufficiency. Lead poisoning, hypoglycemia, and gasoline inhalation would not result from the circumstances in this case. Confusion can result from hypoglycemia, however.

6. The answer is D. (*VII D*) The patient described in the question has presented with psychiatric symptoms of apathy and moodiness. Memory impairment is suggested by his forgetfulness. There is evidence of neurologic impairment. Destruction of the myelin sheaths could explain all of these symptoms, phenomena that are seen in both multiple sclerosis and vitamin B_{12} deficiency. However, without a relapsing, remitting course, vitamin B_{12} deficiency is the more likely diagnosis.

7. The answer is A. (*VIII A 2*) Key elements in this history are the episodic nature of the disturbance, the age of onset, the association between abdominal pain and confusion, and the use of birth control pills. Acute intermittent porphyria is an episodic disorder that first gains expression in young adults in the age group of 20–40 years. Anxiety and emotional lability may be chronic. Abdominal pain accompanies exacerbations. The use of estrogens may precipitate episodes of disturbance.

8. The answer is A. (*IV F 2*) This patient has experienced relapsing and remitting symptoms, a course that is characteristic of multiple sclerosis (MS). Different areas of the brain have been involved—the optic nerve, the parietal lobe, and unspecified areas related to mood. Optic nerve involvement is the most common finding in MS and would be uncommon in any of the other disease processes listed. The patient's age is also consistent with the diagnosis of MS, a disease with a peak incidence around the age of 30 years.

9. The answer is A (1, 2, 3). (*III A 1, 2*) Delirium is an acute process in which brain functioning is severely compromised. Widespread deficits result from delirium, which is defined as a global disorder. Emotional expression fluctuates rapidly. If an individual cannot remember or think clearly, maintaining orientation becomes difficult or impossible. Delirium arises suddenly and must be addressed quickly as a true medical emergency. Emotions typical of delirium are fear and anxiety; depression is not a feature. Depression is commonly seen in dementia, however.

10. The answer is A (1, 2, 3). (*V F 2 d, G 1, 4 a; X A*) The patient presents with a picture of delirium, and the fever and tachycardia may be clues to the etiology of the delirium. Certainly, a systemic infection is possible following major surgery, and sepsis often leads to delirious behavior, usually associated with a high fever. If this patient is alcoholic, she has been withdrawn suddenly. Intercurrent illnesses, such as fractures and infections, predispose an individual to severe alcohol withdrawal or delirium tremens. Penicillin is an antibacterial agent that has produced an acute psychosis characterized by agitation, anxiety, and hallucinations, all of which are present in this case. General anesthetic agents are volatile gases. They are excreted within hours, and an effect after 2 or 3 days is not possible.

11. The answer is B (1, 3). [*III C 2; V B 1 d (2), C 1, F 1 a, 3*] The boy is paranoid and disturbed enough to predicate his actions on paranoid ideation. Evaluation of any episode of psychotic behavior must include consideration of organic factors. In this case, drugs should be of particular concern, and physical safety should be emphasized. Therefore, a toxicologic screen for drugs, such as phencyclidine (PCP), cocaine, and amphetamines, is indicated. Physical restraints and seclusion insure safety until the diagnosis is made and specific treatment can be prescribed. A pentobarbital tolerance test is administered to assess the degree of addiction to barbiturates or other drugs in planning a withdrawal regimen. There is no evidence that this patient is an addict, and such a test could easily worsen his condition. Likewise, naloxone is administered in different circumstances: Specifically, if narcotics addiction is suspected in an unresponsive patient, naloxone can reverse the effect of the narcotic. This boy's agitation, however, is not typical of a narcotics overdose.

12. The answer is C (2, 4). (*IV A 3 b, B 1–4, D 1–3; V E 1*) Alzheimer's disease and intracranial neoplasm may present in a variety of ways. Some patients have pronounced neurologic signs and symptoms, while others have marked changes in personality. One common change in personality is a loss of inhibitions, leading to coarse language or sexually inappropriate behavior. Petit mal seizures are brief in duration, usually lasting 5–30 seconds. The individual stares into space. The normal flow of thought is interrupted, and the individual experiences a disruption in consciousness. Muscular tone may decrease, or twitching may occur. No organized behavior, such as exposing oneself, would be evident. Digitalis toxicity presents a varied picture. Restlessness and apathy may be apparent. With severe toxicity, a delirious state develops. Cognitive impairment, irritability, and psychotic symptoms are observed. Although indiscreet behavior may occur, other, more pronounced signs of disturbance will be present.

13. The answer is E (all). (*IV D 1–3, E 1–7; V C 2 b; VIII B 5*) Oxygenation of the blood is compromised by impaired alveolar gas exchange in chronic obstructive pulmonary disease. At her best, the patient described in the question may barely get enough oxygen to her brain; at night, most individuals hypoventilate. She has no margin of safety; if she hypoventilates, she no longer delivers enough oxygen to her brain. Hypoxia produces confusion, impairment of judgment, erratic behavior, and irrational thinking. Aminophylline is an analeptic agent chemically related to sympathomimetic amines. Intoxication with aminophylline can produce a delirious, confused state. Senile dementia presents in a variety of ways: A change in behavior in an elderly woman may be the first sign of the dementing process. A demented individual may suffer acute disturbances in behavior if an acute insult, such as hypoxia, is present. Cerebrovascular disease is common in the elderly, and an early sign is confusion. Nocturnal confusion may be particularly prominent. Judgment is impaired, and erratic behavior occurs.

14. The answer is B (1, 3). (*V C 1; VI C 5; IX C 1, E 1*) Hyperthyroidism can lead to an agitated, excited state characterized by pressured, erratic behavior. Although delusions and hallucinations may occur in hyperthyroidism, as they do in this case, the mechanism is unknown. Amphetamines have potent effects on the central nervous system. With chronic use, an organic delusional syndrome may develop, which resembles paranoid schizophrenia. The individual becomes suspicious and paranoid; he or she experiences hallucinations. Unpredictable and dangerous behavior is predicated upon irrational fears and beliefs. Acute arsenic intoxication, if severe, leads to serious medical symptomatology. Chronic intoxication typically leads to apathy and lethargy, and the individual would appear to be depressed, ill, or both. Addison's disease results from chronic adrenal insufficiency. In a state of chronic corticosteroid depletion, an individual becomes depressed, lethargic, and easily fatigued: The energetic and psychotic behavior that is seen in this case is highly unlikely.

15. The answer is E (all). (*V F 3 a–c*) Users of cocaine often feel that they perform better in many areas when intoxicated. This misperception probably results from the overriding effects of euphoria and stimulation caused by the drug. Chronic cocaine use can lead to erectile and ejaculatory dysfunction in men as well as hypersomnia. Acutely, cocaine can cause severe anxiety with paranoia and hallucinations.

16. The answer is D (4). (*IX D 2*) One complication of neck or thyroid surgery is inadvertent removal of the parathyroid glands. If this is done, the serum concentration of calcium falls, leading to the symptoms that this woman is experiencing. Although adrenal insufficiency, hypoxia, and anemia might produce similar symptoms, there is no reason to suspect any of these conditions from this history.

17–20. The answers are: 17-C, 18-A, 19-A, 20-B. (*IV A 3 c; B 2*) As does temporal lobe epilepsy, temporal lobe neoplasms cause outbursts of symptoms. Onset is sudden and unpredictable. Various mood states arise without warning, or a trance-like condition appears. Symptoms last for 2 minutes or less and then remit. The individual may not recall the paroxysm.

Frontal lobe neoplasms usually present as a gradual, insidious change in personality. A normally active and involved individual may slowly become passive. Interest in work, hobbies, and family diminishes until apathy and indifference are marked. Another personality change observed in frontal lobe disease is a loss of inhibitions. The socializing functions of the brain are carried out in the frontal lobes. People act in ways that are appropriate to social norms when these functions are intact. Neoplasms disrupt this.

The visual cortical areas of the brain are located in the occipital lobes. A neoplasm disrupts the structural integrity of these areas, which can result in misperceptions or simple visual hallucinations.

21–24. The answers are: 21-A, 22-B, 23-D, 24-A. *(V F 2 a, d–f)* Hallucinations occur in both delirium tremens and alcohol hallucinosis. The sensory modality is critical. Typically, auditory hallucinations are present in hallucinosis. Visual and tactile hallucinations, such as spiders crawling over the skin, are much more likely to occur in delirium tremens.

Blackouts refer to transient periods of amnesia that result from intoxication. They stand out because the individual has no trouble with memory when he or she is not drinking. The individual has a memory gap of a few hours and may be painfully aware of it. Amnestic periods of different types appear in delirium tremens, Wernicke's encephalopathy, and Korsakoff's psychosis.

Memory is grossly impaired in Korsakoff's psychosis. Amnesia is severe and persistent. Confabulation is common. Stories are told with an air of certainty, even though no memory of events is present. This typically occurs without the confabulator being aware of the process. It is an attempt to adapt in the face of overwhelming deficits.

Delirium tremens is a condition in which an individual is often febrile and agitated. Loss of water may be enormous. Furthermore, the delirium interferes with the capacity for appropriate response to thirst and dehydration. Careful monitoring and replenishment of fluids is crucial in this disorder.

5
Substance Use Disorders

Steven L. Dubovsky

I. **INTRODUCTION.** Because terms such as drug abuse, addiction, and dependence evoke social disapproval and are variously defined within different cultures, they must be carefully defined at the outset.

A. **Pathologic use of centrally acting substances** is divided into the categories of dependence and abuse.

1. **Psychoactive substance dependence** (*DSM-III-R*)* is diagnosed when three of the following physical and behavioral consequences of use of a psychoactive substance are present for at least 1 month or recur intermittently over a longer period of time:
   a. Use of the substance in larger amounts or for longer periods of time than the patient desires
   b. Inability to control substance use
   c. Intoxication or withdrawal at work or school, while fulfilling important roles (e.g., taking care of children) or when intoxication or withdrawal are dangerous (e.g., while driving)
   d. Spending an excessive amount of time obtaining or taking the substance or recovering from its effects
   e. Interference with important activities by use of the substance
   f. Continued use of the substance despite knowledge of the adverse social, physical, and psychological effects of the substance
   g. Development of tolerance (i.e., decreased effect of the same amount of the substance or increased amount of the substance is necessary to produce the same effect)
   h. Development of withdrawal symptoms when the substance is reduced in dose or discontinued
   i. Use of the substance to prevent or relieve withdrawal symptoms

2. **Psychoactive substance abuse** (*DSM-III-R*) is diagnosed if either of the following two manifestations of dependence are present for at least 1 month or recur intermittently over a longer period of time:
   a. Continued substance use in spite of knowing that it is harmful
   b. Use of the substance in situations in which use is dangerous or impairs role performance

B. **Addiction** is a term used by some researchers to refer to overwhelming involvement with seeking and using drugs or alcohol and a high tendency to relapse after withdrawal. It is, therefore, a quantitative description of the degree to which drug use pervades an individual's life rather than a condition that can be clearly defined. Insofar as total preoccupation with a drug is a severe form of dependence, addiction may be said to be a form of substance abuse and dependence as defined in section I A.

1. It is possible to develop tolerance and withdrawal and not be addicted in that an individual's life is not organized around finding and using the drug. This is common in patients who become physically dependent on narcotics or tranquilizers during treatment of prolonged illness.

2. It may be possible to be addicted in the sense that drug-seeking behavior is paramount in an individual's life without being physically dependent.

---

*Terms followed in this chapter by the designation *DSM-III-R* are defined as they are in the American Psychiatric Association's *Diagnostic and Statistical Manual of Mental Disorders*, 3rd ed., revised, Washington, D.C., American Psychiatric Association, 1987.

C. Categories of substance abuse and dependence in the *DSM-III-R* depend on whether they involve one or more of 11 specific substances, all of which produce dependence and abuse except nicotine, which causes dependence only. The standard list includes:

1. Alcohol

2. Sympathomimetics

3. Cannabis

4. Cocaine

5. Hallucinogens

6. Inhalants

7. Narcotics

8. Arylcyclohexylamines (e.g., phencyclidine)

9. Sedative-hypnotics

10. Anxiolytics

11. Nicotine

II. **INTOXICATION SYNDROMES.** Since the manifestations and treatment of the intoxication syndromes produced by different drugs vary drastically, it is crucial to be able to recognize the symptoms of intoxication produced by the commonly abused prescription and nonprescription drugs.

A. **Alcohol** is frequently combined with other substances. The odor on the patient's breath that is characteristically associated with alcohol intoxication is caused by impurities in the preparation used and is extremely unreliable in diagnosing intoxication. In addition, head injuries and metabolic encephalopathies are frequently mistaken for alcohol intoxication. Blood and urine screens are reliable means of diagnosis.

1. **Mild intoxication** is characterized by disorganization of cognitive and motor processes. The first functions to be disrupted are those that depend on training and previous experience. Central nervous system concentrations of alcohol parallel its concentrations in the blood. As intoxication becomes more noticeable, the following changes occur:
   a. **Overconfidence.** Only if performance is initially impaired by psychological inhibitions may an individual function more effectively after ingestion of small amounts of alcohol. Otherwise, all aspects of physical and mental performance are decreased by alcohol. Nevertheless, the intoxicated individual tends to feel more efficient.
   b. **Mood swings, emotional outbursts, and euphoria** may occur.
   c. **Initial enhancement of spinal reflexes** as they are released from higher inhibiting circuits, followed by progressive general anesthesia of central nervous system functions, may develop.
   d. **An increased pain threshold** may be evident while other sensory modalities are unaffected.
   e. **Nausea, vomiting, restlessness, and hyperactivity** may be present.

2. **Severe intoxication** is characterized by:
   a. Stupor or coma
   b. Hypothermia
   c. Slow, noisy respiration
   d. Tachycardia
   e. Dilated pupils (may be normal in some intoxicated individuals)
   f. Increased intracranial pressure
   g. Death (rare in the absence of ingestion of additional drugs, trauma, infection, or unconsciousness, lasting longer than 12 hours)

3. **Treatment** depends on whether or not the patient is conscious.
   a. **The conscious patient** needs little to be done except wait for the alcohol to be metabolized.
      (1) Stimulants and caffeine do not hasten sobriety.
      (2) Restraint for severe agitation is safer than administration of tranquilizers or sedatives, which may potentiate the central nervous system depressant effects of alcohol.
      (3) Antipsychotic drugs, such as haloperidol, in low doses may decrease hyperactivity without increasing sedation.

   b. The stuporous or unconscious patient should be kept warm. It may also be necessary to:
     (1) Prevent aspiration, especially if gastric lavage is performed.
     (2) Treat increased intracranial pressure with mannitol or by other measures (e.g., steroids), in addition to the normal management of overdoses of central nervous system depressants.
     (3) Remove alcohol by hemodialysis in extreme situations.

B. Central nervous system depressants other than alcohol

  1. Specific substances
    a. Benzodiazepine tranquilizers (e.g., diazepam, oxazepam, chlordiazepoxide, lorazepam, prazepam, chlorazepate, and alprazolam)
    b. Benzodiazepine hypnotics [sleeping pills] (e.g., flurazepam, temazepam, and triazolam)
    c. Barbiturates (e.g., phenobarbital, amobarbital, pentobarbital, and secobarbital). Barbiturates and related compounds should not be used routinely because they:
     (1) Produce abuse, tolerance, and dangerous abstinence syndromes
     (2) Are not as effective as benzodiazepines
     (3) Are lethal when taken in overdose
    d. Drugs related to barbiturates [e.g., ethchlorvynol, glutethimide, propanediols (e.g., meprobamate), methyprylon, and paraldehyde]
    e. Chloral compounds (e.g., chloral hydrate)

  2. Mild to moderate intoxication with barbiturates and related compounds and benzodiazepines causes:
    a. Euphoria
    b. Hyperalgesia (increased pain threshold)
    c. Increased seizure threshold
    d. Sedation or paradoxical excitement in:
     (1) Susceptible individuals
     (2) The elderly
     (3) Children
     (4) The presence of organic brain disease
    e. Nystagmus, dysarthria, and ataxia
    f. Postural hypotension

  3. Severe intoxication is usually due to purposeful overdoses in suicide attempts and accidental overdoses by addicts. A few patients, especially those with preexisting brain disease, may take too much medication because of drug automatism (i.e., confusion that is worsened by the drug), which results in the patient not remembering how much has been taken and continuing to take more pills, usually in an effort to get to sleep. Severe intoxication can cause:
    a. Stupor and coma
    b. Respiratory depression
    c. Depressed reflexes
    d. Hypotension
    e. Decreased cardiac output
    f. Hypoxemia
    g. Bullous skin lesions and necrosis of sweat glands
    h. Hypothermia
    i. Death
     (1) Barbiturate intoxication that causes death is usually due to complications, such as pneumonia and renal failure.
     (2) Short-acting preparations, such as amobarbital, are more lethal at lower doses than long-acting compounds, such as phenobarbital.
     (3) Death from an overdose of benzodiazepines alone is extremely rare.

  4. Treatment of central nervous system depressant intoxication involves emesis, if the ingestion has occurred within ½ hour of admission and the gag reflex is intact, and gastric lavage, if these conditions have not been fulfilled. A cathartic should then be given to decrease intestinal absorption of the drug. For severe poisoning, the following steps are taken:
    a. Protection of the airway
    b. Oxygen administration
    c. Ventilation when necessary
    d. Prevention of further loss of body heat
    e. Correction of hypovolemia and maintenance of blood pressure with dopamine

     f. Forced diuresis with maximal alkalinization of the urine
     g. Hemodialysis

C. Central nervous system stimulants

  1. Specific substances
     a. Amphetamines. Medical indications for amphetamines include:
       (1) Hyperactivity in children
       (2) Depression in the elderly
       (3) Medically ill patients with time-limited depression who cannot tolerate antidepressants
       (4) Augmentation of antidepressants in treatment-resistant depression
     b. Pemoline. Medical indications are the same as for amphetamines.
     c. Methylphenidate. Medical indications are the same as for amphetamines.
     d. Cocaine, which is used to treat nosebleeds
     e. Phenmetrazine
     f. Phenylpropanolamine
     g. Antiobesity drugs. Long-term treatment of obesity with stimulants is almost always unsuccessful due to tolerance.

  2. Mild to moderate intoxication produces:
     a. Elevated mood
     b. Increased energy and alertness
     c. Decreased appetite
     d. Talkativeness
     e. Anxiety and irritability
     f. Insomnia
     g. Increased ability to perform repetitive tasks when the individual is tired or bored
     h. Hypertension in susceptible individuals
     i. Tachycardia
     j. Hyperthermia

  3. Severe intoxication may produce a toxic psychosis. Although tolerance develops to many of the effects of stimulants, there is no tolerance to the tendency to develop psychotic symptoms, which may be indistinguishable from those of schizophrenia. Signs and symptoms include:
     a. Visual, auditory, and tactile hallucinations
     b. Delusions, especially of being infested with parasites
     c. Paranoia and loose associations in a clear sensorium
     d. Mania
     e. Fighting
     f. Hypervigilance
     g. Dilated pupils
     h. Elevated blood pressure and pulse (may be normal in some chronic abusers)
     i. Arrhythmias
     j. Seizures
     k. Exhaustion
     l. Coma (in very severe cases)
     m. Intracranial hemorrhage (has been reported)

  4. Treatment
     a. Hypertension and hyperthermia can be treated with phentolamine.
     b. Psychotic symptoms can be treated by haloperidol, which antagonizes the dopaminergic properties of stimulants.

D. Hallucinogens and cannabis substances

  1. Specific substances
     a. Lysergic acid diethylamide (LSD)
     b. Psilocybin
     c. Mescaline
     d. Phencyclidine (PCP)
     e. 2,5-Dimethoxy-4-methylamphetamine (STP)
     f. Marijuana
     g. Hashish
     h. Δ-Tetrahydrocannabinol (THC)

2. **Intoxication** depends on the substance.
   a. Most hallucinogen intoxications produce:
     (1) Dilated pupils
     (2) Increased heart rate and blood pressure
     (3) Increased temperature
     (4) Paranoia in a clear sensorium
     (5) Illusions
     (6) Hallucinations
     (7) Depersonalization
     (8) Anxiety
     (9) Distortion of time sense
    (10) Inappropriate affect
   b. **PCP intoxication** can also cause:
     (1) Violent behavior
     (2) Extreme hyperactivity
     (3) Coma
     (4) Mutism
     (5) Echolalia
     (6) Analgesia
     (7) Nystagmus
     (8) Ataxia
     (9) Seizures
    (10) Hypervision
    (11) Intracranial hemorrhage (rare)
   c. **Intoxication by marijuana and related substances** rarely produces hallucinations. More common characteristics include:
     (1) Euphoria
     (2) Anxiety
     (3) Increased appetite
     (4) Increased suggestibility
     (5) Distortion of time and space
     (6) Injected conjunctivae
     (7) No change in pupils

3. **Treatment** of intoxication and "bad trips" also depends on the substance.
   a. The psychological effects of the cannabis group of drugs and most hallucinogens are usually decreased by reassurance in a quiet setting. Oral administration of diazepam is sometimes a useful adjunct.
   b. Patients intoxicated with PCP may react violently to any environmental stimulation, including attempts at reassurance. They generally should be left alone in a quiet area. If they become violent, they may be sedated with intravenously administered haloperidol or diazepam. Seizures should be treated with intravenous administration of diazepam.

E. **Narcotics.** Many street preparations are adulterated with quinine, procaine, lidocaine, lactose, or mannitol and are contaminated with bacteria, viruses, or fungi.
  1. **Specific substances**
   a. Morphine
   b. Heroin
   c. Hydromorphone
   d. Oxymorphone
   e. Levorphanol
   f. Codeine
   g. Hydrocodone
   h. Oxycodone
   i. Methadone
   j. Meperidine
   k. Alphaprodine
   l. Propoxyphene
   m. Pentazocine, which has both narcotic antagonist and agonist properties

  2. **Mild to moderate intoxication** may produce:
   a. Analgesia without loss of consciousness
   b. Drowsiness and mental clouding
   c. Nausea and vomiting
   d. Apathy and lethargy

e. Euphoria
f. Itching
g. Constricted pupils
h. Constipation
i. Flushed, warm skin due to cutaneous vasodilation

3. **Severe intoxication** is associated with:
   a. Miosis
   b. Respiratory depression, which may recur up to 24 hours after apparent recovery from an overdose with most narcotics and up to 72 hours after apparent recovery from a methadone overdose
   c. Hypotension or shock
   d. Depressed reflexes
   e. Coma
   f. Pulmonary edema
   g. Seizures (with propoxyphene or meperidine)

4. **Treatment**
   a. Severe intoxication is primarily treated by supportive reassurance.
   b. Naloxone, a narcotic antagonist, can:
      (1) Reverse coma and apnea; however, the effects of concomitantly self-administered drugs, such as barbiturates, are not altered, and detoxification from these drugs should also be undertaken.
      (2) Precipitate a severe abstinence syndrome in narcotic-dependent patients
      (3) Cause vomiting

F. **Anticholinergic drugs.** Some anticholinergic substances grow wild, and some are included in various herbal medications.

   1. **Specific substances**
      a. Most over-the-counter cold and sleeping preparations
      b. Atropine
      c. Belladonna
      d. Henbane
      e. Scopolamine
      f. Antiparkinsonian drugs (e.g., trihexyphenidyl and benztropine)
      g. Tricyclic antidepressants
      h. Some neuroleptics (especially low-potency neuroleptics, such as thioridazine)
      i. Jimson weed
      j. Mandrake
      k. Propantheline

   2. **Intoxication** may produce:
      a. Confusion
      b. Delirium
      c. Hallucinations
      d. Amnesia
      e. Body image distortions
      f. Drowsiness or coma
      g. Tachycardia
      h. Decreased bowel sounds
      i. Fever
      j. Warm, dry skin
      k. Fixed, dilated pupils

   3. **Treatment** is primarily directed toward protecting the patient and waiting for the drug to be metabolized. Intravenous administration of physostigmine can temporarily reverse coma or severe hyperpyrexia but should be used cautiously because of serious side effects, including vomiting.

III. **ABSTINENCE SYNDROMES** are substance-specific, physiologically determined syndromes that appear after abrupt withdrawal or decrease in dosage of the drug. Withdrawal from some compounds produces mild syndromes; withdrawal from others produces phenomena that are uncomfortable but not dangerous, and from a few substances, life-threatening abstinence syndromes result. Blood levels are often zero in abstinence syndromes.

A. Alcohol abstinence syndromes

1. **Alcohol withdrawal ("the shakes")** [*DSM-III-R*] usually appears within a few hours of stopping or decreasing alcohol consumption and lasts for 3–4 days and occasionally as long as 1 week.

   a. **Signs and symptoms** include:
   (1) Tachycardia
   (2) Tremulousness
   (3) Diaphoresis
   (4) Nausea
   (5) Orthostatic hypotension
   (6) Malaise or weakness

   b. **Treatment**
   (1) Tapering doses of a benzodiazepine, such as chlorazepate, are given, beginning with a 60-mg divided dose on the first day, a 30-mg divided dose on the second day, a 15-mg divided dose on the third day, and none on the fourth day.
   (2) Thiamine is usually administered parenterally at 100 mg/day for 3 days.

2. **Major motor seizures ("rum fits")**
   a. **Symptoms.** Major motor seizures occur during the first 48 hours of withdrawal in a small percentage of cases of alcohol withdrawal.
   b. **Treatment** is by means of intravenous administration of diazepam. Phenytoin is not administered unless the patient is an epileptic.

3. **Alcohol withdrawal delirium (delirium tremens)** [*DSM-III-R*] begins on the second or third day, rarely later than 1 week, after withdrawal or decrease in intake of alcohol. It occurs in fewer than 5% of alcohol-dependent patients, usually after they have been drinking heavily for 5–15 years. If seizures occur too, they always precede the development of delirium. With appropriate treatment, mortality is extremely rare.

   a. **Symptoms** of delirium tremens include:
   (1) Delirium
   (2) Autonomic hyperactivity (increased pulse rate, blood pressure, and sweating)
   (3) Agitation
   (4) Vivid hallucinations
   (5) Gross tremulousness

   b. **Treatment**
   (1) Hydration
   (2) Parenteral administration of thiamine for 3–4 days
   (3) A benzodiazepine (e.g., chlordiazepoxide) administered in a divided dose (i.e., 200–400 mg/day)
   (4) A neuroleptic, such as haloperidol, in severe cases of agitation or psychosis

4. **Alcohol hallucinosis** (*DSM-III-R*) is a rare condition that develops within 48 hours of cessation of drinking or at the end of a long binge with gradual decreases in blood levels.

   a. **The principal symptom** is vivid auditory hallucinations without gross confusion. Usually, the patient hears threatening or derogatory voices that discuss the patient in the third person or speak directly to him or her. Command hallucinations are absent. Symptoms usually last a few hours or days but persist for weeks or months in about 10% of cases. Occasionally, the syndrome may become chronic, in which case it may be indistinguishable from schizophrenia.

   b. **Treatment.** Neuroleptics may relieve agitation and hallucinations in patients who do not improve spontaneously.

B. Withdrawal from barbiturates, benzodiazepines, and related tranquilizers and sleeping pills produces syndromes that are similar in symptomatology but not in time of onset and duration to alcohol withdrawal. Abstinence syndromes are likely to occur after chronic use of 400–600 mg/day of pentobarbital, 3200–6400 mg/day of meprobamate, and 40–60 mg/day of diazepam or their equivalents. Withdrawal syndromes, which are usually less severe, have appeared in individuals taking lower doses for longer periods of time.

1. **Symptoms** usually begin within 12–24 hours, peak at 4–7 days, and last about 1 week after withdrawal from short-acting barbiturates. Withdrawal from long-acting barbiturates and benzodiazepines begins later (i.e., 4–10 days after drug discontinuation) and reaches its peak more slowly (i.e., around the seventh day). Signs and symptoms include:
   a. Anxiety and agitation
   b. Orthostatic hypotension
   c. Weakness and tremulousness

d. Hyperreflexia and clonic blink reflex

e. Fever

f. Diaphoresis

g. Delirium (appears on the fourth to seventh day as the syndrome peaks)

h. Seizures (may appear as late as the seventh day with withdrawal from short-acting barbiturates; later with long-acting preparations)

i. Cardiovascular collapse

2. Treatment. Withdrawal from central nervous system depressants can be life-threatening, and treatment is mandatory whenever the syndrome is suspected. Even if the patient seems only mildly anxious, he or she must be hospitalized to ensure adequate coverage if the condition worsens and to ensure compliance with the treatment protocol. A known compound (pentobarbital or phenobarbital) is substituted for the offending substance and is gradually withdrawn to suppress the abstinence syndrome. Treatment is not as effective if it is initiated after the appearance of delirium.

a. Since all central nervous system depressants produce cross-tolerance, the amount of barbiturate or related compound to which the patient is tolerant can be calculated by administering 200 mg of pentobarbital or 60–100 mg of phenobarbital when the patient no longer appears to be intoxicated (usually within 12–16 hours after discontinuation of the offending substance).

(1) If the patient becomes severely intoxicated or falls asleep with the test dose, he or she is not tolerant and does not need further treatment.

(2) If the patient develops moderate symptoms after the test dose (e.g., dysarthria, nystagmus, and ataxia without sleepiness), he or she is moderately tolerant and requires 200–300 mg of pentobarbital or 60–90 mg of phenobarbital a day.

(3) Absence of symptoms, or nystagmus without other signs of intoxication in response to the test dose, indicates significant tolerance. The patient should then be administered a total daily (divided) dose of 600–1000 mg of pentobarbital or 180–300 mg of phenobarbital every 6 hours to suppress withdrawal.

(4) Tolerance may also be tested by giving successive 60–100-mg doses of phenobarbital every 1–4 hours until the patient is intoxicated. The amount necessary to produce definite signs of intoxication, or a maximum of 500 mg/day, should then be administered in a divided dose every 6 hours to suppress the abstinence syndrome.

b. Once the patient is stabilized, the dose of pentobarbital is decreased by 10% every 1–2 days. Phenobarbital, which is longer acting, may be withdrawn more quickly. Reappearance of abstinence phenomena indicates that the dose needs to be reduced more gradually.

c. Since cross-tolerance exists between barbiturates and alcohol, phenobarbital or pentobarbital can also be used to suppress alcohol abstinence syndromes.

C. Stimulant withdrawal. There is no observable physiologic disruption; thus, gradual withdrawal is not necessary.

1. Symptoms

a. Increased sleep

b. Nightmares due to rapid eye movement (REM) rebound

c. Fatigue

d. Lassitude

e. Increased appetite

f. Depression, which may be severe

2. Treatment

a. Imipramine is indicated for withdrawal depression, which is also called the "cocaine blues."

b. Hospitalization may be necessary if the patient is suicidal.

D. Cessation of hallucinogens does not produce a significant abstinence syndrome.

1. Symptoms. Flashbacks (brief re-experiences of the hallucinogenic state) may be precipitated by marijuana or antihistamine intake.

2. Treatment. Reassurance that symptoms will subside and administration of a benzodiazepine are usually sufficient therapy.

E. Narcotic withdrawal is not life-threatening; however, it may be extremely uncomfortable.

1. Symptoms usually appear 8–10 hours after cessation of morphine. The onset is slower when long-acting drugs, such as methadone, have been used. Symptoms peak at 48–72 hours

and disappear in 7–10 days. Disturbances include:
  a. Lacrimation and rhinorrhea
  b. Yawning and sweating
  c. Restlessness and sleepiness
  d. Gooseflesh
  e. Dilated pupils
  f. Irritability
  g. Violent yawning
  h. Insomnia
  i. Coryza

2. **Treatment**
  a. Narcotic withdrawal is ameliorated by methadone substitution. When the patient demonstrates objective signs of withdrawal, a sufficient dose of methadone to suppress abstinence or a maximum dose of 20–50 mg/day is administered. The dose of methadone is then decreased by 10%–20% a day.
  b. Clonidine, administered at 0.1–0.3 mg three times a day for 2 weeks may help to suppress withdrawal symptoms, although it may cause hypotension. Clonidine should be tapered rather than abruptly discontinued.

F. Anticholinergic drugs occasionally produce influenza-like syndromes, depression, mania, or seizures when they are withdrawn abruptly. Discontinuation of clinically significant doses taken for more than 1 month should, therefore, be gradual.

IV. PRINCIPLES OF TREATMENT OF SUBSTANCE USE DISORDERS. Certain approaches are useful for treatment of abuse and dependence with all substances.

A. Detoxification. It is impossible to address the causes of substance abuse and dependence while the patient continues to use the substance. The first goal of treatment, therefore, is to withdraw the substance.

B. Insistence on abstinence. There may be a few individuals who can use addicting substances in moderation after successful treatment of a substance use disorder, but it is impossible to identify them. Complete abstinence from all substances on which the patient could become dependent is preferred.

C. Involvement of the family. Family members may encourage use of the substance in the patient, especially if there is family strife that everyone is able to ignore because all attention is focused on the identified patient. A spouse may also be drug dependent. The family can also be important allies in insisting that the patient deal with the problem.

D. Toxicology screens. Despite technical problems that may reduce reliability, periodic urine screens are often essential in identifying relapse and noncompliance.

E. Self-help groups. Peer support groups provide credibility and encouragement from individuals who have had similar problems and who are adept at dealing with common resistances to treatment.

F. Sanctioned treatment. When a patient is forced to remain in therapy by a legal sanction (e.g., loss of driver's license or professional license for relapse), the outcome is likely to be better than when the patient is free to withdraw from therapy at any time.

G. Contingency contracting. This approach provides a powerful negative contingency for leaving treatment or relapsing or a positive contingency for remaining drug-free. In the most widely used form of contingency contracting, the patient agrees in advance (in writing) that the therapist will notify an employer or licensing body if relapse occurs. The patient may leave a letter with the therapist outlining the problem, which is to be mailed if a urine screen is positive or the patient does not keep an appointment. Some patients deposit a sum of money with the therapist; a certain amount is then paid back to the patient for each week of abstinence.

V. ALCOHOLISM affects about 10% of the population. Alcohol abuse or dependence usually develops during the first 5 years of regular use of alcohol.

A. **Three patterns of chronic alcohol abuse**

1. Regular daily excessive drinking

2. Regular heavy drinking on weekends only

3. Long periods of sobriety interspersed with binges that last weeks or months

B. **Genetic influences** seem to play a role in the development of alcoholism. Individuals are at an increased risk of being alcoholic if they have:

1. A family history of alcoholism

2. A family history of teetotalism

3. An alcoholic spouse

C. **Diagnostic clues** to alcoholism include:

1. Inability to decrease or discontinue drinking

2. Binges lasting at least 2 days

3. Occasional consumption of a fifth of spirits or the equivalent in wine or beer

4. Blackouts (transient amnesia for events that occur while the patient is intoxicated)

5. Continued drinking despite a physical illness that is exacerbated or caused by drinking

6. Drinking a nonbeverage alcohol (e.g., shaving lotion)

7. Drinking in the morning

8. Abstinence syndromes

9. Apparent sobriety in the presence of an elevated alcohol level in the blood, indicating tolerance to the sedative effects of alcohol

D. **Physical, psychiatric, and social complications**

1. **Physical complications**, which may be caused by associated nutritional deficiencies or by a direct toxic effect of alcohol, are not uncommon in patients who drink more than 3–6 oz of whiskey a day or the equivalent. More familiar syndromes include:
   a. Cerebral atrophy
   b. Wernicke's encephalopathy
   c. Korsakoff's psychosis
   d. Nicotinic acid deficiency encephalopathy
   e. Polyneuropathy
   f. Cardiomyopathy
   g. Hypertension
   h. Skeletal muscle damage of uncertain clinical significance
   i. Gastritis
   j. Peptic ulcer
   k. Constipation
   l. Pancreatitis
   m. Cirrhosis
   n. Impotence
   o. Various anemias
   p. Teratogenicity. The fetal alcohol syndrome of mental retardation, microcephaly, slowed growth, and facial abnormalities may be a risk even if moderate amounts of alcohol are consumed during pregnancy. Since safe quantities have not been established, abstention from alcohol during pregnancy is recommended. If the patient does drink, she should be advised to do so on a full stomach to minimize rapid rises in blood levels.

2. **Psychiatric complications**
   a. Seventy-five percent of alcoholics have no other primary psychiatric diagnoses, although they may become depressed after withdrawing from alcohol when they realize that they have caused serious problems for themselves. Major depressive syndromes may also be caused by alcohol. **The major psychiatric complication of alcoholism is suicide:** More than 80% of individuals who kill themselves are depressed, alcoholic, or both.

b. Alcoholism may be an attempt at self-treatment of another psychiatric disorder—usually depression, anxiety, or psychosis. This may be a possibility if psychiatric symptoms clearly preceded heavy drinking. However, the history is often undependable, and only a trial period of abstinence reliably distinguishes between primary alcoholism and alcohol abuse that is secondary to another condition. If psychological distress resolves after a period of abstinence, alcoholism is likely to have been a cause rather than a result of the psychiatric disorder.

3. **Social complications** accompany the use of all psychoactive substances. The accident rate on the job is increased 3–4 times in workers who use psychoactive substances. Alcohol and other drugs cause sexual and marital problems.

E. **Specific treatment approaches** are geared toward the patient's preferences. In all therapeutic modalities, about one-third of patients remain sober, one-third enjoy a period of sobriety followed by relapse, and one-third continue drinking. Useful interventions include the following:

1. **Confrontation of denial.** The major obstacles to therapeutic success are the patient's denial of the severity of the problem and his or her wish to continue drinking. Repeated statements that the patient is not in control of the drinking and repeated confrontation with the complications of the alcoholism may be necessary before the patient agrees to treatment.

2. **Insistence on abstinence.** Since it is not possible to identify in advance the very few patients who may be able to succeed with controlled drinking, total abstinence is the only realistic goal.

3. **Assessment of motivation.** The patient who is willing to consider abstaining completely for at least 1 month is usually sufficiently motivated to give up alcohol completely. If the patient insists on some continued alcohol intake (usually with the assurance that he or she will be able to keep from drinking excessively), it is unlikely that the patient will be able to control his or her intake. Further therapeutic efforts may be unsuccessful until the patient is willing to give up alcohol completely for at least a brief period of time.

4. **Disulfiram (Antabuse).** Many alcoholics' efforts at abstinence are supported by disulfiram, which causes severe nausea and vomiting when it interacts with alcohol. Even if the patient does not need the drug, his or her willingness to take it is a favorable prognostic sign. The only contraindications to the use of disulfiram are organic brain syndromes or other conditions that might interfere significantly with compliance. The usual dose is 500 mg at bedtime for 5 days followed by 250 mg at bedtime for at least 6 months. Vitamin C and antihistamines may abort the alcohol–disulfiram reaction.

5. **Involvement of family.** The patient's family can be an important source of support, or they may openly or covertly encourage the patient to go on drinking. Occasionally, a statement by a spouse that he or she will not remain with the patient unless the patient stops drinking is the only force strong enough to convince the patient to agree to a trial of abstinence. Such threats should be mobilized only rarely and only when they are a true expression of the involved individual's feelings. Employers and other important individuals in the patient's life should also be involved in treatment whenever possible.

6. **Referral to specialized services.** Alcoholics Anonymous is the most effective treatment for patients who prefer a spiritual therapeutic approach. Other counseling programs also provide peer support and encouragement for the patient to stop drinking. Behavior therapy, which consists primarily of punishing drinking and rewarding sobriety, is useful for patients who consider their drinking a bad habit. Psychotherapy is appropriate for patients who feel that their drinking is motivated by unresolved emotional conflicts.

7. **Ongoing emotional support by the primary physician** is probably the most important factor in helping the patient to confront the problem and to maintain sobriety. The physician should accept periodic relapses in a nonjudgmental manner. If the patient refuses specific therapy for alcoholism, the physician should continue to be available to the drinking patient in case a psychosocial crisis precipitates a wish to become involved in treatment.

VI. NARCOTIC (OPIOID) DEPENDENCE AND ABUSE is a major public health problem. The incidence of heroin use increased during the 1960s, and use of this substance is now a problem in smaller communities in the United States as well as in the large cities.

A. **The epidemiology** of narcotic use, particularly heroin, deserves careful consideration. Two to three percent of adults aged 18–25 years have tried heroin at some time in their lives; additionally, abuse of narcotics usually occurs in the context of abuse of other drugs. Using "soft" drugs, such as marijuana, seems to break down a psychological barrier to using "hard" drugs. About 50% of the individuals who abuse narcotics become physically dependent on the drugs. Most addicts tend to abstain increasingly with time. They often finally discontinue drug dependence about 9 years after its onset.

1. **Patterns of narcotic abuse vary widely.** Some addicts, particularly those who are maintained on methadone, lead productive lives and enjoy good health. The need to obtain illicit drugs increases the incidence of prostitution and other crimes in order to support addiction; however, the behavior of the individual, once he or she is a narcotic abuser, is at least partially determined by his or her behavior and personality prior to drug use. Many narcotic abusers lead an antisocial life-style that persists until the drug is withdrawn. These individuals are different from those with antisocial personality disorder who are also narcotic abusers in that the antisocial behavior antedated substance abuse. Because of physical complications of abuse and a life-style associated with violence, the death rate is 2–20 times higher in addicts (10/1000) than it is in the general population. Patterns of narcotic use and dependence are as follows.

   a. **Medical treatment.** A very small percentage of the addicted population becomes dependent in the course of medical treatment. If these individuals continue to receive narcotics from the physician, they are less likely to encounter the problems faced by other dependent individuals, who must obtain the drugs illicitly.

   b. **Recreational use.** More commonly, narcotic abuse develops when an adolescent or young adult who is engaged in experimental or recreational drug use progresses to more intensive use. Since 60%–90% of adolescents experiment to some extent with drugs (experimentation with drugs has been reported in children as young as 5 years of age), the number who actually develop a major drug abuse problem is not great. Problems are more likely to develop with use of central nervous system stimulants and depressants. Two determining factors appear to be the context in which drug use takes place and the psychopathology of the abuser.

   c. **Methadone maintenance.** A significant number of individuals who have become dependent on narcotics now are receiving methadone from organized treatment programs.

   d. **Health care personnel.** The incidence of narcotic addiction is much higher in physicians, nurses, and other health care personnel than in any other group of individuals with comparable education and socioeconomic class. Most physician-addicts initially use a narcotic to relieve depression, fatigue, or a physical ailment rather than for pleasure. The pattern and consequences of the addiction are no different than they are for other addicts, except that health care personnel are more likely to make drugs available to themselves through prescriptions and through use of narcotics ordered for patients in hospitals.

2. **Epidemic transmission.** Heroin abuse tends to be transmitted in an epidemic fashion among individuals who know each other. These epidemics begin slowly, peak rapidly, and then decline quickly. They tend to abate completely after 5–6 years.

   a. Populations at risk have varying susceptibilities to heroin addiction. Young black males are at highest risk, and women seem to be at lowest risk.

   b. Abuse is initiated in a susceptible individual by someone personally known to him or her who is already addicted. The risk of such initiators exposing their acquaintances to heroin abuse continues for about 1 year. Drug "pushers" actually cause few new cases of dependence, although they obviously are a major source of the drug.

   c. Heroin abuse tends to spread until all susceptible individuals within a given group have been exposed. New addicts then tend to expose their friends in other circles, who produce a third generation of abusers.

3. **Drug cultures.** When cultural norms support heroin use and relatively pure preparations are available, a large percentage of users become dependent.

   a. More than 40% of the United States Army enlisted men stationed in Vietnam reported trying narcotics at least once, and about one-half of these became physically dependent at some time during their stay in Vietnam. However, very few individuals who became dependent on narcotics in Vietnam continued drug abuse when they returned to the United States, suggesting that removal of peer group support for drug abuse, removal of the easy availability of drugs and, possibly, removal of major environmental stresses, leading to intense anxiety, ended the reasons for continued abuse.

   b. Most individuals in this country who become dependent on narcotics tend to remain in a peer group that encourages abuse and tend to be psychologically predisposed to develop abuse. Most of these individuals develop a chronic behavioral disorder that may remit when access to the drug is denied but has a high tendency to relapse when the individuals return to an environment in which drugs are available and friends and colleagues condone abuse.

   4. Psychiatric illness. Approximately 50%–87% of drug abusers suffer from another psychiatric illness, especially depression, anxiety states, and borderline and antisocial personality disorders. Individuals from disorganized social backgrounds are also more susceptible to abuse. A combination of a susceptible psychosocial constellation, availability of narcotics, an environment that encourages abuse, and friends or colleagues who already are users may be necessary for the development of addiction.

B. Medical complications of narcotic abuse may result from contaminants of illicit preparations and the patient's life-style.

   1. Venereal disease. Female drug abusers have a high incidence of venereal disease because of the need to engage in prostitution to obtain the narcotic.

   2. Fatal overdose due to fluctuations in the purity of available compounds is not uncommon.

   3. Anaphylactic reactions may be caused by the intravenous injection of impurities.

   4. Hypersensitivity reactions to impurities may also cause the formation of granulomata and neurologic, musculoskeletal, and cutaneous lesions.

   5. Infections commonly caused by contaminated products and shared needles include hepatitis, endocarditis, septicemia, tetanus, and formation of pulmonary, cerebral, and subcutaneous abscesses. Up to two-thirds of individuals in narcotic treatment centers test positive for human immunodeficiency virus (HIV).

   6. Suicide and death at the hands of associates are more common in narcotic abusers than in the general population.

C. Treatment of narcotic abuse requires a multidisciplinary approach.

   1. Methadone maintenance
   a. If the patient has strong psychosocial supports available and is highly motivated to discontinue drug use, he or she can be withdrawn immediately using methadone (see section III E 2).
   b. If supports are weak or motivation to undergo withdrawal is uncertain, a period of methadone maintenance is instituted to strengthen supports, motivation, and the relationship with the treatment team. The usual dose of methadone in this setting is 40–80 mg/day.
      (1) Although methadone can be prescribed for acute or chronic pain by any appropriately licensed physician, methadone maintenance for the treatment of addiction can only be carried out by a federally approved program. Methadone maintenance is only permissible if the patient has clearcut signs of addiction, such as intoxication, needle tracks, and medical or psychosocial consequences of abuse.
      (2) Periodic unscheduled urine and blood screens are performed to test compliance with the program. Persistent noncompliance (i.e., continued self-administration of narcotics) results in dismissal.
      (3) Very gradual withdrawal from methadone is attempted when the patient seems ready. Most addicts note some abstinence symptoms when the dosage is reduced below 20 mg/day, and reduction in dosage by as little as 1 mg/week below this level may be necessary for the treatment of long-term methadone users.

   2. *l*-α-Acetylmethadol (LAAM), also known as methadyl acetate, a long-acting preparation, suppresses narcotic withdrawal for 72 hours. When it is used instead of methadone for maintenance, less frequent administration of the drug is necessary. However, more patients drop out of LAAM treatment programs than methadone treatment programs.

   3. Therapeutic communities play an important role in the treatment of narcotic addiction. Confrontation by fellow addicts has more credibility to an addict than therapies that are administered by professionals.

   4. Residential treatment. If outpatient therapy is not successful, residential treatment is necessary to remove the patient from easy access to the drug and from associates who encourage continued abuse. Group confrontation and support are used extensively in these settings. Compliance with treatment is higher when it is mandated by the courts than when it is voluntary and the patient is free to withdraw at any time.

5. **Licensure restrictions.** Narcotic-abusing physicians increasingly are being identified by state licensing bodies and medical societies. Treatment programs have been extremely successful when the problem is identified early and when continued licensure for medical practice is made contingent on ongoing treatment and surveillance.

6. **Prevention of addiction in a medical setting.** It is extremely important that health care providers not permit fears of addiction from interfering with the administration of appropriate doses of narcotics to patients in pain. The following guidelines apply.

   a. Adequate doses of narcotics should be administered to patients with bona fide pain syndromes. Addicts generally require higher doses than other patients.

   b. Narcotics should be administered regularly rather than as needed. This approach prevents the patients from becoming preoccupied with pain and its relief and provides a constant blood level that results in lower individual doses being necessary.

   c. An addict should not be withdrawn when he or she is physically ill.

   d. Prescriptions should not be written for outpatients with suspicious complaints or those with a high abuse potential, as indicated by:

      (1) Losing prescriptions or running out of medication early
      (2) Requests for a specific drug
      (3) History of abuse of alcohol or other drugs
      (4) Physician shopping
      (5) Claims that a physician who originally wrote a prescription is unavailable
      (6) Threats when narcotics are not prescribed
      (7) Dishonesty with the physician for any reason

VII. ABUSE OF AND DEPENDENCE ON TRANQUILIZERS AND SLEEPING PILLS, unlike problems with other centrally acting drugs, may be created or encouraged in everyday medical practice.

A. **Manifestations of abuse.** Barbiturates and related compounds are particularly prone to abuse. Benzodiazepines are more effective and less habituating than barbiturates. While benzodiazepines may relieve anxiety or insomnia temporarily, tolerance quickly develops to their antianxiety or sedative effects. Tolerance to the hypnotic effects of benzodiazepines is also common. Dependence may only first be suspected when an abstinence syndrome that responds to phenobarbital or pentobarbital appears in a patient who is admitted to the hospital and is denied access to the abused substance.

   1. Because they suppress REM sleep, barbiturates and related sedatives, such as secobarbital, glutethimide, and ethchlorvynol, subject the patient who uses them to a rebound of REM sleep, usually in the form of nightmares, when the drug is discontinued. Although it seems to the patient that he or she cannot sleep without the drug, continued drug use serves only to prevent withdrawal and suppress REM rebound, and escalating doses often are needed to accomplish this result.

   2. When barbiturates and related compounds are used as tranquilizers, drug withdrawal tends to be mistaken for a return of anxiety, occasioning an increase in dosage to suppress the symptoms. Fear of withdrawal symptoms then leads to continued drug use and an inability to function without the drug as well as other manifestations of abuse.

   3. Sedative abuse often complicates abuse of other substances.

B. **Identification and management of abuse.** Abuse of sedatives and tranquilizers can be minimized if barbiturates are not prescribed routinely for insomnia and anxiety and benzodiazepines are not prescribed for patients with a high abuse potential. Identification and management of abuse are facilitated by the following:

   1. A detailed history of amounts and kinds of all prescription and nonprescription drugs that have ever been taken should be obtained. Often the patient continues to take drugs that were prescribed by a physician that he or she is no longer seeing.

   2. Prescriptions for a patient who has terminated treatment must be discontinued.

   3. Drug screens in patients who abuse any drug should be performed to identify mixed abuse. Drugs will not be present in the blood of a patient who is experiencing an abstinence syndrome.

   4. Regular appointments should be scheduled for the patient who has been taking barbiturates for years and who is reluctant to discontinue them. When the patient is assured

of an ongoing relationship with a physician whom he or she trusts, he or she may be willing to taper drug intake gradually.

5. All patients with severe or mixed dependence who agree to be detoxified should be hospitalized. This permits adequate treatment of what may be a life-threatening withdrawal and ensures compliance with the withdrawal protocol.

VIII. COCAINE ABUSE AND DEPENDENCE have become extremely serious public health problems. One-fourth of young adults have used cocaine, and adverse consequences are common.

   A. Routes of administration. There are three routes of self-administration of cocaine.

   1. Nasal administration is associated with the onset of euphoria, over about 20 minutes, which lasts about an hour.

   2. Intravenous administration produces immediate euphoria.

   3. Crack, an easily synthesized compound that is not inactivated by high temperature, is smoked. Euphoria with crack is almost as rapid as it is following intravenous injection.

   B. Addictive potential. Contrary to the popular wisdom of a few years ago, cocaine is highly addictive. The advent of crack and the flooding of the market with cheap cocaine has made cocaine a drug of abuse at all socioeconomic levels.

   1. Animals will choose self-administration of cocaine over food and water until they die.

   2. Some patients report feeling addicted from the very first dose of cocaine.

   3. Crack is the cheapest and most addictive form of cocaine.

   4. Cocaine is frequently used in conjunction with other substances, especially alcohol and tranquilizers.

   C. Psychiatric disorders. Cocaine use may be a means of self-treatment for certain psychiatric disorders, especially depression and attention-deficit disorder. Some manics abuse cocaine in order to achieve a sense of control over excitement that occurs spontaneously without the drug.

   D. Treatment of cocaine abuse and dependence involves three types of medications that appear to reduce cocaine craving and withdrawal symptoms. All three classes of drugs are thought to be mediated by their effects on dopamine metabolism.

   1. Imipramine, desipramine, and maprotiline are the antidepressants that have been used to reduce craving. Other antidepressants have not been studied.

   2. Amantadine decreases cocaine craving in the first few weeks after withdrawal. It may also be useful in long-term treatment.

   3. Bromocriptine is a dopamine agonist that has been reported to be useful in a short-term trial.

STUDY QUESTIONS

Directions: Each question below contains five suggested answers. Choose the **one best** response to each question.

1. The most important feature of addiction is

(A) overwhelming involvement in seeking and using a drug
(B) physical dependence on a drug
(C) use of narcotics
(D) antisocial behavior
(E) tolerance, withdrawal, and abstinence syndromes

2. Effects of amphetamine intoxication include all of the following EXCEPT

(A) tachycardia
(B) depression
(C) suspiciousness
(D) anorexia
(E) insomnia

3. In contrast to most hallucinogens, phencyclidine is more likely to cause

(A) hallucinations
(B) mydriasis
(C) dangerous behavior
(D) depersonalization
(E) anxiety

4. An overdose of narcotics causes all of the following abnormalities EXCEPT

(A) dilated pupils
(B) hypotension
(C) depressed reflexes
(D) coma
(E) respiratory depression

5. Treatment of alcohol abstinence syndromes involves all of the following regimens EXCEPT

(A) thiamine supplementation
(B) benzodiazepine administration
(C) caffeine ingestion
(D) intravenous hydration
(E) neuroleptic administration

6. Which of the following statements best characterizes cocaine?

(A) It is relatively safe when used in moderation
(B) It causes life-threatening abstinence syndromes
(C) It is used primarily in high socioeconomic groups
(D) It is usually used alone
(E) It is highly addictive

7. The percentage of United States Army enlisted men who became dependent on narcotics while in Vietnam was roughly

(A) 10%
(B) 20%
(C) 30%
(D) 40%
(E) 50%

8. The most effective treatment of narcotic abuse is

(A) administration of narcotic antagonists
(B) antidepressant therapy
(C) administration of long-acting agonists
(D) removal of the addict from his or her environment
(E) ongoing psychological support

Directions: Each question below contains four suggested answers of which **one or more** is correct. Choose the answer

A   if **1, 2, and 3** are correct
B   if **1 and 3** are correct
C   if **2 and 4** are correct
D   if **4** is correct
E   if **1, 2, 3, and 4** are correct

9. True statements about hallucinogens include which of the following?

(1) Hallucinogens are not associated with abstinence syndromes
(2) Intoxication causes depersonalization and anxiety
(3) Most "bad trips" can be ameliorated by reassurance
(4) Tolerance develops to hallucinogenic effects

13. True statements concerning narcotic abuse include which of the following?

(1) Narcotic abuse does not increase mortality significantly
(2) Most addicts are introduced to opioids by drug pushers
(3) Narcotic abuse is common in young adults
(4) Narcotic abuse tends to occur in an epidemic fashion

10. The differences between phencyclidine (PCP) and other hallucinogens are characterized by which of the following statements?

(1) PCP is more likely to produce neurologic abnormalities
(2) PCP is more likely to produce hallucinations
(3) An individual intoxicated with PCP is less likely to respond to reassurance
(4) PCP intoxication is less likely to be associated with violence

14. The relationship between alcoholism and depression is characterized by which of the following statements?

(1) Nonbeverage forms of alcohol are most frequently associated with depression
(2) Depression may occur when the patient is sober
(3) Alcohol intoxication provides an easy means of suicide
(4) Suicide is more common in alcoholics

11. Stimulant withdrawal may be associated with

(1) increased appetite
(2) paranoia
(3) suicide
(4) insomnia

15. Narcotic abuse has which of the following characteristics?

(1) It continues indefinitely once it is established
(2) It is more common when it is condoned by others
(3) It is more likely to be initiated by a pusher than a friend
(4) It is associated with an increased mortality rate

12. Characteristics of contingency contracting include which of the following?

(1) Rewards are contingent on abstinence
(2) Contingencies are agreed to in advance (in writing)
(3) Negative consequences are contingent on relapse
(4) Therapy is contingent on paying

Directions: The groups of questions below consist of lettered choices followed by several numbered items. For each numbered item select the **one** lettered choice with which it is **most** closely associated. Each lettered choice may be used once, more than once, or not at all.

Questions 16–20

Match each substance listed below with the characteristic sign of intoxication.

(A) Suggestibility
(B) Insomnia
(C) Decreased pain sensitivity
(D) Violence
(E) Postural hypotension

16. Phencyclidine

17. Marijuana

18. Stimulants

19. Barbiturates

20. Alcohol

Questions 21–25

For each commonly abused substance listed below, select the medication that is used to treat dependence on that substance.

(A) Desipramine
(B) Methadone
(C) Antabuse
(D) Phenobarbital
(E) Diazepam

21. Central nervous system depressants

22. Cocaine

23. Phencyclidine

24. Alcohol

25. Narcotics

ANSWERS AND EXPLANATIONS

1. The answer is A. (*I B*) Although addiction is defined differently by different clinicians, the most popular definition is overwhelming involvement and preoccupation with obtaining and using any type of drug. Addicts often are physically dependent, but it is possible to become preoccupied with drug use even if one is not physically dependent on the substance. Any drug, including alcohol, that acts upon the central nervous system can be addictive. Although antisocial behavior often develops as a result of attempting to obtain drugs, it is not the defining feature of addiction.

2. The answer is B. (*II C 2, 3*) Amphetamine intoxication produces tachycardia, hypertension, a paranoid psychosis, loss of appetite, and sleeplessness. Depression is caused by withdrawal from amphetamines. Amphetamine psychosis may be indistinguishable from schizophrenia; it is treated with haloperidol. Withdrawal depression, which may result in a high risk of suicide, is treated with a noradrenergic antidepressant, such as imipramine.

3. The answer is C. [*II D 2 a, b (1)*] Hallucinogens produce autonomic arousal, increased temperature, illusions, hallucinations, anxiety, depersonalization, and paranoia without clouding of the sensorium. In addition to these effects, phencyclidine intoxication causes violent behavior and neurologic signs.

4. The answer is A. (*II E 2 g*) Like alcohol, barbiturates, and benzodiazepines, narcotics produce central nervous system, respiratory, and cardiovascular depression when they are taken in large amounts. In contrast to many other substances, narcotics cause constricted rather than dilated pupils unless cerebral hypoxia has supervened. Improvement with intravenous administration of naloxone helps to confirm the diagnosis of narcotic intoxication.

5. The answer is C. (*III A 1–4*) Benzodiazepines suppress alcohol withdrawal ("the shakes"), seizures, and delirium tremens. Thiamine is usually given because glucose administered for an alcohol abstinence syndrome in the presence of thiamine deficiency can precipitate Wernicke's encephalopathy. Hydration and sedation are the mainstays of treatment of severe abstinence syndromes, and neuroleptics may ameliorate the few cases of alcohol hallucinosis that do not improve spontaneously. Caffeine is not useful in the treatment of abstinence from or intoxication with alcohol.

6. The answer is E. (*III C 2 a; VIII B*) Cocaine was at one time thought to be a relatively benign drug used primarily by the rich. The fact is that dependence and abuse are very common in all social strata, sometimes beginning with the first dose. Many people progress to cocaine use after experimenting with other drugs and continue to use those drugs along with it. Cocaine withdrawal may produce severe depression, but if the patient does not become suicidal, the withdrawal is not life-threatening.

7. The answer is B. (*VI A 3 a*) Forty percent of enlisted men tried narcotics while they were in Vietnam, and about one-half of these individuals became dependent. The finding that only a minority of men continued to use drugs upon return to the United States suggests that easy availability of drugs and the encouragement of a peer group that supports abuse are necessary for drug abuse to continue.

8. The answer is D. (*II E 4 b; VI C 4*) Narcotic antagonists precipitate severe abstinence syndromes in patients who take narcotics. Satisfactory long-acting antagonists analogous to disulfiram have not been developed. Although narcotic abusers may become depressed or may attempt to treat depression with narcotics (this is especially true of physician-addicts), antidepressants are not helpful unless the patient stops abusing the narcotic. Psychological support may also be helpful, but it is usually an insufficient reason for the patient to abstain from use. Removal of the patient from the environment that supports abuse is the most reliable means of encouraging abstinence.

9. The answer is A (1, 2, 3). (*II D 1, 2 a, 3; III D*) Hallucinogens are not known to produce physical dependence (i.e., tolerance and withdrawal do not occur). The depersonalization, anxiety, hallucinations, and severe dysphoria produced by most hallucinogens can be ameliorated by reassurance in a quiet setting and by administration of benzodiazepines, if necessary.

10. The answer is B (1, 3). (*II D 1–3*) Unlike other hallucinogens, phencyclidine (PCP) may produce neurologic disturbances, such as seizures, coma, analgesia, nystagmus, and ataxia. It is, however, no more likely to produce hallucinations than other drugs in this class. Patients who are intoxicated with PCP are more likely to become violent than those intoxicated with other hallucinogens, and attempts to reassure them may make them even more violent. A more effective treatment of intoxication is to leave the patient alone in a quiet place and sedate or restrain him or her if agitation does not abate.

11. The answer is B (1, 3). (*III C*) Increased appetite, fatigue, depression, and suicidal ideation may occur with stimulant withdrawal. Although nightmares may occur, the patient usually sleeps after being deprived of the stimulant. Paranoia is a symptom of stimulant intoxication, not withdrawal.

12. The answer is A (1, 2, 3). (*IV G*) In contingency contracting, the patient agrees in advance that in the event of relapse or noncompliance, the therapist will notify an employer, a licensing body, or will arrange some other negative consequence. The patient may also deposit a sum of money or other reward with the physician, who then pays the patient a certain amount for each week of continued abstinence. Treatment for substance abuse is available to indigent patients through state and federally funded treatment centers.

13. The answer is D (4). (*VI A, B*) The combined mortality rate for narcotic abuse, suicide, and murder is approximately 10/1000. Although many adolescents and young adults experiment with a variety of drugs, hallucinogens, stimulants, and central nervous system depressants are more popular than narcotics. Two to three percent of this group have tried heroin, and a smaller percentage are addicted to opioids. Most addicts are introduced to the drug by their friends rather than by pushers. Heroin abuse tends to occur in epidemics in which individuals become addicted and then "infect" their friends.

14. The answer is C (2, 4). (*V D 2*) Any form of alcohol may produce depression as a direct effect of abuse. Alcoholics may drink in an attempt to treat an underlying depression; when they are sober, the depression may become more evident, or they may simply appreciate their problems more clearly. Although intoxication with alcohol alone is not commonly fatal, the overall suicide rate is increased in alcoholics.

15. The answer is C (2, 4). (*VI A 1–3, B 6*) Narcotic abusers are usually introduced to the drug by a friend, often after the patient has had experience with other psychoactive substances. Heroin use tends to be transmitted in epidemic fashion, with epidemics "burning out" in 5–6 years. The likelihood of narcotic use increases in settings in which the drug is readily available and social norms support its use. The mortality rate is increased 2–20 times in narcotics users, primarily from infection [especially human immunodeficiency virus (HIV)], overdose, and murder.

16–20. The answers are: 16-D, 17-A, 18-B, 19-E, 20-C. [*II A 1 d, B 2 f, C 2 f, D 2 b (1), c (4)*] Phencyclidine intoxication causes violent behavior much more frequently than other hallucinogens; on the other hand, marijuana is associated with suggestibility, but intoxication rarely produces hallucinations. Stimulants disrupt sleep. Alcohol intoxication, in contrast to that caused by barbiturates, increases the pain threshold. Postural hypotension is commonly a result of barbiturate intoxication.

21–25. The answers are: 21-D, 22-A, 23-E, 24-C, 25-B. (*II D 3 b; III B 2; V E 4; VI C 1 b; VIII D 1*) Detoxification from combinations of central nervous system depressants can be safely accomplished with phenobarbital; reliable patients taking one benzodiazepine can usually be withdrawn by gradual dose reduction. Imipramine, desipramine, and maprotiline appear to reduce cocaine craving and cocaine-induced euphoria. Diazepam is used to treat seizures and severe agitation associated with phencyclidine intoxication. Antabuse, which causes severe nausea and vomiting when it interacts with alcohol, helps patients to avoid impulsive drinking. Methadone maintenance is effective in preventing relapse of narcotic use.

6

Anxiety Disorders

Steven L. Dubovsky

I. OVERVIEW. Anxiety is abnormal fear that is out of proportion to any external stimulus. Significant anxiety is experienced by 10%–15% of general medical outpatients and 10% of inpatients. Of the healthy population, 25% of individuals are anxious at some time in their lives; about 7.5% of these have a diagnosable anxiety disorder during a given month. Until recently, anxiety was viewed primarily as a psychological response to internal or external stress; however, biologic factors are thought to play a role in some types of anxiety.

A. Endogenous and exogenous categories of anxiety

  1. Endogenous anxiety occurs spontaneously without any identifiable precipitating stress. Physical and psychological symptoms of anxiety persist for at least 1 month, and no specific medical or psychiatric disorder explains the symptoms. Eight stages of endogenous anxiety include:
  a. Spontaneous and sudden subclinical (limited symptoms) anxiety attacks
  b. Gradual progression to full-blown panic attacks
  c. Hypochondriacal fears of occult disease
  d. Development of **anticipatory anxiety** that unpredictable anxiety will result
  e. Phobic avoidance of situations in which panic attacks occur or from which escape might be impossible if panic did occur
  f. Generalized phobic avoidance
  g. Abuse of drugs or alcohol to control anxiety
  h. Depression

  2. Exogenous anxiety is precipitated by environmental stress.
  a. Spontaneous anxiety or panic does not occur if the anxiety is truly exogenous.
  b. The anxiety can always be explained by a specific external stress or psychological conflict.
  c. Symptoms are more irregular than those of endogenous anxiety and demonstrate a relatively consistent relationship to psychosocial stressors.

B. Diagnostic categories of anxiety*

  1. Panic disorder
  a. Symptoms. At least three spontaneous panic attacks, characterized by sudden apprehension or fear (see section I C 1–3) and usually accompanied by autonomic arousal, which are not precipitated by physical exertion, a life-threatening situation, or a phobic stimulus, occur within a 3-week period.
  b. Treatment. Panic disorder is treated with antidepressants, alprazolam, and with behavioral therapies.

  2. Generalized anxiety disorder
  a. Symptoms. Unrealistic worry about two or more life circumstances accompanied by at least six symptoms of anxiety is present for at least 6 months.
  b. Treatment. Benzodiazepines and buspirone are the drugs used to treat generalized anxiety disorder. Relaxation therapies, biofeedback, and related treatments are also useful.

  3. Obsessive–compulsive disorder
  a. Symptoms. This disorder is characterized by persistent intrusive, recurrent ideas, thoughts, feelings, images, or impulses (**obsessions**), which are experienced as senseless

---

*Information is taken from the American Psychiatric Association's *Diagnostic and Statistical Manual of Mental Disorders*, 3rd ed., revised (*DSM-III-R*). Washington, D.C., American Psychiatric Association, 1987.

or repugnant and which the patient tries to resist, or repetitive stereotyped actions (**compulsions**), which the patient recognizes as senseless and tries to resist. These actions, which are performed with a subjective sense of necessity to prevent some future event or in response to an obsession, are often a significant source of distress or interfere with the patient's ability to function.

  b. Treatment of obsessive–compulsive disorder is with chlorimipramine, fluoxetine, and in some cases, monoamine oxidase (MAO) inhibitors. Behavioral therapies are important adjuncts.

4. **Post-traumatic stress disorder.** After a psychologically traumatic event, patients continue to experience considerable distress as a result of the trauma.

  a. Symptoms. Some patients with marginal premorbid adjustment may develop psychotic symptoms in association with post-traumatic stress disorder. Differentiation from schizophrenia, mania, and depression may be difficult. Symptoms of post-traumatic stress disorder may appear immediately after the trauma or may be delayed for 6 months or more. In addition to continuing or recurrent preoccupation with the event, the patient experiences:

  (1) Decreased responsiveness to the present environment with diminished interest in usual activities, feelings of detachment or estrangement from others, and constricted emotional responsiveness.

  (2) Signs of distress that were not present before the traumatic event, including hyperalertness, startle reactions, insomnia, nightmares, guilt about having survived or about what actions were necessary in order to survive, difficulty concentrating, avoidance of activities that recall the event, and increased symptoms when the patient is exposed to situations that symbolize or resemble the original trauma

  b. Treatment of this condition can be more difficult than that of a more acute adjustment disorder. Adjunctive techniques (e.g., biofeedback) and medication (especially MAO inhibitors, tricyclic antidepressants, and carbamazepine) may be useful. Peer support groups are also helpful.

5. **Phobias.** The patient has persistent, irrational fears of benign situations, accompanied by a compelling need to avoid them. The patient realizes that this behavior is unreasonable and is disturbed by it. Phobias may develop spontaneously (endogenous) or develop after a specific traumatic event (exogenous).

  a. Symptoms

  (1) Simple phobias. Patients fear and avoid animals, heights, closed spaces, or any specific circumscribed object or situation that does not primarily involve being alone, being in public places, or being in certain social situations.

  (2) Agoraphobia. Patients' lives are increasingly constricted by fear and avoidance of being alone or being in crowds, public places, tunnels, public transportation, or on bridges from which escape might be difficult or help not available in case of sudden incapacitation. Agoraphobia may be a complication of panic disorder. There is some controversy about how frequently it occurs in patients who do not have panic attacks.

  (3) Social phobia. Patients suffer from a persistent, irrational fear that they will humiliate themselves in a social or public situation, leading to what they realize is an irrational avoidance of such situations. The inhibition may be limited (e.g., to public speaking), or there may be more global social avoidance.

  b. Treatment. Phobias are treated with systematic desensitization, exposure, and other behavioral therapies. Atenolol and MAO inhibitors have been used for social phobia.

6. **Primary psychiatric disorders** may be associated with anxiety, which may be prominent or even the presenting complaint.

  a. Depression. About 70% of depressed patients also feel anxious, and 20%–30% of apparent cases of anxiety are caused by an underlying depression. Approximately 40%–90% of patients with panic disorder become depressed, and 20% of depressed patients have panic attacks. Depressed patients with blood relatives who are anxious are more likely to experience anxiety plus depression than those with a family history only of depression.

  b. Psychosis. As control of mental processes is lost, a patient experiencing psychotic disorganization due to mania, schizophrenia, or borderline (brief reactive) psychosis often displays considerable anxiety, which initially may obscure the underlying severe disturbance of thinking, affect, or behavior.

  c. Organic mental syndrome. Anxiety is the most common emotion experienced by patients with acute organic mental syndromes (delirium), who are frightened by a sudden disruption of cognitive abilities, and by demented patients, whose mental syndromes are made worse by an intercurrent illness or by a sudden change in the environment (e.g., a change in the roommate of a hospitalized, demented patient).

    d. Adjustment disorder with anxious mood. Patients experience symptoms in excess of those that would normally be expected or suffer impairment of social or occupational functioning within 3 months of exposure to an obvious stress. In contrast to post-traumatic stress disorder, anxiety and other symptoms appear soon after the onset of the traumatic event and are expected to resolve when the stress abates or when the patient achieves a new level of functioning.

    e. Factitious disorder. Rarely, patients will consciously simulate a mental disorder, including anxiety, for the sole purpose of becoming a patient. The patient often relates an improbable history and has been hospitalized numerous times, often under different names. In contrast, **malingering** refers to the conscious simulation of a condition for some obvious gain. It is more common in a patient with a history of lying, drug abuse, and antisocial behavior.

C. Signs and symptoms. A subjective state of anxiety may be obvious, or it may be masked by physical and other psychological complaints.

  1. Psychological symptoms
    a. Apprehension, worry, fear, and anticipation of misfortune
    b. Sense of doom or panic
    c. Hypervigilance
    d. Irritability
    e. Fatigue
    f. Insomnia
    g. Predisposition to accidents
    h. Derealization (the world seems strange or unreal) and depersonalization (the patient feels unreal or changed)
    i. Difficulty concentrating

  2. Somatic complaints
    a. Headache
    b. Dizziness and lightheadedness
    c. Palpitations and chest pain
    d. Upset stomach and diarrhea
    e. Frequent urination
    f. Lump in the throat
    g. Motor tension or restlessness
    h. Shortness of breath
    i. Paresthesias
    j. Dry mouth

  3. Physical signs
    a. Diaphoresis
    b. Cool, clammy skin
    c. Tachycardia and arrhythmias
    d. Flushing and pallor
    e. Hyperreflexia
    f. Trembling, easy startling, and fidgeting

D. Illnesses that cause anxiety. Before investigating psychological causes of anxiety, it is important to exclude the possibility of physical disorders in which anxiety may be a presenting complaint even before other signs of disease become evident.

  1. Cardiovascular disorders
    a. Arteriosclerotic heart disease
    b. Paroxysmal tachycardia
    c. Mitral valve prolapse
    d. Hyperdynamic β-adrenergic circulatory state

  2. Pulmonary disorders
    a. Pulmonary embolism
    b. Hypoxemia
    c. Asthma
    d. Chronic obstructive lung disease

3. **Disorders of the endocrine system and metabolism**
   a. Hypoglycemia
   b. Hyperthyroidism
   c. Hypocalcemia
   d. Cushing's syndrome
   e. Porphyria

4. **Tumors**
   a. Insulinoma
   b. Carcinoid tumor
   c. Pheochromocytoma

5. **Neurologic disorders**
   a. Multiple sclerosis
   b. Temporal lobe epilepsy
   c. Organic mental syndrome of any etiology
   d. Meniere's disease

6. **Infections**
   a. Tuberculosis
   b. Brucellosis

7. **Drug-related disorders**
   a. Abstinence syndromes (e.g., abstinence from alcohol, tranquilizers and sleeping pills)
   b. Intoxication with sympathomimetics
   c. Akathisia
   d. Caffeinism
   e. Chinese restaurant syndrome, resulting from the ingestion of monosodium glutamate

E. **Anxiety that mimics disease states.** Anxiety may also mimic physical disease. For example, in **hyperventilation syndrome**, the patient who complains of shortness of breath, weakness, paresthesias, headache, and carpopedal spasm is often unaware of the psychological stresses that lead to hyperventilation and may either deny feelings of anxiety or feel that any anxiety that is experienced is secondary to not being able to breathe. Symptoms abate when the patient is calmed and respiratory rate decreases. Treatment consists of instructing the patient to breathe into a paper bag, which is held over the nose and mouth. Carbon dioxide accumulates and reverses the respiratory alkalosis caused by hyperventilation.

II. PSYCHOLOGICAL COMPONENTS OF ANXIETY. Patients who are encountered in nonpsychiatric practice often display anxiety that reflects specific combinations of internal and external conflicts. Although they are not part of the standard diagnostic nomenclature, these types of anxiety are easy to recognize, especially in medical and surgical patients.

A. **Situational anxiety.** Severe stress may temporarily overwhelm anyone's ability to cope. Even minor stress can be traumatic if it has important symbolic meaning.

1. **Symptoms.** When current stress reminds the patient of previous and unresolved conflicts, a relatively minor situation may feel overwhelming because it recalls other situations in which the patient was unable to cope. The intensity and nature of anxiety that evolves from a stressful situation depends upon the patient's previous level of adjustment. A relatively well-adjusted patient may experience only transient symptoms, while an underlying psychosis may be precipitated in a more marginally compensated patient.

2. **Treatment.** When patients must contend with acute, ongoing stress, antianxiety medication, when appropriate, and support should be offered. In addition, patients should be encouraged to talk about what the stress means to them.

B. **Anxiety about death.** Even nonfatal illnesses may remind patients of their mortality.

1. **Symptoms.** Persistent fear of death, even in terminally ill patients, symbolizes concern about loss of control, pain, isolation, helplessness, and the prospect of losing important relationships.

2. **Treatment.** Reassurance that the patients will not be left alone and in pain often decreases the apparent fear of death.

C. **Anxiety about mutilation, loss of prowess, and loss of attractiveness** is especially common in patients who feel that love, approval, and self-esteem are dependent upon their strength or beauty.

1. **Symptoms.** Patients become frightened if an illness threatens their appearance or prowess and express excessive fear of side effects and aftereffects of the illness, complain continuously, or fail to improve as expected. Patients may also attempt self-reassurance by demonstrating attractiveness (e.g., by behaving seductively) or strength (e.g., by exercising conspicuously) in inappropriate or even dangerous ways.

2. **Treatment.** Patients should be reassured that they still possess valued traits. The reaction of their families to the illness or surgery should be evaluated.

D. **Anxiety about loss of self-esteem.** Patients whose self-esteem is fragile are especially vulnerable to experiencing illness as an imperfection, weakness, or failure, which can lead to attempts to bolster a sense of self-worth by boasting about importance and superiority.

1. **Symptoms.** Patients may adopt a self-important air, insisting on being treated only by the most senior or well-known physician and treating others as worthless inferiors. Attempts to convince these patients that they are not as important as they think only increases their insecurity, which is covered up with greater protestations of importance and, by comparison, the unimportance of others.

2. **Treatment.** Patients should be approached with appropriate deference and should be reassured that they are still important. Reasonable requests should be granted.

E. **Separation anxiety.** Children and regressed adults (i.e., those who function psychologically more as children than as adults, a condition that is seen in hospitalized, overly dependent, and some psychotic individuals) may become frightened when they are separated from important caretakers.

1. **Symptoms.** Patients signal distress by becoming anxious, by complaining (e.g., of pain), or by ringing for the nurse whenever they are left alone. They often fear that, once out of sight, the caretaker will never return.

2. **Treatment.** Family and close friends should be encouraged to be with the patient as much as possible; the nursing staff should be encouraged to visit the patient frequently for brief periods of time, and a roommate should be provided. The patient's room should be close to the nursing station to facilitate frequent visits.

F. **Stranger anxiety**

1. **Symptoms.** Patients who suffer from separation anxiety also may react adversely to unfamiliar people, including new physicians, nurses, and visitors. In a hospitalized adult this can lead to distress at changes of shift or in other situations in which there are new caretakers.

2. **Treatment.** As much continuity in personnel as possible should be provided (e.g., the same nurse should be assigned to the patient each day). Unrestricted visiting by those familiar to the patient should be allowed, and unfamiliar visitors should be limited. Changes in roommates should be minimized.

G. **Anxiety about loss of control**

1. **Symptoms.** Because others must make decisions about the patient's life, illness and hospitalization may be threatening to individuals with strong needs to feel in complete control of their lives and their environment. Patients may attempt to regain control by refusing to comply with the physician's advice, by becoming excessively demanding, by making the physician feel helpless, or by otherwise asserting control over the physician in charge.

2. **Treatment.** Patients should be allowed as much control as possible over their own care. For example, patients' opinions about therapeutic decisions should be solicited, or they could be consulted about medication schedules.

H. **Anxiety about dependency.** Patients who fear loss of control also commonly have anxiety about dependency. Often normal dependency needs were not met in childhood (e.g., because of parental illness or unavailability).

1. **Symptoms.** Extremely strong wishes to be cared for, which have been unchanged since childhood, threaten to break through when the patients are put in a dependent position (e.g., as a result of becoming ill). Because patients are afraid that they will not be able to control dependency needs, the attempts of others to be helpful are rejected, and patients

become hostile toward potential caretakers. Patients also may be noncompliant, fail to keep appointments, or otherwise indicate that they do not need care.

    2. Treatment. When possible, patients should be reassured that the illness and the dependency required by it are temporary. They should be helped to maintain as much independent function as possible.

I. Anxiety about intimacy

    1. Symptoms. Patients with concerns about dependency also may be afraid of becoming too close emotionally to caretakers or loved ones, leading to the maintenance of a greater than normal emotional distance, attempts to ward off (e.g., through hostility) people who are nice or express concern, and distress at expressions of friendliness or intimacy.

    2. Treatment. Intimacy must not be forced on the patients who should be allowed to determine interpersonal distance.

J. Anxiety about being punished

    1. Symptoms. Patients with an underlying sense of guilt about real or imagined transgressions may have a conscious or unconscious expectation of punishment. Patients may attempt to relieve this anxiety by self-inflicted punishment (e.g., through an unhappy marriage, repeated accidents, or alcoholism).

    2. Treatment. The suffering of patients should be acknowledged, and attempts should be made to uncover the source of their guilt. Patients with some insight may benefit from expressive psychotherapy.

K. Signal anxiety

    1. Symptoms. When awareness of a previously unconscious, unresolved psychological conflict is stimulated by some external occurrence (e.g., the patient had mixed feelings about a parent and the patient's age is the same as that of the parent at the time of death), anxiety may signal the emergence of the conflict. This anxiety may call forth **psychological defenses**, which are unconscious mechanisms that keep the conflict out of the patient's awareness.

      a. Repression (forgetting) is an automatic process by which memories, thoughts, and feelings are excluded from the patient's awareness.

      b. Rationalization is explaining away a psychological symptom in order to remain unaware of its cause.

      c. Reaction formation is feeling the opposite of an affect in order to avoid an awareness of it (e.g., experiencing excessive affection toward someone who actually elicits hostility).

      d. Isolation of affect is experiencing the content of a thought without its associated emotions.

      e. Denial is ignoring the emotional significance of an event or the event itself.

    2. Treatment. When it is possible and practical, an attempt to resolve the underlying conflict should be undertaken. Behavioral and adjunctive measures, such as relaxation training, that are useful for control of exogenous anxiety may help to ameliorate signal anxiety.

L. Anxiety about the emergence of another affect.
A problem related to signal anxiety occurs when the patients are threatened by the awareness of an unconscious affect (e.g., depression) that they consider bad or intolerable.

    1. Symptoms. Patients may experience anxiety without a specific cause—mimicking endogenous anxiety. When the underlying mental state is intense or psychotic, defenses that tend to distort reality may be necessary for patients to control it.

      a. Denial is remaining unaware of some aspect of reality (e.g., feeling that one does not have to be afraid of the consequences of an illness because one is not really sick).

      b. Projection is attributing one's own motives to someone else.

      c. Projective identification is incompletely projecting an intense emotional state, which is usually anger, onto another individual while inducing the emotion in the object of the projection through provoking behavior. Patients also experience the original emotion but feel that this is only because they are attempting to protect themselves from the other individual's affect.

    2. Treatment. An attempt to uncover the underlying affect must be made. When patients cannot tolerate an awareness of their motives, they should be helped to develop less disabling defenses against them (e.g., isolation of the affect rather than denial of it).

III. TREATMENT OF ANXIETY

A. Psychotherapy is the most effective treatment for exogenous anxiety and anxiety due to identifiable intrapsychic conflict. It is not effective for panic attacks and phobias. Psychotherapy may be facilitated by medication and behavioral techniques.

    1. Supportive therapy. Psychotherapy that is primarily supportive is useful for acutely ill patients, patients under severe stress, and patients with limited emotional and psychosocial resources (e.g., because of organic mental disease or personality disorders).

        a. Development of defenses. The principal therapeutic approach involves encouraging the development of defenses that are as adaptive as possible; for example:

            (1) Patients with acute myocardial infarction should be helped to minimize the immediate danger since intense fear may contribute to the onset of lethal arrhythmias. When symptoms first appear, however, denial may lead to a fatal delay in seeking medical attention.

            (2) Marginally compensated schizophrenic patients might be encouraged not to pay too much attention to psychotic thoughts that cannot be dealt with constructively by directing their attention to problems in everyday living that can be solved.

        b. Reality testing. The continuous assessment of reality through objective evaluation of the world and one's relationship to it should be encouraged, particularly in patients who tend to distort reality.

        c. Advice should be given, especially when the patient attempts to avoid anxiety through destructive or self-destructive behavior. For example, the patient might be advised to stop attempting to relieve anxiety by arguing with a spouse and to go for a walk instead.

        d. Adaptive behavior by the patient should be reinforced (encouraged).

    2. Expressive psychotherapy. Patients whose anxiety reflects intrapsychic conflicts and who are able to and are interested in understanding themselves may gain more control of their symptoms by learning more about the psychological meaning of the anxiety. Before applying expressive psychotherapy, it is important to assess the ability of the patients to be aware of emotions without acting on them and to handle frustration as well as their willingness and ability to look into themselves. Components of expressive psychotherapy include:

        a. Clarification of the patients' statements in order to make them more comprehensible.

        b. Confrontation of aspects of reality or the patients' emotions that they are ignoring (e.g., "You say that you are not anxious, but you look very nervous").

        c. Interpretation of unconscious thoughts and feelings in order to bring them into the patients' awareness (e.g., "Do you think that you are anxious around your boss because he is so much like your father?").

B. Behavior therapy is very effective for phobias, especially those that develop after a frightening experience (exogenous phobic avoidance).

    1. In systematic desensitization, patients are taught deep muscle relaxation, which is incompatible with anxiety. Situations that cause anxiety are imagined by the patients while relaxed in this way. When these patients can imagine the most anxiety-provoking scene while still feeling relaxed, they will experience much less anxiety in the corresponding real-life situation. In vivo exposure is usually necessary to solidify these gains.

    2. Graduated in vivo exposure involves the patients, usually with a family member, friend, or physician for reassurance, in situations in which they have become increasingly phobic. Systematic desensitization may be necessary first if the patients are too frightened to face the phobic situations.

    3. Adjunctive behavioral techniques may be useful for patients who suffer from any type of anxiety.

        a. Relaxation techniques. Since an individual cannot feel tense and relaxed at the same time, any method that decreases tension tends to relieve anxiety.

        b. Hypnosis is an altered state of consciousness in which the patient is helped to concentrate on calming thoughts, that is, those that do not provoke anxiety. Patients with excessive fear of loss of control or with an organic mental syndrome often cannot be hypnotized.

        c. Biofeedback is a technique that is useful for patients who prefer to learn to relax with a machine or alone. It also has been used to treat migraine and tension headaches and mild essential hypertension. The level of muscular tension, usually in the forearm or frontalis muscles is "fed back" through a visual or auditory stimulus to help patients learn to decrease motor tension and, with it, anxiety.

C. Psychopharmacology. Medication is indicated for the treatment of endogenous anxiety and associated phobias that are complications of panic attacks, not responses to specific trauma or conflict. It is also indicated if a 3-month trial of psychotherapy and behavior therapy for treatment of exogenous anxiety is unsuccessful. Adjunctive use of antianxiety medication may facilitate psychotherapy and behavior therapy in patients with acute stress reactions or chronic anxiety. Conversely, if endogenous anxiety or phobic avoidance are still present after primary drug therapy, behavior therapy should be added to the drug regimen. If complete recovery does not follow appropriate drug therapy, the diagnosis may be incorrect (e.g., the patient may be psychotic or have an organic mental syndrome). However, 30% of chronically anxious patients do not recover.

1. **Benzodiazepines** are the safest and generally most effective antianxiety drugs. They are most useful for acute situational anxiety, anticipatory anxiety associated with panic attacks, and chronic generalized anxiety that is unresponsive to other forms of treatment or that afflicts patients who are unable to resolve the cause of anxiety.

   a. **Uses**

   (1) **Endogenous anxiety.** For the treatment of endogenous anxiety, some clinicians prefer to begin alprazolam (Xanax), a triazolobenzodiazepine, or clonazepam, a benzodiazepine anticonvulsant. Recovery should be apparent after 4 weeks of treatment with a dose of 2–10 mg/day of alprazolam or 1–5 mg/day of clonazepam. If the patient recovers, the medication should be continued for 6–12 months and then gradually discontinued for a drug-free trial. If recovery is not apparent after 4–6 weeks, another medication should be tried (see section III C 2). High doses of other benzodiazepines may be effective for panic disorder.

   (2) **Exogenous anxiety.** All benzodiazepines are commonly prescribed for exogenous anxiety. The benzodiazepine antianxiety drugs differ mainly in their half-lives and potency.

   (a) **Long-acting benzodiazepines** include diazepam (Valium), chlordiazepoxide (Librium), chlorazepate (Tranxene), and prazepam (Centrax). Long-acting preparations can be given less frequently during the day, although they are usually administered at least twice daily to minimize peaks in blood level.

   (b) **Short-acting benzodiazepines** include lorazepam (Ativan) oxazepam (Serax), alprazolam (Xanax), and halazepam (Paxipam). Short-acting drugs must be given more frequently—that is, as often as every 2–3 hours for some patients taking alprazolam. Abstinence syndromes are more severe and abrupt but last a shorter period of time with short-acting benzodiazepines, especially the high-potency preparations.

   (3) **Insomnia.** Benzodiazepines, such as flurazepam (Dalmane), temazepam (Restoril), and triazolam (Halcion), are preferred medications for insomnia. All other benzodiazepines can be used to treat insomnia as well as generalized anxiety.

   b. **Administration.** Benzodiazepines generally should be prescribed for acute exogenous anxiety. The best results are obtained with treatment of time-limited anxiety that occurs in response to clear-cut stress, and treatment ideally should last less than 8 weeks. Occasionally, chronically anxious patients or patients with limited intrapsychic or external resources need long-term therapy.

   c. **Addiction** to benzodiazepines is rare in medical patients. However, individuals with a history of alcohol or drug abuse, physician shopping, and antisocial behavior as well as those who request a specific drug are at high risk.

   d. **Abstinence syndromes** (withdrawal symptoms) may appear up to 10 days after abrupt discontinuation of moderate doses of benzodiazepines that have been taken for more than 1 month. Signs and symptoms of withdrawal include anxiety, insomnia, irritability, and, at times, delirium and seizures. Some patients may experience prolonged attenuated withdrawal symptoms lasting up to a year. Withdrawal is more abrupt and severe after discontinuation of short-acting benzodiazepines.

   e. **Common side effects** include sedation, memory problems, and impaired psychomotor performance. Tolerance develops to the sedative effects but not to the anxiolytic effects or impaired performance. Benzodiazepines may cause or aggravate depression.

2. **Heterocyclic and antidepressant drugs**

   a. **Uses.** All antidepressants except bupropion have been shown to be effective for panic disorder and agoraphobia.

   b. **Administration.** Standard antidepressant doses should be used (e.g., 150–300 mg/day of imipramine or its equivalent). If effective, antidepressants should be continued for 6–12 months before an attempt is made to stop them.

3. MAO inhibitors

  a. Uses
- **(1)** MAO inhibitors are medications that are used to treat atypical depression, depression that does not respond to other drugs, and post-traumatic stress disorder. They may be effective when standard antidepressants do not work.
- **(2)** They may also be effective in relieving endogenous forms of anxiety and phobias when the other medications discussed above are ineffective.

  b. Administration. Phenelzine has been found to improve social phobia. Phenelzine (45–90 mg/day) and tranylcypromine (20–80 mg/day) are used most frequently in the United States. If a MAO inhibitor is effective, it should be continued for 6–12 months, followed by a drug-free trial.

  c. Side effects. MAO inhibitors may produce hypertensive crises when given with a variety of foods and medications and may have a higher incidence of side effects than cyclic antidepressants.

4. Buspirone (Buspar)

  a. Uses. Buspirone is a nonbenzodiazepine azospirodecanedione antianxiety drug that is used for the same indications as the benzodiazepines.

  b. Administration. Buspirone must be given in a divided dose (10–40 mg/day) for a month before it is effective.

  c. Side effects. It does not cause sedation, physical dependence, or abstinence syndromes and does not raise the seizure threshold. It has few clinically important interactions. Since higher doses cause dysphoria, patients do not escalate the dose. Because it is not a central nervous system depressant, it will not suppress withdrawal from benzodiazepines and cannot be directly substituted for them.

5. Barbiturates

  a. Uses. Barbiturates should not be prescribed for anxiety or insomnia except for the very rare patient who has been taking them for years and cannot be withdrawn.

  b. Side effects. Barbiturates (e.g., phenobarbital and secobarbital), propanedioles (e.g., meprobamate) and related compounds (e.g., glutethimide) cause addiction and severe abstinence syndromes and are extremely dangerous if they are taken in overdose.

6. Antihistamines (e.g., hydroxyzine and diphenhydramine) are especially useful as antianxiety drugs and hypnotics for elderly patients and for those in whom addiction may be a problem. They are not as predictably effective as other antianxiety drugs.

7. Neuroleptics (antipsychotic drugs)

  a. Uses
- **(1)** Neuroleptics are indicated for schizophrenia, mania, and psychotic depression.
- **(2)** Low doses of neuroleptics may stabilize some patients with borderline personality disorder.

  b. Side effects. The danger of long-term side effects, especially tardive dyskinesia, precludes long-term administration to nonpsychotic patients.

8. Beta-blocking agents (e.g., propranolol) are indicated for anxiety that is accompanied by signs of adrenergic stimulation. They are not as predictably effective in relieving anxiety as benzodiazepines, however. High doses can diminish assaultiveness in the brain-injured patient. One dose may be useful in relieving stage fright. Atenolol has been shown to reduce social phobia and avoidance in some patients, even though it does not cross the blood–brain barrier.

STUDY QUESTIONS

Directions: Each question below contains five suggested answers. Choose the **one best** response to each question.

1. A patient with endogenous anxiety can become phobic if

(A) the phobic trait is inherited along with the anxiety trait
(B) the patient becomes frightened of situations in which anxiety attacks were experienced
(C) the patient has experienced some sort of environmental stress resulting in phobia
(D) the anxiety attacks symbolize deep-seated conflicts that frighten the patient
(E) the phobias are side effects of drug therapy for endogenous anxiety

2. Before a diagnosis of panic disorder can be made, all of the following conditions must exist EXCEPT

(A) the occurrence of at least three discrete episodes in a 3-week period
(B) the presence of symptoms for at least 1 month
(C) identification of an environmental stressor
(D) onset in early adulthood
(E) the occurrence of spontaneous anxiety attacks

3. An example of a simple phobia is fear of

(A) horses
(B) public transportation
(C) bridges
(D) social situations
(E) crowds

4. Agoraphobia is best characterized by which of the following statements?

(A) It is caused by a specific trauma
(B) It is treated with β-blockers
(C) It involves a fear of heights
(D) It is a symptom of schizophrenia
(E) It commonly accompanies panic attacks

5. *Both* post-traumatic stress disorder and adjustment disorder with anxious mood are characterized by all of the following statements EXCEPT

(A) the disorders can be seen in veterans
(B) impairment of social functioning can occur
(C) the disorders persist long after the stress has abated
(D) obsessive rumination about the stress by patients is common
(E) the disorders may be accompanied by depression

6. A 25-year-old woman who recently had an extramarital affair feels that her physician disapproves strongly of her behavior. This probably represents

(A) denial
(B) repression
(C) reaction formation
(D) isolation
(E) projection

7. Correct statements about diazepam include all of the following EXCEPT

(A) addiction is rare in medical practice
(B) it is an effective treatment for endogenous anxiety in usual doses
(C) it should not be prescribed for more than 6–8 weeks
(D) it is an effective hypnotic
(E) it is an effective sedative

8. Correct statements about buspirone include all of the following EXCEPT

(A) it is not addicting
(B) it has the same indications as the benzodiazepines
(C) it can be substituted directly for benzodiazepines
(D) it has a delayed onset of action
(E) it is given in a divided dose

9. Anxiety is a common symptom of all of the following illnesses EXCEPT

(A) hypoglycemia
(B) hypothyroidism
(C) pheochromocytoma
(D) porphyria
(E) hypocalcemia

10. A patient with endogenous anxiety is most likely to respond to which of the following drugs?

(A) Diazepam
(B) Buspirone
(C) Trifluoperazine
(D) Imipramine
(E) Secobarbital

Directions: Each question below contains four suggested answers of which **one or more** is correct. Choose the answer

A   if **1, 2, and 3** are correct
B   if **1 and 3** are correct
C   if **2 and 4** are correct
D   if **4** is correct
E   if **1, 2, 3, and 4** are correct

11. Correct statements concerning anxiety that arises in the context of an obviously stressful situation include which of the following?

(1) It may result from the stimulation of previously unresolved conflicts
(2) It may respond to antianxiety drugs
(3) It may be of mild to psychotic intensity
(4) It may be accompanied by exogenous anxiety

12. A 30-year old man complains of dizziness, palpitations, feelings of unreality (derealization) and altered states of consciousness that are not associated with any obvious stress. The differential diagnosis should include which of the following conditions?

(1) Partial complex seizures
(2) Depression
(3) Panic disorder
(4) Hypercalcemia

13. A middle-aged man complains of chest pains and palpitations for which careful examination and follow-up reveal no apparent cause. Which of the following symptoms might suggest that his condition is related to anxiety?

(1) Constipation
(2) Feelings of unreality
(3) A conviction of having cancer
(4) Circumoral paresthesias

14. Soon after his admission to the coronary care unit after experiencing his first myocardial infarction, a 45-year-old businessman refuses to be examined by the house officers and demands to see the most senior cardiologist in the hospital immediately. He then insists that his secretary be permitted unrestricted visiting privileges because he has many important business deals that require prompt attention. He adopts a condescending attitude toward the physicians and nurses working with him. Reasonable acute management approaches might include

(1) telling the patient that he is very ill and must cooperate with his physicians or risk serious consequences
(2) restricting visits by the secretary until the patient has recovered
(3) discussing with the patient the impact of the illness on his self-esteem
(4) agreeing that the patient is an important person who needs good care from all concerned

15. Management of a hospitalized patient who becomes hostile whenever his feelings about his illness are questioned or other attempts to get to know him are made might include which of the following approaches?

(1) Telling the patient that his hostility is interfering with the physician–patient relationship
(2) Helping the patient to see that his anger is really due to anxiety
(3) Attempting to behave in a more friendly manner
(4) Allowing the patient to determine the degree of interpersonal distance

SUMMARY OF DIRECTIONS

A	B	C	D	E
1, 2, 3 only	1, 3 only	2, 4 only	4 only	All are correct

16. A 30-year-old chronic schizophrenic individual who is maintained on antipsychotic drugs develops anxiety and increased psychotic symptoms. Approaches to management might include

(1) reality testing
(2) support of defenses
(3) advice
(4) insight therapy

17. A 25-year-old man becomes anxious whenever he must work closely with an authority figure. Which of the following factors should be evaluated to assess his candidacy for expressive psychotherapy?

(1) Frustration tolerance
(2) Social class
(3) Interest in self-awareness
(4) The nature of the conflict

18. Appropriate management of phobias includes which of the following techniques?

(1) Systematic desensitization
(2) Expressive psychotherapy
(3) Monoamine oxidase inhibitor therapy
(4) Biofeedback

19. Correct statements about the use of medication in the treatment of anxious patients include which of the following?

(1) It may improve most forms of endogenous anxiety
(2) It may be adjunctive to the treatment of posttraumatic stress disorder
(3) It may ameliorate phobias
(4) It may undo the effectiveness of psychotherapy

20. A 30-year-old man complains of panic attacks and anticipatory anxiety. Which of the following drugs would be effective treatment for his condition?

(1) Haloperidol
(2) Imipramine
(3) Meprobamate
(4) Diazepam

21. Appropriate indications for propranolol in the treatment of anxiety include

(1) stage fright
(2) panic attacks
(3) sympathetic arousal
(4) phobias

Directions: The group of questions below consists of lettered choices followed by several numbered items. For each numbered item select the **one** lettered choice with which it is **most** closely associated. Each lettered choice may be used once, more than once, or not at all.

Questions 22–26

Match each statement below with the type of medication that it describes.

(A) Benzodiazepines
(B) Antihistamines
(C) Barbiturates
(D) Neuroleptics
(E) Tricyclic and tetracyclic antidepressant drugs

22. These drugs may cause tardive dyskinesia if taken chronically

23. There is low incidence of toxicity, but these drugs are not always effective

24. Addiction rarely occurs with these drugs

25. These drugs are indicated for endogenous anxiety and phobias

26. There is high danger of tolerance, abstinence syndromes, and addiction

ANSWERS AND EXPLANATIONS

1. The answer is B. (*I A 1 e*) Patients with endogenous anxiety become progressively more phobic of situations in which they experienced spontaneous anxiety attacks. Although biologic factors seem to be strongly implicated in spontaneous anxiety attacks and some phobias, there is no evidence that these conditions are inherited together. Phobias that develop after exposure to a frightening situation are called exogenous phobias and are not associated with endogenous anxiety. Patients may become phobic of benign situations that stimulate unconscious conflicts; however, the symbolism of the phobia is usually apparent, and exogenous rather than endogenous anxiety occurs. While psychological therapies are generally ineffective in endogenous anxiety and many phobias, drug treatment often is effective for both of these conditions.

2. The answer is C. (*I A 1, B 1)*) Panic disorders occur spontaneously without a precipitating event and tend to acquire a life of their own independent of psychosocial stressors. Diagnosis of this condition requires that symptoms be present for at least 1 month and that at least three anxiety attacks occur within a 3-week period. Anxiety that begins later in life frequently indicates a covert medical illness, use of central nervous system depressants, or a reaction to an acute stress.

3. The answer is A. (*I B 5 a*) Irrational fear of a situation in which help might not be immediately available or from which escape might be difficult, such as being in crowds, on public transportation, and crossing bridges, are types of agoraphobia. Fear that one will humiliate oneself in certain social situations indicates a social phobia. Simple phobias, such as fear of horses, include fears of any specific circumscribed objects or situations that are not primarily associated with being alone, in public places, or in certain social situations.

4. The answer is E. [*I B 5 a (2)*] Agoraphobia is fear of being away from home in situations in which escape might be difficult or help unavailable if the patient became incapacitated; agoraphobia is usually a complication of panic disorder. Specific traumas produce more circumscribed phobias. Antidepressants, alprazolam, and clonazepam, which ameliorate panic attacks, usually reduce agoraphobia as well. However, systematic desensitization may be necessary to treat residual phobic avoidance.

5. The answer is C. (*I B 4, 6 d*) Post-traumatic stress disorder tends to have a delayed onset and may persist for years after the stress has abated. Although the clinical significance of this syndrome was initially appreciated in veterans, it may develop after any severe stress. A soldier, under the stress of battle, may develop the more acute adjustment disorder, which resolves when the stressful situation ceases. Many patients who become anxious immediately or long after a severe stress tend to become preoccupied with the event in an attempt to master it in their minds. The more severe the symptoms of either disorder, the more likely is impairment of social functioning to result. Patients with acute or delayed stress reactions frequently become depressed.

6. The answer is E. (*II K 1, L 1*) Projection is attributing to others one's own feelings, thoughts, or impulses that are personally unacceptable. Denial involves ignoring elements of external reality, while repression involves forgetting memories, thoughts, and feelings that cause internal conflict. Reaction formation, which involves adopting the opposite attitude or interest of an unconscious psychological state, and isolation, which involves repressing the affect that is associated with the mental state, are defenses that help support repression.

7. The answer is B. (*III C 1*) Alprazolam and antidepressants are more effective treatment for endogenous anxiety than diazepam, which is indicated for the short-term treatment of exogenous anxiety. Diazepam and other benzodiazepines are safe when prescribed appropriately for anxiety and insomnia, although the resulting sedation may bother some patients.

8. The answer is C. (*III C 4*) Buspirone is a new nonbenzodiazepine antianxiety drug that has the same indications as the benzodiazepines. It is not habituating or sedating and has no major interactions. It is given in a divided dose (10–40 mg/day) and may not produce a clinical effect for up to a month. If it is directly substituted for a benzodiazepine, patients may develop a benzodiazepine abstinence syndrome.

9. The answer is B. (*I D 3, 4*) Hypothyroidism is more likely to cause depression than anxiety. Hypocalcemia may produce anxiety accompanied by increased neuromuscular irritability. Anxiety due to hypoglycemia and pheochromocytoma may be accompanied by signs of increased adrenergic activity, such as sweating and tachycardia. Porphyria may produce a variety of psychiatric complaints, including psychosis and anxiety.

10. The answer is D. (*III C 1 a*) The benzodiazepines and buspirone may be used for patients with exogenous anxiety or with anticipatory anxiety with endogenous panic attacks; however, in usual doses, buspirone and the benzodiazepines, except alprazolam and clonazepam, do not usually resolve panic attacks. Antidepressants, such as imipramine, may ameliorate endogenous anxiety or endogenous phobias. Because of the danger of addiction and abstinence syndromes, barbiturates, such as secobarbital and related compounds, should not be prescribed for any form of anxiety or insomnia. Neuroleptics, such as trifluoperazine, may help some anxiety patients who are bothered by sedation; however, they are not specifically useful in endogenous anxiety.

11. The answer is E (all). (*I A 2; II A 1; III C 1*) Although most individuals might suffer in a situation that evokes exogenous anxiety, the subjective meaning of the stress, the way in which the individual has handled similar circumstances in the past, and overall adjustment (i.e., whether the individual has an underlying psychosis or is fundamentally healthy psychologically) determine the extent of the anxiety. Antianxiety drugs are most appropriately used during short-term stresses.

12. The answer is B (1, 3). (*I B 1, C 1, D*) Feelings of unreality, detachment, and light-headedness that may proceed to fainting, along with symptoms of autonomic arousal, often accompany panic attacks. If they are not also markedly anxious, depressed patients usually do not complain of these symptoms. Hypercalcemia causes depression and lethargy; hypocalcemia can cause anxiety and agitation. Partial complex seizures may produce anxiety symptoms along with the symptoms of the seizure disorder.

13. The answer is C (2, 4). (*I C 1, 2, D 1*) Anxious patients may experience feelings of unreality in two different forms: depersonalization (the patient has changed) and derealization (reality has changed). When hyperventilation occurs, light-headedness, paresthesias, and carpopedal spasm may occur. Diarrhea is more common than constipation in anxiety. While preoccupation with heart disease might be understandable in a patient with chest pain, an unrealistic conviction of having cancer is more likely to indicate a delusion.

14. The answer is D (4). (*II D*) An attempt to frighten the patient into submission is likely to increase his fear that his illness will have disastrous consequences, and his attempt to reassure himself through protestations of his importance may increase. Since the patient seems to need his secretary both as an indicator of his importance and possibly as a familiar, reassuring person, restricting his access to her also may increase his panic. Unless the patient gives a clear indication that he wishes to discuss his underlying fears, attempts to uncover his insecurities at this stage may further threaten his fragile sense of self-worth. Support of the patient's attempts to increase his self-esteem, especially while he is acutely ill, is more likely to ensure his compliance and decrease the possible adverse physiologic effects of anxiety on the heart.

15. The answer is D (4). (*II I*) Although a few acutely ill patients who fear closeness may benefit from understanding the reasons for their reactions, most are made more anxious by attempts to decrease interpersonal distance, which include greater friendliness, attempts to understand them too deeply, or attempts by physicians to force themselves on the patient.

16. The answer is A (1, 2, 3). (*III A 1*) Psychotherapy that is primarily supportive is useful to a patient with limited psychosocial resources, such as a schizophrenic. Reality testing, support of adaptive defenses, and advice may help to suppress psychotic anxiety, while patient insight into deeper conflicts may exacerbate the symptoms.

17. The answer is B (1, 3). (*III A 2*) Expressive psychotherapy may be helpful to patients whose unresolved conflicts are stimulated by an external event if these patients can keep themselves from acting on impulses and strong emotions that can be stimulated by this form of treatment and who are interested in gaining self-awareness. Although patients must be willing to make a commitment to treatment, social class and the nature of the conflict (as opposed to the patients' personalities) do not determine the response to therapy.

18. The answer is B (1, 3). (*III B, C*) Systematic desensitization helps the phobic patient feel comfortable in anxiety-provoking situations. Monoamine oxidase inhibitors may be effective drug therapy. Biofeedback is a useful nonspecific technique for reducing anxiety, but it is not particularly helpful in the treatment of phobias. Expressive psychotherapy has not been shown to be effective in treating phobias.

19. The answer is A (1, 2, 3). (*III C*) Alprazolam, antidepressant drugs, and monoamine oxidase (MAO) inhibitors may ameliorate endogenous anxiety and phobias, while MAO inhibitors have been used successfully to treat some patients with post-traumatic stress disorder. When used appropriately, medication facilitates, rather than interferes, with psychotherapy.

20. The answer is C (2, 4). (*III C 1, 2*) Imipramine and similar antidepressant drugs may abort spontaneous panic attacks, while diazepam and related benzodiazepines are helpful for the treatment of the associated anticipatory anxiety. Haloperidol is occasionally helpful to the patient who fears sedation, but it should not be prescribed as the first drug or on a long-term basis. The dangers of addiction and withdrawal preclude the use of meprobamate as an antianxiety drug.

21. The answer is B (1, 3). (*III C 8*) Treatment with propranolol may be helpful when anxiety is accompanied by marked arousal. Propranolol may also ameliorate stage fright when it is taken shortly before a performance. Panic attacks and phobias should be treated with alprazolam, antidepressants, or monoamine oxidase inhibitors.

22–26. The answers are: 22-D, 23-B, 24-A, 25-E, 26-C. (*III C*) Recent evidence indicates that few medical patients become addicted to benzodiazepines when the drugs are prescribed appropriately. Barbiturates, on the other hand, tend to cause tolerance, abstinence syndromes, and addiction. Antihistamines can be particularly useful as antianxiety drugs or hypnotics in the elderly, but they are not as predictably effective as other medications and may cause anticholinergic side effects. In low doses, nonsedating neuroleptics (antipsychotic drugs) may help to relieve anxiety in patients who fear sedation, but the danger of tardive dyskinesia must not be ignored. Antidepressants may be very effective in the treatment of endogenous anxiety and phobias.

7
Somatoform Disorders

Janice L. Petersen

I. INTRODUCTION

A. Theories concerning psychological factors that affect physical conditions. The extent to which psychological factors contribute to medical disorders is indicated by the term "psychological factors affecting physical conditions." This term is preferred to the terms "psychosomatic" and "psychophysiologic" disorders, which are no longer accurate. Disorders with a demonstrable organic pathology are differentiated from somatoform disorders, which present with physical symptoms with no known physiologic abnormalities. One-third of all patients seen by physicians have a mixture of psychological and physical distress, and these psychological problems are thought to contribute to the medical disorder in some causal way.

1. **Specificity theory.** The theory of emotional specificity (i.e., the physiologic expression of blocked emotions) has led to personality studies of patients with peptic ulcers, coronary artery disease, and cancer. Although these studies have lent some support to the theory, it has, in general, lost favor as a comprehensive explanation.
   a. **Freud** and his followers studied somatic involvement in psychological conflict and were particularly interested in **conversion reactions**, in which a psychological problem is symbolically manifested physically, although physiologic tissue damage cannot be demonstrated.
   b. **Dunbar** suggested that **specific conscious personality traits** cause specific psychosomatic diseases.
   c. **Alexander** theorized that **specific unconscious conflicts** cause specific illnesses in organs innervated by the autonomic nervous system. This occurs because prolonged tension can produce physiologic disorders, leading to eventual pathology. He also believed that there are constitutional predisposing factors involved. Alexander's theory led to the concept of the classic psychosomatic diseases, including:
      (1) Bronchial asthma
      (2) Rheumatoid arthritis
      (3) Ulcerative colitis
      (4) Essential hypertension
      (5) Neurodermatitis
      (6) Thyrotoxicosis
      (7) Duodenal peptic ulcer

2. **Nonspecificity theory.** Whatever event is perceived by the patient as stressful can produce **stress**, whether this event is the death of a loved one, divorce, financial loss, or illness. Psychological reactions to stress can lead to a failure of adaptive physiologic responses, which can lead to a **nonspecific cause of disease**. Hormones, especially cortisol, are released in response to stress and act on different organs to produce a variety of changes.
   a. **Neurophysiologic reactions** to stress activate the pituitary–adrenal axis and are known as the **general adaptation syndrome**. The nonspecific systemic reactions of the body to stress include:
      (1) **Alarm reaction** (shock)
      (2) **Resistance** (adaptation to stress)
      (3) **Exhaustion** (resistance to prolonged stress cannot be maintained)
   b. **Physiologic reactions** to stress include the following:
      (1) **Fight–flight response** is arousal of the sympathetic nervous system, resulting in increased production of epinephrine and norepinephrine with an increase in pulse and muscle tension. When an affected individual can neither fight nor flee, this

state of arousal can lead to organic dysfunction.

  (2) **Withdrawal–conservation.** Engel and coworkers showed that when an individual is threatened with loss (real or imagined), the metabolism can slow down. The individual withdraws, which has the effect of conserving energy. Pulse and body temperature decrease, and the individual may become susceptible to illness, particularly infection. Studies on the psychophysiologic effects of bereavement support this hypothesis: Morbidity and mortality rates are higher during the first year after death of a spouse in a bereaved group compared to those rates in an age-controlled nonbereaved group. The theory of withdrawal–conservation may also explain sudden death from hexes and curses.

B. Major illnesses with psychological factors

  1. **Gastrointestinal disorders.** Emotional states have long been known to cause a reaction in the gastrointestinal tract. Vague complaints of nausea, indigestion, diarrhea, constipation, and abdominal pain are common.
    a. **Peptic ulcers**
      (1) **Etiology.** Gastric, duodenal, and acute post-traumatic stress ulcers all have different etiologies. The Mirsky study of army recruits showed that several factors are necessary for the development of ulcers, including high stress, the constitutional factor of high pepsinogen secretion, and psychological (dependency) conflict. Although conflicts involving dependency are noticeable in ulcer patients, not all individuals affected by these conflicts are prone to developing ulcers.
      (2) **Treatment.** Patients who comply with good medical management do not usually require psychotherapy. The physician should help the patient identify those areas of life that seem to cause stress. Also, it may be useful to teach the patient relaxation techniques, in which an individual tenses all of his or her muscles and then relaxes them in groups (e.g., arms, hands, legs, and feet), notes the resultant feeling, and practices the technique. Antianxiety agents are occasionally indicated along with antispasmodics.
    b. **Ulcerative colitis**
      (1) **Etiology.** A large proportion of familial occurrence of ulcerative colitis would suggest a genetic cause; however, the exact etiology is unknown. It has been demonstrated clearly that exacerbation of ulcerative colitis is associated with psychological stress and remission is associated with psychological support. Stress, such as unresolved grief on the anniversary of a death, can precipitate the disorder. Associated psychological features include:
        (a) Immaturity
        (b) Indecisiveness
        (c) Conscientiousness
        (d) Covertly demanding behavior
        (e) Fear of loss of an important individual
      (2) **Treatment.** Although psychotherapy cannot guarantee that the condition will not recur, it is useful when it is focused on helping patients develop mature ways of expressing needs as well as helping them deal with any unresolved losses.
    c. **Irritable bowel syndrome** (also termed spastic colon and nervous diarrhea) is disordered bowel motility, including both hyper- and hypomotility.
      (1) **Etiology.** Although the syndrome is usually associated with environmental stress, patients tend to have other psychological symptoms, such as anxiety and depression.
      (2) **Treatment.** Brief psychotherapy to help the patient identify environmental stress and to effect changes where possible usually aids in decreasing symptoms. Tricyclic antidepressants have also been found to be effective in this disorder.

  2. **Cardiovascular disorders.** There is much evidence that the cardiovascular system reacts to the emotional state of the patient.
    a. **Coronary artery disease** is by far the most common cause of death in the United States.
      (1) **Etiology.** Multiple nonpsychiatric elements are implicated in the development of coronary artery disease, including genetics, diet, smoking, high blood pressure, obesity, and amount of physical activity. A personality type has also been implicated, according to some studies. The **type A behavior pattern** is only one risk factor out of many, and its exact role in the development of coronary artery disease is unclear, although men who fall into this type of behavior pattern are at twice the risk for coronary artery disease as those who do not. Characteristics of the type A personality include:
        (a) Competitiveness
        (b) Ambition

(c) Drive for success
(d) Impatience
(e) A sense of time urgency
(f) Abruptness of speech and gesture
(g) Hostility

(2) Treatment. Behavioral methods designed to decrease environmental stress and modify life-style when mutable are increasingly common.

b. Essential hypertension

(1) Etiology. The causes of essential hypertension are unknown, but psychological factors were initially thought to involve conflicts between passive–dependent and aggressive tendencies in patients who repressed their hostility. Unfortunately, there is no reliable evidence to support this theory. On the other hand, a common reaction to stress is an elevation of blood pressure. Patients who have a biologic susceptibility to essential hypertension may react to a stressful situation by exacerbating that hypertension rather than, for instance, increasing gastrointestinal motility.

(2) Treatment of hypertension may involve biofeedback, in which the patient is attached to a machine that provides information about ordinarily unnoticed biologic parameters; for example, a tone sounds when the patient's blood pressure goes up, and the patient learns to relax to decrease the tone as well as the blood pressure. Biofeedback therapy, however, tends not to be long lasting and must be repeated to maintain the effect.

c. Arrhythmias

(1) Etiology. Even in the absence of heart disease, psychological factors can influence the normal rhythm of the heart beat. **Stress** may cause arrhythmias by arousal of the sympathetic nervous system (as is evident in the fight–flight reaction). Sinus tachycardia, a paroxysmal atrial tachycardia (PAT), and ventricular ectopic beats are the most common arrhythmias to arise in reaction to stress. These reactions may be more common in patients who are already fearful of heart disease.

(2) Treatment involves questioning the patient about unreasonable fears of heart disease and helping the patient identify environmental stresses that precipitate the reaction. The condition may be part of an anxiety disorder, which should be treated. Benzodiazepines may be useful for a limited time as may blocking agents, such as propranolol.

3. Respiratory disorders. Changes in respiration in the normal individual may correspond to an emotional state (e.g., the sigh of boredom and the gasp of surprise). The strongest psychological reactions associated with respiratory disease, however, are those that develop secondary to the illness. The panic associated with shortness of breath can be quite disabling.

a. Hyperventilation syndrome

(1) Etiology. This disorder is often associated with **anxiety** (see Chapter 6, "Anxiety Disorders"), which may cause an increased depth or rate of breathing. In turn, this leads to **respiratory alkalosis** and then to lightheadedness, paresthesias, and carpopedal spasms. These symptoms increase the anxiety in the patient, resulting in a vicious circle of increased hyperventilation and respiratory alkalosis.

(2) Treatment. Educating the patient about the syndrome once the acute event is past may be sufficient treatment; however, if underlying anxieties continue to provoke the syndrome, psychotherapy is indicated. If the patient meets the criteria for panic disorder, pharmacotherapy can be considered as well.

b. Bronchial asthma

(1) Etiology. Once thought to be caused by psychological factors, asthma attacks now are believed to be the result of a genetic vulnerability exacerbated by allergies and infections. Nevertheless, stress and an ambivalent relationship between the asthmatic child and an overly protective mother may be a factor in the onset. Both overly dependent patients who react to any slight changes of symptoms and overly independent patients who deny symptoms are at greater risk for hospitalization than are psychologically normal patients.

(2) Treatment. Psychotherapy is usually indicated when anxiety, which may precipitate an asthma attack, is not relieved by the supportive care of a physician. Family therapy may be helpful in separation issues, which may also exacerbate asthma symptoms.

4. Migraine headache

a. Etiology. Over 90% of chronic, recurrent headaches are either migraine, tension, or mixed migraine–tension. Although anxiety and stress commonly precipitate all three types of headache, the theory that specific psychological dynamics, such as repressed hostility, lead to migraine headaches has not been proven. Depression should be ruled out as a cause and treated if present.

    b. Treatment of migraine headache includes:
       (1) Drug therapy
         (a) Ergotamine
         (b) Propranolol
         (c) Tricyclic antidepressants
         (d) Calciuim channel blockers (verapamil)
       (2) Biofeedback
       (3) Psychotherapy in cases where stresses are chronic

  5. Immune disorders. Psychological states affect immune response in complex, not yet fully understood, ways. Stress may depress cell-mediated (via T lymphocytes) immune response. It also affects neuroendocrine systems; for example, some depressed patients have increased levels of corticosteroids and do not suppress the production of these when challenged with dexamethasone (cortisol levels are normally lower following dexamethasone administration). Disorders of immune response may involve susceptibility to the following:
    a. Autoimmune diseases, including:
       (1) Systemic lupus erythematosus
       (2) Rheumatoid arthritis
       (3) Pernicious anemia
    b. Allergic disorders
    c. Cancer. Studies show that the patient who reacts to stress with feelings of hopelessness or depression is at higher risk for cancer.

II. SOMATOFORM DISORDERS, including somatization, conversion, somatoform pain disorder, hypochondriasis, and body dysmorphic disorder present with physical symptoms; however, no clear physical etiology can be demonstrated. The symptoms of somatoform disorders are not under voluntary control nor is the patient aware of possible gains derived.

  A. Somatization disorder

    1. Clinical presentation. This disorder presents with a history of recurrent multiple physical complaints of several years' duration, beginning before the age of 30 years, generally in adolescence. The description of the symptoms may often be vague, but the presentation is often dramatic. The *Diagnostic and Statistical Manual of Mental Disorders*, 3rd ed., revised (*DSM-III-R*) requires complaints of at least 13 of the 35 listed symptoms for the diagnosis. These symptoms involve complaints in many organ systems, including:
      a. Conversion symptoms
        (1) Paralysis or weakness
        (2) Seizures
        (3) Urine retention and difficulty in urinating
        (4) Difficulty in swallowing
        (5) Blurred vision and double vision
        (6) Blindness
        (7) Fainting or other loss of consciousness
        (8) Loss of voice
        (9) Stiffness
      b. Menstrual symptoms
        (1) Pain
        (2) Irregularity
        (3) Excessive bleeding
      c. Gastrointestinal symptoms
        (1) Nausea and vomiting
        (2) Abdominal pain
        (3) Diarrhea
        (4) Bloating
        (5) Food intolerance
      d. Pain, usually ill-defined in:
        (1) Various joints
        (2) The back
        (3) Extremities
        (4) Urination

e. Psychosexual symptoms
   (1) Lack of sexual drive
   (2) Lack of pleasure during intercourse
   (3) Pain during intercourse
f. Cardiopulmonary symptoms
   (1) Shortness of breath
   (2) Palpitations
   (3) Chest pains
   (4) Dizziness

2. **Epidemiology.** Approximately 1% of women have somatization disorder, and the ratio of women to men is 10:1. It is thought to be less common in individuals with higher education.

3. **Etiology**
   a. Recent studies suggest that there is a significant genetic component to somatization disorder. It has been linked to a high incidence of:
      (1) Alcoholism in first-degree male relatives
      (2) Sociopathy in first-degree male relatives
      (3) Somatization disorder in first-degree female relatives
   b. Adoption studies of female children of somatizing women showed a markedly increased rate of somatization disorder compared to control groups.
   c. Environmental influences are suggested by an increased rate of somatization disorder when the child is raised in chaotic circumstances, involving parental divorce, poverty, and alcoholism.
   d. Evidence of dysfunction on neuropsychiatric tests has led some investigators to hypothesize that patients have an impaired ability to screen out somatic sensations.
   e. Secondary gains of the sick role may provide a learned component of the disorder.

4. **Complications**
   a. Excessive medical evaluations due to frequent consultation with multiple physicians
   b. Unnecessary invasive diagnostic procedures and surgery
   c. Anxiety and depressive symptoms, which are common in this population
   d. A wide range of associated interpersonal difficulties, including marital and parenting problems
   e. Substance abuse, including prescribed medications
   f. Suicidal ideation, particularly in patients with substance abuse problems and depression

5. **Differential diagnosis** of somatization disorder is discussed in section II F.

6. **Treatment** of somatization disorder is often frustrating for the physician. Physicians should expect and accept their own feelings of frustration and anger when managing this condition. This disorder is best conceptualized as a lifelong character style rather than a curable condition. Symptoms tend to fluctuate with stress in the patient's life. General principles of treatment include:
   a. Regular appointments so that the patient is assured of an ongoing supportive relationship with the physician, focusing on life stresses and the patient's functioning rather than symptoms. Recent studies have shown that supportive treatment reduces utilization of health services, such as emergency room visits, hospital days, and physician charges.
   b. Consolidation of care with one physician to minimize medications and diagnostic evaluations
   c. Avoidance of unnecessary surgery. Surgical procedures should be considered only for clear indications. The physician should thoughtfully consider the expected gains as compared to the potential complications.
   d. Avoidance of habit-forming medications and little or no medications for questionable indications
   e. Appropriate evaluation of new symptoms when they do occur as patients with somatization disorder are still at risk for organic illness

B. Conversion disorder (Table 7-1)

1. **Clinical presentation**
   a. Associated features. Conversion disorder involves the unconscious "conversion" of a psychological conflict into a loss of physical functioning, which suggests a neurologic disease. The symptom is temporally related to a psychosocial stressor.
      (1) An additional psychiatric diagnosis can be made in 30%–50% of patients, such as adjustment disorder, schizophrenia, and personality disorder.

Table 7-1. The Five S's of Conversion Disorder

Stress
The formation of a symptom helps the patient deal with a psychological stress or an acute conflict.

Sensory-Motor Symptoms (Special Senses)
The symptoms that develop are, by definition, pseudoneurologic. These include blindness, paralysis, paresthesias, and seizures.

Significant Other
The patient identifies with someone who has a similar symptom, which is due to an organic neurologic illness.

Secondary Gains
Most illnesses have secondary gains; for example, the patient is cared for by others and may avoid unpleasant duties.

Symbolic Nature of Symptom
Although the symptom may be symbolic (e.g., an arm becomes paralyzed because the patient has an unconscious wish to strike out), symbolism may be difficult to uncover.

---

    (2) Conversion disorders are also seen in cases in which there is real organic physical illness; for example, a patient with seizures may also have conversion seizure disorder.

    (3) "La belle indifference" in which the patient exhibits little concern over the symptoms is sometimes present; however, it is not a reliable sign of conversion alone since a patient with a physical illness may be stoic about his or her condition.

    (4) Modeling is common; that is, patients may unconsciously imitate the symptoms observed in important individuals in their lives.

  b. Symptoms. While most conversion symptoms are transient, some can have a chronic course and result in significant disability. Also, symptoms may be inconsistent with known pathophysiology, such as a stocking–glove anesthesia. The patient classically presents with an acute loss of function, which suggests neurologic disease. Symptoms may be bizarre or unusual, including:

    (1) Paresthesias and anesthesias
    (2) Gait disturbances (e.g., astasia and abasia)
    (3) Paralysis
    (4) Loss of consciousness and seizures
    (5) Aphonia
    (6) Vomiting
    (7) Fainting
    (8) Visual disturbances (e.g., blindness and tunnel vision)

2. Incidence and prevalence are not known with certainty; however, conversion disorder seems to be less common now than in the past, and it may present with less classic symptomatology than was seen previously. Conversion disorder is seen more frequently in low socioeconomic classes, and most cases are found on neurology wards. Although the disorder occurs more commonly in women, it is seen in men. Usually onset is in adolescence through the twenties; however, it can occur at any age.

3. Etiology is thought to be psychological.

  a. Two mechanisms have been described that explain the gains experienced by the patient in conversion disorder.

    (1) The primary gain is that the internal conflict is kept from consciousness. Stress from the external environment stimulates internal conflict, and the symptoms of the disorder symbolize this conflict (e.g., paralysis of the arm stops the patient from striking out).

    (2) The secondary gain is reinforcement from the environment, such as the patient avoiding unpleasant duties because of the symptoms. Some secondary gain is seen in almost all illnesses, however.

  b. Other etiologies that have been postulated include the following:

    (1) The less powerful individual gains control over his or her environment by the elaboration of symptoms (i.e., the concern and attention of others are focused on the patient).

(2) The symptoms are learned and are then reinforced by the reactions of those around the patient.

(3) For some patients, physiologic contributions are suggested by the fact that the symptoms are seen more frequently in patients with brain injuries and other neurologic defects.

4. Differential diagnosis. It is important to note that 15%–30% of patients diagnosed as having conversion disorder have an undiagnosed physical illness, such as multiple sclerosis and other neurologic conditions.

5. Prognosis. A good prognosis is associated with:
  a. Good premorbid functioning
  b. Acute onset
  c. An obvious stressful precipitant
  d. The absence of other forms of psychopathology

6. Treatment
  a. Stressful events in the patient's life should be evaluated and appropriate intervention made, such as psychotherapy or marital or family therapy. Associated psychiatric illness, such as depression, should be treated, which may involve pharmacologic approaches.
  b. Confronting the patient with the fact that the symptoms are psychologically based is not helpful. While some patients come to understand the symbolic aspect of the symptom and gain conscious mastery of the conflict, most patients are receptive to the explanation that the disorder is a reaction to stress and to reassurance that the condition will resolve over time. These interventions may allow the patient to let go of symptoms without losing face.
  c. Suggestion during hypnosis or an amobarbital (Amytal) interview that the symptoms will improve can result in dramatic resolution.

C. Somatoform pain disorder

  1. Clinical presentation. The patient complains of pain for which there is no demonstrable physical cause or that is excessive given the known organic pathology. Generally, this disorder results in significant impairment and inability to function.
  a. To qualify for this diagnosis, the symptom must be present for at least 6-months.
  b. In some cases, psychological factors appear to play a role in the symptoms, such as:
    (1) Secondary gain due to financial compensation
    (2) Avoidance of objectionable work
    (3) Control of significant others
  c. In other cases, there is little indication of psychological factors.
  d. Most cases of chronic pain involve both physical and psychological contributions, which can lead to:
    (1) Problems with the physician–patient relationship
    (2) Multiple physical examinations
    (3) Unnecessary surgery
    (4) Substance abuse

  2. Incidence and prevalence are unknown; however, it is a common condition in a primary care setting. The disorder occurs more frequently in women than in men.

  3. Etiology
  a. Psychological factors
    (1) Patients may have learned as children to express emotions physically instead of verbally.
    (2) Patients may be unconsciously reinforced by the sick role.
    (3) When compensation for injury is an issue, patients may be consciously or unconsciously reinforced for illness behavior.
    (4) Many patients report histories of deprivation, neglect, or abuse, which may make them more vulnerable as adults.
    (5) Many patients have a history of working at an early age, holding physically demanding jobs, and centering their lives around work.
  b. Physical theories
    (1) Endogenous opiate substances (endorphins) in the brain, which raise pain threshold, may be altered either genetically, developmentally, or secondarily to stress, making these individuals more prone to continued pain.
    (2) Monoamine neurotransmitters (particularly serotonin) appear to be involved in pain inhibitory fibers in the brain stem. This neurotransmitter system may be altered

genetically, developmentally, or secondarily to stress, resulting in continued pain perception. This hypothesis is supported by the responsiveness of this disorder to tricyclic antidepressants.

(3) A possible genetic component to this disorder is suggested by the increased incidence of first-degree relatives with:
   (a) Chronic pain
   (b) Depression
   (c) Alcohol dependence

4. **Differential diagnosis** is discussed in section II E. This disorder requires a thorough diagnostic workup to rule out organic pathology. Other disorders to be ruled out are hypochondriasis, somatization, depression with somatic symptoms, and schizophrenia. When secondary gain is evident, such as financial compensation, conscious simulation of the pain symptom (**malingering**) must be considered. Also, personality and cultural attributes must be taken into consideration; for example, an overly dramatic, histrionic presentation of organic pain should not be confused with somatoform pain disorder.

5. **Prognosis**
   a. **Duration of illness.** The longer the duration, the less likely the chance of functional recovery. Very few patients with chronic pain of greater than 5 years duration improve.
   b. **Age.** The older the patient, the less likely the chance of recovery.
   c. **Secondary gain.** The more reinforcement—financial, social, or otherwise—for the symptom, the less likely the chance of recovery.
   d. **Co-existing personality disorder** is also a negative prognostic factor.

6. **Treatment.** This condition is notoriously difficult to treat, and although many patients can make significant improvements in functioning, few are cured.
   a. **Medications**
      (1) **Chronic narcotic use**, paradoxically, is not helpful in chronic pain because the patient becomes habituated to the narcotics, resulting in a loss of the analgesic effect and a vulnerability to withdrawal symptoms. Because of the peaks and valleys of short-acting narcotic blood levels, these agents can actually exacerbate chronic pain symptoms. Detoxification can result in improvement in pain symptoms. For a minority of chronic pain patients who appear to require chronic narcotic treatment, a long-acting preparation, such as methadone, is preferable.
      (2) **Sedative-hypnotics** depress the nervous system and increase pain perceptions as well as inactivity. Thus, they should be avoided.
      (3) **Antidepressants.** Fifty to sixty percent of patients report an improvement in sleep, sense of well-being, and pain perception with tricyclic antidepressants. These effects occur shortly after starting treatment and on lower doses (50–100 mg) than required for the treatment of depression. Responsiveness to antidepressants is independent of overt symptoms of depression.
   b. **Therapy**
      (1) **Psychotherapy.** Supportive approaches are useful in helping the patient deal with life stresses that may exacerbate pain symptoms.
      (2) **Behavioral therapy** focuses on reinforcing wellness instead of sick role behavior. Although this approach may not affect the patient's perception of pain, it is effective in improving the patient's level of functioning.
      (3) **Family therapy** is a useful adjunctive approach when family dynamics reinforce the patient's sick role and undermine attempts to improve functional capacity.
      (4) **Group therapy**, where available, is a useful adjunct in supporting the patient's efforts to improve functional capacity.
   c. **Multidisciplinary approaches**, which are usually available in pain clinic settings, allow a comprehensive treatment plan, which may be necessary for some patients to maximize their functioning. It may involve the above-mentioned strategies as well as:
      (1) Physical therapy
      (2) Occupational therapy
      (3) Biofeedback training
      (4) Relaxation techniques

D. Hypochondriasis

1. **Clinical presentation.** Patients are chronically preoccupied with fears that they have an illness despite thorough evaluation and reassurance from the physician that no organic problems can be found.

    a. Normal physical sensations, such as sweating and bowel movements, are misinterpreted, and minor ailments, such as cough or backache, are exaggerated.

    b. "Physician shopping" is common and is a frustration for both the patient and physician.

    c. Anxious and depressed mood, as well as obsessive–compulsive features are commonly observed.

    d. Impairment can be mild or so severe as to result in invalidism.

    e. In general, these patients do not accept the idea that this is a psychiatric disorder.

2. Incidence and prevalence

    a. As many as 1% of the population may be hypochondriacal, and it is commonly seen in medical practice. Equal numbers of men and women are affected.

    b. Usual age of onset is 20–30 years of age, but patients most commonly present to the physician in their forties and fifties.

3. Etiology. Psychological theories focus on possible developmental contributions. Patients with this disorder may have been raised in homes where there was excessive concern about illness or where there was little parental warmth except when the child was ill. The patient may be unable to express emotion in other than physical terms.

4. Differential diagnosis. Other conditions that must be ruled out are:

    a. Depression

    b. Panic attacks

    c. Schizophrenia

5. Treatment

    a. Physician reaction to hypochondriacal patients is often negative. If the physician is unaware of such feelings, he or she may act on them in an antitherapeutic way, such as overprescribing medication or performing unnecessary diagnostic procedures.

    b. It is not helpful to tell the patient that his or her problems are psychologically caused. The fact that the patient is concerned and desires assistance should be acknowledged early in treatment. Regular follow-up appointments legitimize the patient's need to be sick.

    c. It may be necessary to prescribe medication; however, the patient should be told that it will only help and not "cure" the ailment. Narcotics and other habit-forming drugs should not be prescribed in order to preclude addiction.

E. Body dysmorphic disorder

1. Clinical presentation. The hallmark of this disorder is preoccupation with some imagined defect in the body, usually of the face. There is usually a history of frequent visits to doctors, especially dermatologists or plastic surgeons. Depressive mood and obsessive–compulsive traits are common.

2. Incidence and etiology are unknown.

3. Differential diagnosis

    a. If the symptom is of delusional intensity, it should be classified as a delusional disorder, somatic subtype—a disorder that may be responsive to antipsychotic medication.

    b. Major depression and schizophrenia should be ruled out.

4. Treatment

    a. Invasive diagnostic procedures or unnecessary surgery should be avoided.

    b. There are few data on the treatment of this disorder, but empirical approaches involving tricyclic antidepressants, antipsychotic agents, and psychotherapy can be considered.

F. Differential diagnosis of the somatoform disorders. The possibility exists in all of the somatoform disorders that the patient may have an undiagnosed physical disorder with inconsistent, vague, or confusing symptoms. Several illnesses should be considered.

1. Systemic lupus erythematosus is associated with multiple organ systems and is characterized by exacerbation and remissions. The illness begins in late adolescence or the early twenties, and women are nine times more likely to have systemic lupus erythematosus than men. The onset may be vague, and psychiatric symptoms, such as mood disorders and even schizophreniform disorder, may be present.

2. Endocrine disorders

    a. Hyperthyroidism (thyrotoxicosis) may be present with complaints of fatigue, palpitations, dyspnea, and anxiety.

    b. Hypothyroidism also may present with fatigue and anxiety. Mood disorders, including depression, are possible. Menstrual problems are commonly seen and may be dismissed as a somatization problem.

   c. Hyperparathyroidism may present with severe anxiety, gastrointestinal symptoms, polyuria, and some pain.

3. Neurologic disorders. Any physical illness that begins early in life and that is associated with an insidious or intermittent onset of symptoms should be considered in the differential diagnosis of a somatoform disorder.

   a. Multiple sclerosis may have transient, remitting neurologic symptoms associated with dysphoric mood and anxiety and often is misdiagnosed as a psychiatric illness early in its course.

   b. Temporal lobe or **complex partial seizures** may cause a distorted body image as well as mood disorders and changes in personality.

   c. Acute intermittent porphyria is rare, but it may mimic somatization disorder with its gastrointestinal pain and neurologic complaints.

4. Psychiatric disorders

   a. Acute adjustment reactions can present with multiple vague somatic symptoms or preoccupation with symptoms.

   b. Schizophrenia occasionally presents with multiple somatic complaints or delusions.

   c. Major depression can present with multiple somatic complaints as well as delusions about dying, rotting inside, or other morbid apprehensions.

   d. Panic disorders can present with multiple somatic complaints and extreme preoccupation with symptoms.

   e. Personality disorders frequently co-exist with somatoform disorder and should be discriminated.

III. FACTITIOUS DISORDER

A. Clinical presentation. Patients are in voluntary control of their symptoms of physical illness in that, although their behavior is deliberate, what precipitates this behavior is not.

1. Symptoms may range from complaints of pain when patients feel no pain to self-inflicted infection, such as that arising from self-injection with feces or saliva, which can develop into life-threatening illness. The medical knowledge of patients is often highly sophisticated, and by complaining of bizarre or unusual symptoms, they may encourage invasive diagnostic procedures, such as laparotomy and angiography. Patients may lie about any aspect of their history with a dramatic flair (**pseudologia fantastica**). Narcotic abuse and addiction are associated findings in about one-half of these patients.

2. History. Upon hospital admission, patient behavior is disruptive and demanding. Symptoms change as workups prove negative. Eventually, patients are confronted with evidence of faking, and they usually react angrily and leave against medical advice. This pattern of behavior can become chronic and involve multiple admissions to different hospitals, and it is then called **Munchausen syndrome**. Other names for factitious disorder with physical symptoms include the following:

   a. Polysurgical addiction

   b. Hospital hoboes

   c. Hospital addiction

B. Incidence and prevalence. The disorder may seem to be more common than it actually is because a single patient may interact with many physicians in different hospitals. It usually begins in adult life and is a lifelong condition.

C. Etiology. Although an illness or operation in early childhood may be a contributing factor, the disorder is considered to be entirely psychological. There may have been an experience with a physician in early life either through a family relationship or through illness. A significant proportion of these patients are employed in the health care field as paraprofessionals. Masochism has been considered to be an important feature in a patient who seeks unnecessary surgery. The illness has also been conceptualized as a variant of the borderline syndrome in that the physician becomes the perpetual object of transference; the patient continually re-enacts with the physician the disordered relationship with his or her parents.

D. Differential diagnosis

1. Physical illness. A patient with a true physical disorder may present symptoms with an unusual or dramatic flair, which makes the physician suspicious of faking and which is more

likely to occur if the patient also has a personality disorder, including one of the following types:
   a. Histrionic
   b. Borderline
   c. Schizotypal

   2. Somatization disorder. The symptoms are not under the patient's voluntary control, and
   the patient does not usually insist on hospitalization. Conversion disorder also may be
   present.

   3. Hypochondriasis. The essential feature of this disorder is the patient's preoccupation with
   illness in general rather than symptoms. The symptoms are not under the voluntary control
   of the patient. Hypochondriasis starts later in life than factitious disorder, and the patient
   is less likely to insist on hospital admission or submit to dangerous diagnostic procedures.

   4. Malingering. Although it is difficult to differentiate malingering from factitious disorder,
   the goals in malingering are clear to both patient and physician, and the symptoms can be
   stopped when they no longer serve an end (Table 7-2).

E. Treatment. A patient with factitious disorder with physical symptoms rarely receives psychiatric
treatment. The physician's reactions are usually strongly negative, which also prevents psychiatric evaluation. Until the patient is willing to face the fact that he or she has a psychiatric
illness and agrees to psychiatric hospitalization or treatment, the prognosis is likely to be poor.
The approach to the patient is one of management rather than cure, and unnecessary diagnostic procedures should be avoided. The patient should be confronted in a calm, non-
condemning manner, and the cost of the illness emotionally as well as financially should be
discussed.

IV. MALINGERING

A. Clinical presentation. Malingering is not considered a mental disorder. Malingering individuals
willfully and deliberately fake or exaggerate illness with the conscious intent to deceive others.
Their reasons for faking illness (e.g., monetary and legal concerns) can be understood by
examining the circumstances affecting these individuals rather than their psychological make-
up. Individuals are often evasive and uncooperative upon examination, and there is a marked
discrepancy between their claimed disability and the physical findings. Individuals who
malinger may have an antisocial personality disorder (see Chapter 11, "Personality Disorders").

B. Incidence and prevalence. True malingering is rarely seen. A physician is more likely to diagnose this condition incorrectly in a patient with one of the somatoform disorders because of
a negative reaction to the patient and the inability to see that another disorder, such as hypochondriasis, is not consciously faked by the patient.

C. Differential diagnosis. In **factitious disorder** with physical symptoms, the goals of the patient
cannot be clearly understood, as they can in the case of malingering, even though the patient
is voluntarily causing the symptoms of illness.

D. Treatment. Since **malingering is not an illness**, there is no medical or psychiatric treatment.

V. PLACEBO RESPONSE has been defined as any effect attributable to a medication, procedure,
or other form of therapy but not to the specific pharmacologic property of that therapy. For
instance, 30%–40% of patients in pain respond equally well to placebos as to morphine. There
is no particular personality type that responds to a placebo (e.g., a histrionic patient is no more
likely to have a placebo response than is any other patient). Physicians use the placebo response

Table 7-2. Patient Control of Symptoms

Illness	Control of Symptoms	Motive
Somatization disorder	Involuntary	Unconscious
Conversion disorder	Involuntary	Unconscious
Psychogenic pain disorder	Involuntary	Unconscious
Hypochondriasis	Involuntary	Unconscious
Factitious disorder	Voluntary	Unconscious
Malingering	Voluntary	Conscious

(mistakenly) to help differentiate "real" from "psychological" symptoms in their patients. The placebo response is a powerful aspect of most medical care. It operates commonly, even when the physician is unaware of it. However, it does not differentiate physical from psychological symptoms.

Recent findings suggest that the placebo response to pain is a **physiologic phenomenon.** Placebo response can be blocked by a narcotic antagonist, naloxone, which suggests that the analgesic effect of a placebo may be based upon the action of endorphins, the naturally occurring opioid substances in the brain, which raise the pain threshold.

BIBLIOGRAPHY

Alexander F, French T, Bacon C, et al: *Studies in Psychosomatic Medicine.* New York, Ronald Press, 1984

American Psychiatric Association: *Diagnostic and Statistical Manual of Mental Disorders,* 3rd ed, revised. Washington DC, American Psychiatric Association, 1987

Breuer J, Freud S: Studies in hysteria. In *Standard Edition of Complete Psychological Works of Sigmund Freud,* vol 2. London, Hogarth Press, 1955

Dunbar F: *Psychosomatic Diagnosis.* New York, Harper and Row, 1948

Engle G: *Psychological Development in Health and Disease.* Philadelphia, Saunders, 1962

Mirsky IA: Physiologic, psychologic, and social determinants in the etiology of duodenal ulcer. *Am J Dig Dis* 3:285, 1958

STUDY QUESTIONS

Directions: Each question below contains five suggested answers. Choose the **one best** response to each question.

1. Patients with psychological factors contributing directly to their medical problems are commonly patients seen by physicians. What percentage of all patients do these patients with psychological factors represent?

(A) 10%
(B) 25%
(C) 33%
(D) 50%
(E) 90%

2. All of the following physiologic changes are a result of the withdrawal–conservation reaction to stress EXCEPT

(A) decrease in heart rate
(B) decrease in body temperature
(C) decrease in immunologic suppression
(D) decrease in metabolism
(E) none of the above

3. All of the following statements about conversion disorder are true EXCEPT

(A) concurrent psychiatric diagnoses are frequent
(B) the symptoms are involuntary
(C) incidence is decreasing
(D) the symptoms are consistent with pathophysiology
(E) it is seen more commonly in women

Questions 4–6

4. A 38-year-old woman has a 10-year history of pelvic pain, which is partially relieved by narcotics. Extensive workup, including laparotomy, has revealed no organic pathology. The patient denies feelings of depression and other psychiatric problems but expresses anger at physicians for being unable to cure her. The most likely diagnosis for this disorder is

(A) depressive disorder
(B) somatization disorder
(C) malingering
(D) factitious disorder
(E) somatoform pain disorder

5. All of the following disorders should be considered in the differential diagnosis of this case EXCEPT

(A) malingering
(B) schizophrenia
(C) bipolar illness
(D) organic illness
(E) conversion disorder

6. Although the psychological mechanisms of this disorder are not fully known, all of the following etiologic theories concerning this case are possible EXCEPT

(A) the pain may enable the patient to avoid an untenable situation
(B) the patient did not learn to verbalize her emotions as a child
(C) the patient had a painful illness as a child
(D) the patient needs to deceive her physicians in order to feel better about herself
(E) the pain may arise from a central nervous system response to stress

(end of group question)

7. Preoccupation with the idea or fear of having an illness is termed

(A) hypochondriasis
(B) phobia
(C) conversion disorder
(D) somatization disorder
(E) factitious disorder

8. All of the following are characteristics of hypochondriasis EXCEPT

(A) physician shopping
(B) higher occurrence in women than in men
(C) increased complaints after reassurance by the physician
(D) exaggeration of minor ailments
(E) presentation in the fourth and fifth decades of life

9. The most common associated finding in patients with factitious disorder is

(A) relatives in health-care professions
(B) narcotic abuse and addiction
(C) depressive disorder
(D) poor health in childhood
(E) a criminal record

10. Which of the following personality types is most likely to respond to a placebo?

(A) Obsessive–compulsive
(B) Histrionic
(C) Narcissistic
(D) Paranoid
(E) None of the above

Directions: Each question below contains four suggested answers of which **one or more** is correct. Choose the answer

A	if **1, 2, and 3** are correct
B	if **1 and 3** are correct
C	if **2 and 4** are correct
D	if **4** is correct
E	if **1, 2, 3, and 4** are correct

11. The classic psychosomatic diseases described by Alexander in the 1940s include which of the following?

(1) Asthma
(2) Coronary artery disease
(3) Peptic ulcer disease
(4) Migraine headache

12. The "fight–flight" behavioral response includes which of the following physiologic reactions?

(1) Increased arousal
(2) Cardiac arrhythmias
(3) Increased muscle tension
(4) Exhaustion

13. Mirsky's work on the development of duodenal ulcers showed that risk factors include

(1) high stress
(2) dependency conflicts
(3) constitutional factors
(4) developmental history of neglect

14. Symptoms that are commonly present in patients with somatization disorder include

(1) painful menstruation
(2) heart palpitations
(3) anxiety
(4) nausea

15. Complications that are likely to be associated with somatization disorder include

(1) psychiatric hospitalization
(2) unnecessary surgery
(3) factitious disorder
(4) substance abuse

16. Effective treatment of somatization disorder commonly involves

(1) gradual reduction in unnecessary medication
(2) regular visits to a physician
(3) consolidation of care with one primary physician
(4) antianxiety medication

17. Characteristics that are specific to conversion reaction include

(1) symbolic nature of symptoms
(2) somatization
(3) stress
(4) stereotyped behavior

18. Correct statements about the use of narcotic medication in somatoform pain disorder include which of the following?

(1) It is usually combined with sedative-hypnotics
(2) It is essential for the treatment of stress-related exacerbations
(3) It is the cornerstone of treatment
(4) It can exacerbate pain symptoms because of habituation and withdrawal

19. Medical illnesses that are misdiagnosed as somatoform disorders, particularly early in the disease course, include

(1) multiple sclerosis (MS)
(2) systemic lupus erythematosus
(3) thyrotoxicosis
(4) rheumatoid arthritis

20. Malingering differs from somatoform disorders in which of the following ways?

(1) It occurs rarely
(2) Patient gains are obvious
(3) It is not a mental disorder
(4) It involves multiple organ systems

Directions: The group of questions below consists of lettered choices followed by several numbered items. For each numbered item select the **one** lettered choice with which it is **most** closely associated. Each lettered choice may be used once, more than once, or not at all.

Questions 21–26

Match each statement listed below with the physical disorder that it describes.

(A) Ulcerative colitis
(B) Cardiovascular disease
(C) Migraine headache
(D) Immune disorder
(E) Bronchial asthma

21. Psychological features of the disorder include immaturity, covertly demanding behavior, and sensitivity to the threat of loss

22. Overly independent as well as overly dependent patients are at higher risk for hospitalization than are those who are psychologically "normal"

23. Some studies have shown that patients who react to stress with feelings of hopelessness or depression are at higher risk for this disorder

24. A behavior pattern that features competitiveness, ambition, and impatience is considered to be predisposing

25. Unresolved grief on the anniversary of the death of a loved one can be a precipitating event

26. The theory that specific psychological conflicts, such as repressed hostility, are causal has not been proven

ANSWERS AND EXPLANATIONS

1. The answer is C. (*I A*) While many physicians feel that all of their patients have a major psychological component to their illnesses, others feel that none of their patients do. Clearly all patients have a psychological reaction to their illnesses, but here we are considering those patients whose psychological conflicts are more than a reaction to the illnesses and actually contribute to them. In many cases, it is believed, at least partially, that psychological conflicts are involved in the pathophysiology of an illness even if the mechanisms are not fully understood; this represents by most estimates about one-third of all patients.

2. The answer is C. [*1 A 2 b (2)*] When heart rate, body temperature, and metabolism in general decrease, it has been noted that the immune system is less reactive and that patients may be more susceptible to illness, particularly infections, in a generalized state of withdrawal–conservation. They also may be susceptible to bradycardia and arrhythmias, which develop secondary to this, so that susceptibility to illness increases rather than decreases.

3. The answer is D. (*II B 1 b*) Often symptoms in a conversion disorder are inconsistent with the normal anatomy of the nervous system (e.g., a stocking–glove type of anesthesia). Concurrent psychiatric diagnoses are common, and the patient may be unaware that the symptoms are caused by psychological conflict. Incidences of conversion disorder seem to be decreasing rather than increasing, particularly as our population becomes more psychologically sophisticated. Although conversion disorder tends to be more common in women than in men, this predominance is not exclusive.

4. The answer is E. (*II C 1*) The primary issue in this case seems to be one of a somatoform pain disorder since pain is the major complaint of the patient. Depression may be present, but it is not the fundamental problem. Also, the physician should be wary of malingering to obtain narcotics, but there is, with the information given, no strong evidence of this. The diagnosis of somatization disorder requires the existence of multiple symptoms, and diagnosis of factitious illness is determined by the patient's awareness that the symptoms are not real.

5. The answer is B. (*II C 4, F 4*) The least likely diagnosis in this case is schizophrenia, the diagnosis of which requires that the patient exhibit some disorders in thinking beyond that in the information given. In malingering, the patient would be faking an illness for a clear gain, which is possible in this case. A bipolar illness involving somatic symptoms is also possible as is conversion disorder, which involves pseudoneurologic symptoms. The question of an undiagnosed organic illness must always be raised in patients with somatoform disorders.

6. The answer is D. (*II C 3*) The psychological mechanisms are not fully understood in any of the somatoform disorders. Some researchers speculate that children who do not learn how to express their emotions verbally are more at risk for developing somatoform disorders. Also, patients with somatoform disorders tend to have a history of illness in childhood. Part of the mechanism may also be that they simply have a different kind of central nervous system response to stressful stimuli. In Munchausen syndrome (factitious disorder), patients seem to have a need to fool the physician and fake an illness to that end.

7. The answer is A. (*II D 1*) Hypochondriasis is defined as the preoccupation with the idea of or fear of illness. Phobias, which are also fears, involve specific reactions to external stimuli rather than preoccupation with ideas. Conversion disorder involves a loss of function, and somatization disorder is associated with multiple symptoms rather than a fear of illness. Factitious disorder involves the voluntary production of symptoms.

8. The answer is B. (*II D 1, 2*) Hypochondriasis is seen equally in both sexes. Women are more commonly diagnosed as having other somatoform disorders than are men. Physician shopping results often from a patient's reaction to being told that there is nothing wrong. Exaggeration of minor ailments is a hallmark of the illness and, unlike many other psychiatric illnesses, hypochondriasis is more likely to present in the fourth and fifth decades of life.

9. The answer is B. (*III A 1*) Although associated findings in a patient with factitious disorder may include relatives in health-care professions, depression, and poor health in childhood, the most common complication is narcotic abuse, occurring in over one-half of patients.

10. The answer is E. (*V*) Placebo response is unrelated to personality type. It is often incorrectly thought that patients who respond to placebos must have a psychiatric disorder or at least have an hysterical or histrionic personality. The reaction to a placebo does not help to determine if the symptoms are organic in nature, and it should not be used as a test for proving that patient symptoms are psychogenic in nature.

11. The answer is B (1, 3). (*I A 1 c*) Alexander theorized that specific unconscious conflicts caused specific illnesses in organs innervated by the autonomic nervous system, including asthma, arthritis, colitis, hypertension, neurodermatitis, thyrotoxicosis, and peptic ulcer disease. Coronary artery disease is not considered a psychosomatic disease. While migraine headache can be considered a psychosomatic disease because of its association with stress, it was not one of the illnesses considered by Alexander in the 1940s.

12. The answer is A (1, 2, 3). (*I A 2 b, B 2 c*) The "fight–flight" response is arousal of the sympathetic nervous system, which may result in an increased production of epinephrine and norepinephrine with an increase in pulse and muscle tension and cardiac arrhythmias, even in the absence of heart disease. While exhaustion may be a neurophysiologic reaction to stress as in the general adaptation syndrome, it is not characteristic of the "fight–flight" response.

13. The answer is A (1, 2, 3). (*I B 1 a*) Mirsky's studies of army recruits showed that several factors are necessary for the development of ulcers, including high stress, constitutional factors, such as high pepsinogen secretion, and psychological conflict (dependency). While a history of parental neglect is associated with several of the somatoform disorders, it is not a finding in peptic ulcer disease.

14. The answer is E (all). (*II A 1 b, c, f, 4 c*) Painful menstruation, palpitations, and nausea all may be present in patients with somatization disorder, which is more common in women; multiple somatic symptoms are the hallmark of the disorder. Anxiety, while not a somatic symptom, is a commonly associated finding in this disorder.

15. The answer is C (2, 4). (*II A 4*) Patients with chronic physical complaints for which there are no clear diagnoses commonly elicit strong feelings of frustration and helplessness in their physicians. If the physician is unaware of these strong reactions, he or she is likely to prescribe unnecessary procedures, such as surgery, as well as stronger and stronger drugs, leading to iatrogenic substance abuse. While these patients may require psychiatric hospitalization, this is less likely to occur than unnecessary surgery or substance abuse. Factitious illness, in which the patient is faking the illness for an unknown reason, is a separately diagnosed disorder.

16. The answer is A (1, 2, 3). (*II A 6*) Treatment of somatization disorder is often frustrating for the physician. This disorder is best seen as a lifelong character style, rather than a curable condition. Consolidation of care with one physician to minimize medications and diagnostic evaluations and regularly scheduled visits so the patient is assured of an ongoing supportive relationship with the physician appears to reduce the overall use of health services. Avoidance of habit-forming medications and little or no medication for questionable indications are the tenets of pharmacologic therapy. Antianxiety medication is not routinely used unless a diagnosis of an anxiety disorder is made.

17. The answer is B (1, 3). (*II B; Table 7-1*) While it may be difficult to discover at first, the majority of the symptoms with which a patient presents in a conversion reaction tend to have some symbolic meaning. For example, an individual with an angry, aggressive impulse may find his or her arm paralyzed. Conversion reactions are always reactions to acute stress and are a way of dealing with the stress. Somatization occurs in all of the other somatoform disorders and not specifically in a conversion reaction. Stereotypic behavior is not a feature of a conversion reaction, but it is seen in other disorders, such as schizophrenia.

18. The answer is D (4). (*II C 6 a*) Paradoxically, chronic narcotic use is not helpful for chronic pain because habituation results in a loss of the analgesic effect, and a vulnerability to withdrawal symptoms. Sedative-hypnotics depress the nervous system and increase pain perceptions as well as inactivity and, therefore, should be avoided.

19. The answer is A (1, 2, 3). (*II F*) Multiple sclerosis (MS), systemic lupus erythematosus, and thyrotoxicosis (hyperthyroidism) are illnesses that present in their early stages with vague symptoms and often are associated with psychiatric complaints, such as anxiety, mood disorders, and occasionally psychotic episodes. Because of these vague, transient symptoms and the associated psychiatric complaints, patients are often misdiagnosed. Rheumatoid arthritis, while associated with psychiatric complaints, is less commonly misdiagnosed due to the physical findings of swollen and painful joints.

20. The answer is A (1, 2, 3). (*IV A, B*) Malingering is rarer than physicians usually realize. They often diagnose malingering in patients with somatoform disorders because they have difficulty accepting the fact that a patient's production of symptoms when there is no organic illness is not voluntary. Physicians should discover obvious patient gains from the production of a faked symptom. Malingering is not a mental disorder since it is under the control of the individual and is done for felonious or other reasons. Malingering may involve more than one system; it may involve as many as the malingerer feels are necessary to fool the examiner.

21–26. The answers are: 21-A, 22-E, 23-D, 24-B, 25-A, 26-C. (*I B 1 b, 2 a, 3 b, 4, 5*) A significant number of patients with ulcerative colitis have concerns of unresolved grief and fears about the threat of future loss. The death of a loved one can be a precipitating event of the disease. The physician should attend to this in terms of treatment. They also tend to have more image or personality developmental problems. Whether this is a causative factor of the illness is unclear.

It has been shown that individuals who are overly independent or overly dependent may be, for the most part, the same kind of asthma patient. In the case of the overly independent patient, there is a denial of the early symptoms of illness, which leads to improper care and the need for hospitalization as a last resort, whereas symptoms in the overly dependent patient are overattended, which leads to early hospitalization. In both cases, there is more hospitalization than occurs in a psychologically normal patient.

There seems to be a connection between affective states of depression, in particular those associated with feelings of hopelessness, and the immune function. Where there is depression of the emotional state, there may also be depression of the immune state. This may be a factor in the development of cancer.

Individuals with a type A behavior pattern with competitiveness, ambition, and particularly time pressure and impatience seem to show a risk two times greater for coronary artery disease than those who do not exhibit this behavior. This increased risk exists even taking into account other important causative factors, such as smoking, lack of exercise, the state of blood lipids, and so forth.

The understanding of migraine headaches has been changing in recent years. It is questioned now whether or not there is a spectrum disorder involving a combination of both tension and migraine headaches. Other factors, such as allergies and chemical factors, may be more important than issues of psychological conflict.

8
Sexual Issues
Janice L. Petersen

I. NORMAL SEXUAL RESPONSE

A. General issues. Sexuality is a part of the human condition and involves all aspects of the biologic, psychological, and social framework. It concerns not only the mental and physical aspects of an individual's life but the cultural, social, and religious aspects as well.

1. **Assessment of sexual functioning** by the physician ought to be a part of every complete medical evaluation and often is not because of the physician's attitude and anxiety. In order to understand sexual disorders, the physician must understand normal sexual function, including the **stages of sexual response**, that is, desire, excitement, plateau, orgasm, and resolution. Physiologic studies have greatly increased the understanding of both healthy and impaired sexual functioning.

2. **Sexual arousal by physical or psychic stimuli**
   a. Physical stimulation of the genitals, bowel, and bladder may produce an involuntary sexual response via spinal reflex.
   b. Psychic stimuli are mediated through the limbic system, the hypothalamus, and the lateral spinal cord.
   c. Erection and lubrication depend on parasympathetic response. Arousal of the sympathetic nervous system, as in situations of fear and anxiety, inhibits this response.

B. Excitement stage

1. **Men.** About 20–30 seconds after stimulation, erection of the penis begins due to increased blood flow into the erectile tissue. The urethral meatus dilates, the testes elevate slightly, the heart rate increases to 100–180 beats per minute, and diastolic pressure increases by 20–40 mm Hg.

2. **Women.** The breasts increase in size, and the nipples stand out. The labia majora and minora engorge with blood and spread. The clitoris lengthens. Heart rate and blood pressure increase.

C. Plateau stage

1. **Men.** The testicles elevate and become engorged with blood. Secretions from Cowper's gland appear on the glans of the penis. The scrotum thickens and looses all the folds. There is general muscle tension and hyperventilation.

2. **Women.** The clitoris becomes very sensitive and retracts. The labia deepen in color. The orgasmic platform develops, in which the outer one-third of the vagina narrows due to swelling and muscle tension and the inner two-thirds lengthen and widen. The vagina becomes lubricated. General muscle tension increases, and there is hyperventilation.

D. Orgasm stage

1. **Men.** The sensation of ejaculating inevitably occurs before orgasm. The muscles of the perineum contract rhythmically, and the prostate gland, seminal vesicles, and urethra also contract, causing the emission of semen.

2. **Women.** There may be a variety of experiences in women. The orgasmic platform contracts rhythmically, and the rectal and urethral sphincters close.

E. Resolution stage

1. **Men.** Detumescence of the penis occurs. There is general muscle relaxation. The testes become uncongested and descend. There is a refractory period during which the male cannot have an erection. The length of the refractory period increases from a minute or so in adolescents to hours in older men.

2. **Women.** There is a general relaxation. Vasocongestion is lost, and the labia return to their original size and shape. The inner vagina remains distended for several minutes. Women do not have a refractory period and are able to achieve another orgasm immediately.

II. NORMAL SEXUAL FUNCTION

A. Gender identity

1. Gender identity is one's sense of being masculine or feminine rather than the biologic state of being masculine or feminine. Sexual identity is the term that refers to biologic sexual characteristics, such as genitalia, hormonal composition, and secondary sexual characteristics. An infant is assigned a sex, usually on the basis of genitalia, and is reared with all of the parents' and society's attitudes regarding that sex. By about 2½–3 years of age, gender identity appears to be set.

2. The early embryo is undifferentiated sexually (i.e., it is bisexual). The Y chromosome is necessary for the development of male genitalia. Androgens are produced by the fetal testicles. The androgens influence the organization of the developing brain, which later influences "male" behavior. This behavior is not totally fixed, however, because human beings are the most sensitive of all animals to environmental forces.

B. Theories about gender identity. Behavior that is masculine or feminine appears to be determined much more by learning and culture than by biology. The theories about the development of sex roles have undergone major revisions in recent years.

1. **Sigmund Freud** initially reported on the importance of sexuality in the psychological development of children; however, his theory of psychological development has been challenged. A wider concept of psychosexual development is now used.

   a. **Prenatal factors.** The sex chromosones (XX or XY) in the fetus determine whether embryonic gonadal tissue develops into testes or ovaries. Testes begin to develop at the fetal age of 6 weeks if fetal testicular androgens are present. External genitalia are morphologically complete by 14 weeks of fetal life. Fetal androgens also have an effect on the organization of the developing brain, especially in the limbic system.

   b. **Infancy (0–18 months).** During the period of infancy, the child is highly dependent on the caretaker, usually the mother. Basic trust develops along with a sense of pleasure in the body and bodily functions, such as feeding, sucking, and tasting. Masturbation is common and normal at 15–19 months. Parental attitudes (whether conscious or not) about the infant's sex influence their interaction with the infant. Encouragement of aggressive behavior, physical activity, roughness of play, and so on are all affected by attitudes regarding sexual roles. Freud called this period the oral phase.

   c. **Toddler (1½–3 years).** By this age, core gender identity is set. Major development tasks of this phase include emergence of control over bodily functions. Children become aware of the anatomic differences between the sexes. Socialization also begins. Toilet training generally occurs during this time and represents the struggle for control over bodily functions as well as the acceptance of social restrictions on behavior. Children begin to experience themselves as separate individuals, a process called separation–individuation. Language readiness occurs and is crucial in the development of normal healthy ego functions. Freud called this the anal phase.

   d. **Preschool (3–6 years).** Gender role development is powerfully influenced during these years. Children are very aware of their genitalia. Freud call this interest in the genitalia and the self the phallic phase.

      (1) Masturbation becomes more obviously pleasurable. Recent child observation studies indicate that a girl's sense of femininity is primary in that her "feminine" behavior, such as interest in infants, often occurs before awareness of genital differences.

      (2) Fear of bodily injury is common during this period (fear of castration in boys and fear of genital penetration and mutilation in girls).

      (3) In the fourth and fifth years, strong sexual feelings about the opposite sex parent are common (oedipal phase). In normal development, if the same sex or "rival" parent does not overreact and remains accepting to the child, the child will accept

the reality of his or her position in the family and develop a healthy identification with the same sex partner.

2. The early mother–infant relationship can be conceptualized as **symbiotic**, that is, the infant experiences him- or herself and the mother as merged. There is no clear difference between masculine and feminine behavior prior to 1 year of age.

3. The development of masculine behavior in boys is related to separation and individuation. Failure of separation may lead to problems of gender identity and sexual perversions.

4. It has been suggested that the quality of "masculinity" is more fragile and susceptible to traumatic disruption than that of "femininity." Men are at a much higher risk for gender identity disorders than are women.

III. TRANSSEXUALISM

A. General issues. Transsexualism is a gender identity disorder. There is a persistent belief on the part of affected individuals that, despite being normal, they belong to the opposite sex. Transsexual individuals wish to be rid of their own genitals and live as members of the other sex. This disorder invariably begins in childhood. Because these individuals are unable to live in the role of the "right" sex, psychological symptoms, such as anxiety and depression, are common.

1. **Crossdressing.** In men, there is a history of crossdressing before the age of 4 years in 75% of individuals with this disorder.

2. **The transsexual boy** believes that he will grow up to be a woman and lose his penis and testicles. Occasionally, men attempt to mutilate or castrate themselves out of frustration. Men seek help for this disorder more frequently than women.

3. **The transsexual girl** tends to be masculine in appearance and behavior. She believes that she will grow up to be a man with a penis and will not develop breasts. Women tend to have a more stable course and are more likely to be homosexual.

B. Etiology. The etiology of transsexualism is not known; no biologic factors have been identified.

1. **Men** who develop this condition often have excessively close physical and emotional ties to their mothers and fathers who were absent during childhood. Their mothers crossdressed them and treated them as girls.

2. **Women** with this disorder often have a history of mothers who were distant and unavailable either physically or emotionally during childhood. These girls apparently identified with their fathers.

C. Treatment

1. **Primary transsexualism**
   a. **Surgical.** Primary transsexualism in men, in which the patient has always felt that inside he has been a woman, has been treated by **sexual reassignment surgery**. When surgery is successful, some patients describe a good readjustment to life. However, some patients have had significant difficulty with adjustment. Woman-to-man sexual reassignment has had similarly mixed results.
   b. **Family therapy.** When transsexuality is identified in a child, family therapy to improve the relationship with the parent of the same sex and reinforce gender congruent behavior has been helpful.
   c. **Behavior modification.** In adults, behavior modification approaches have reported some success in supporting gender congruent identity in some patients.

2. **Secondary transsexualism** is the development of a gender identity problem later in life, after there have been periods of apparently normal sexual identity.
   a. **Extended psychotherapy** to explore the meanings of the wish to change sex is indicated.
   b. **Behavior modification** approaches to stabilize the primary gender identity can be considered.

IV. PARAPHILIAS

A. Overview. Previously referred to as **sexual deviations**, these disorders consist of marked and repetitive behavior that involves nonhuman objects for sexual arousal, human beings in activities that are humiliating or involve suffering, and human beings who do not consent to the sexual activity (as occurs in rape). Paraphilic imagery is necessary for masturbation in these disturbances.

Patients are usually unable to become sexually aroused in normal ways and are unable to control the deviant impulses. Although affected individuals may be distressed by the impulses, they often do not see themselves as "sick" and may come to medical attention only after legal difficulties. Patients may feel shame or guilt about this behavior, and depression is common, especially when the patients' interpersonal relationships suffer because of their sexual problems.

B. Etiology. Although not fully understood, the paraphilias are thought to result from problems in early development rather than from genetic or biologic factors. Men are almost exclusively at risk for these disorders. An exception is sadomasochism, which often involves women.

1. It is speculated that problems in the mother–child relationship lead to a poor body image, especially with regard to the genitals. The child becomes unsure and anxious about his penis and its function. "Normal" sexual desire and behavior are too threatening, and this leads to "abnormal" choices for the expression of sexuality. Once the abnormal choice has been made, individuals learn to associate sexual gratification with this behavior and, thus, are reinforced for it.

2. Paraphiliac patients often have a history of being sexually abused as children. People with one paraphiliac disorder may suffer from others as well.

C. Specific paraphilias

1. **Fetishism.** The patient needs a nonliving object, such as women's clothing, for sexual arousal. This does not include objects designed for sexual stimulation, such as vibrators.

2. **Transvestism.** The patient, who is generally heterosexual and not transsexual, must dress in women's clothes in order to become sexually aroused.

3. **Frotteurism.** This disorder involves sexually arousing urges to touch or rub against a non-consenting person.
   a. The act usually takes place in a crowded setting where detection can be avoided.
   b. Most of this behavior is carried out by men 15–25 years of age.

4. **Pedophilia.** In this disorder, the sexual activity or fantasy involves prepubertal children of either sex.
   a. By definition, the adult must be at least 16 years of age and at least 6 years older than the victim. If the patient is a late adolescent, diagnosis requires clinical judgment as to the relative maturity of both the patient and the child.
   b. This disorder should be distinguished from an organic mental syndrome, mental retardation, or alcohol intoxication in which an impaired individual with a problem in impulse control has some sexual activity with a child. In these cases, the sexual behavior is not prominent but is a part of a picture of overall disability.
   c. Sexual abuse of children may be a great deal more common than has been appreciated in the past. Incest as a specific issue is covered in Chapter 10, "Child Psychiatry."

5. **Exhibitionism.** In this disorder, the affected individual exposes his genitals in order to obtain sexual gratification.
   a. Exhibitionists are psychologically immature men who become sexually aroused only by exposing themselves, either during or after the event. Sometimes they masturbate while exhibiting themselves. The "victims" of this behavior are almost always women or girls.
   b. Hostility is usually present. The person wishes to shock the stranger. The act usually occurs in socially inappropriate places. However, despite the wish to frighten, most of these individuals are not dangerous nor do they take further action.
   c. Occasionally, exhibitionism is part of a more pervasive personality disorder, which also includes pedophilia.

6. **Voyeurism** involves the urges and fantasies about seeing unsuspecting people naked or in the act of disrobing.
   a. It is usually heterosexual in nature.
   b. The voyeur does not seek contact with the observed person and achieves orgasm by masturbating while looking. The excitement is heightened by the idea that the victim would feel humiliated knowing that someone is watching.
   c. The "Peeping Tom" is usually male.
   d. This disorder must be differentiated from watching pornography or normal sexual play in which the individuals being watched are willing.

     e. Exhibitionism often occurs with voyeurism.

  7. Masochism. This disorder, which commonly coexists with sadism, involves the achievement of sexual pleasure only through physical pain or suffering.
- **a.** In the sexual disorder of masochism, individuals prefer or require bondage, beatings, humiliation, or other physical suffering to achieve sexual excitement. If individuals have intentionally participated in even a single episode in which they were physically harmed or their lives were threatened in order to achieve sexual excitement, the diagnosis can be made.
- **b.** Fantasies of being bound, raped, or hurt that lead to sexual excitement are not sufficient for the diagnosis.
- **c.** Moral masochism, in which a person takes on the martyr's role of psychological suffering and sacrifice in ongoing interpersonal relationships, is also a different disorder.
- **d.** **Hypoxyphila** is a relatively new and dangerous form of sexual masochism. Sexual excitement is achieved by using a mechanism, such as a noose or a plastic bag of chemicals (nitrates), to produce temporary oxygen deprivation. The behavior may be done alone or with partners. Deaths do occur and are thought to be accidental rather than suicidal.
- **e.** About 30% of sexual masochists also exhibit features of sexual sadism.

  8. Sexual sadism. Individuals with this disorder are sexually aroused by the pain and suffering of others. The suffering may be either physical or psychological.
- **a.** Psychologically, the sadist wants to feel in complete control of his victim.
- **b.** Repeated and intentional physical or psychological pain is inflicted on a partner. Sadistic behavior can range from verbal humiliation to beating, torture, rape, and murder.
- **c.** The partner may be consenting (masochist) or nonconsenting.
- **d.** About 10% of rapists are sexual sadists.

D. Treatment

1. The physician should assess all areas of the patient's level of functioning. Many of these patients have other psychological deficits as well, and they should be referred for treatment to qualified specialists.
- **a.** **Long-term psychotherapy**, including psychoanalysis, has been effective for some patients, but it is expensive, time-consuming, and limited to patients with a relatively high level of functioning.
- **b.** **Behavior modification** has also been successful in the treatment of severe and driven perversions.
- **c.** **Antiandrogen drugs**, such as medroxyprogesterone, have been used with some success in male patients with severe antisocial paraphilias.

2. Patient motivation is extremely important. Paraphilias involve sexual gratification, and it is difficult for anyone to give up an area of sexual pleasure, even when there is legal risk involved. Recidivism rates remain high; for example, the only treatment shown to decrease recidivism rates in pedophilia has been the prolonged use of antiandrogen drugs.

V. SEXUAL DISORDERS

A. Overview. Most types of psychosexual disorders, whether affecting men or women, have certain features in common. The disorder may be primary, that is, lifelong, or secondary, acquired after a period of normal functioning. The disorder may be generalized or situational, that is, it exists only in certain situations or with specific partners. Finally, the disorder may be either total or partial, that is, to a degree or frequency that is less than total.

    The *DSM-III-R* diagnoses of sexual disorders are reserved for sexual dysfunctions due to psychological factors; sexual dysfunctions due solely to physical factors are excluded. Sexual dysfunctions involving both psychological and physical factors are given dual *DSM-III-R* diagnoses on axis I and III. In order to diagnose sexual dysfunction, the physician must consider:

1. Subjective distress

2. Frequency of occurrence

3. Effect of the condition on other areas of the patient's functioning

B. Sexual history. A review of a patient's sexual functioning during the routine medical history is mandatory. A thorough discussion of sexual functioning is particularly necessary for patients whose medical problems, such as diabetes or heart disease, predispose them to sexual problems.

1. A sexual history should be taken at the time of the complete patient history and physical examination. It should not be delayed until the physician is comfortable discussing sexual matters because that may never happen. The physician's discomfort is the primary reason that an adequate history of sexual functioning is not obtained.

2. If sexuality is related to the presenting illness, the physician should ask, "How has your sexual functioning been affected by the illness?" or "Many patients experience changes in sexual functioning as a result of this problem. How has it affected you?" The physician should convey openness and a willingness to discuss the subject of sex.

3. If sexuality is not addressed during the history of the present illness, it can be reviewed during the review of systems.
   a. Pathology involving the genital organs, such as venereal disease, pain, and discharge should be evaluated as well as interest in and capacity of sexual functioning.
   b. If a sexual dysfuntion is present, a detailed sexual history is needed for further evaluation, addressing the following points:
      (1) First childhood awareness of sexuality, including attitudes and punishment
      (2) Problems with gender identity
      (3) First sexual experience, including masturbation
      (4) Age of and reaction to puberty, including menarche in women
      (5) History of sexual abuse
      (6) Patient knowledge about sex and how it was acquired
      (7) First experience with a sexual partner, including intercourse
      (8) Homosexual experiences and interest. Does the patient see these as problems?
      (9) Current sexual functioning, including frequency and satisfaction
      (10) Questions about extramarital partners if the patient is married
   c. Problems that may be uncovered in the sexual history include:
      (1) Concern about normal sexuality or sexual development secondary to the patient's lack of knowledge or misinformation
      (2) Sexual aspects of a pervasive problem in the relationship with the sexual partner
      (3) Sexual problems that result from the presenting medical or surgical problem
      (4) Primary sexual dysfunction that needs further evaluation and treatment

C. Specific sexual disorders

1. **Hypoactive sexual desire disorder**
   a. **Criteria for the diagnosis** of hypoactive sexual desire in the *Diagnostic and Statistical Manual of Mental Disorders*, 3rd ed., revised (*DSM-III-R*) are persistent and pervasive inhibition of sexual desire. Patients with this disorder have very little or no desire for sex. Additionally, the patient has little or no fantasies about sex.
      (1) The clinician must take into account many factors that can affect sexual desire, such as age, health, intensity and frequency of sexual desire, and the norms of sexual behavior in the context of the patient's life. The diagnosis applies only if there is distress from this lack of desire on the part of either partner. This diagnosis is not used if the cause is solely organic.
      (2) In one study of stable marriages, 2% of couples reported never having intercourse, and 8% had intercourse less than once a month. Another study of young married couples found that one-third had definable periods of no sex starting around 8 weeks after marriage. Multiple reasons were given to explain the cessation of sexual activity, but the most common reason was **marital discord**.
   b. **Etiology**
      (1) **Testosterone deficiency.** Testosterone is necessary for normal libido in both men and women. This is shown by the improvement in sexual desire reported by testosterone deficient men or women (secondary to adrenalectomy or occasionally secondary to oophorectomy or menopause) who are given testosterone replacement.
      (2) **Prolactinemia** secondary to pituitary adenomas is rare but can suppress sexual desire.
      (3) **Chronic illness**, such as chronic renal failure and severe endocrine or liver problems, is often associated with decreased sexual desire.
      (4) **Major depression** is one of the most common causes of secondary disorders of sexual desire.
      (5) **Pharmacologic factors.** Alcohol, narcotics, β-adrenergic blockers, hypertensive agents, and sedative hypnotics can cause decreased libido.
      (6) **Psychological factors** include a history of negative parental sexual attitudes, which

can lead to the unconscious inhibition of sexual arousal, chronic marital discord, and high levels of stress.
- **c. Differential diagnosis.** The possibility of testosterone deficiency, pituitary disease, chronic illness, depression, and pharmacologic side effects must be evaluated before concluding that the symptom is due to psychological causes.
- **d. Treatment**
  - **(1) Testosterone replacement** is appropriate only when a true deficiency exists. When normal testosterone levels are present, testosterone supplementation provides only placebo effects.
  - **(2) Management of any contributing illness** is necessary if the inhibited sexual desire is related to such an illness.
  - **(3) Psychotherapy** is useful to help patients to understand the role of early experiences in constricting sexual activity and overcoming inhibition. It is also useful for learning stress management techniques.
  - **(4) Marital therapy** is useful in determining and addressing interactive factors in the couple that contribute to the inhibition (see section VI).

2. Sexual aversion disorder
- **a. Diagnosis.** Patients with sexual aversion disorder suffer from a persistent or recurrent extreme aversion to genital sexual contact with a sexual partner. Thus, they avoid sex completely. The clinician must take into account all of the factors that can affect sexual desire, including health, age, and norms of sexual behavior, in considering the diagnosis. The patient may show aversion to one but not other partners. The diagnosis applies only if there is distress from this aversion to sex on the part of either partner. The diagnosis is not appropriate if the cause is organic.
- **b. Etiology.** Although there is little research in this area, it is thought that attitudes and conflicts from early development contribute to this problem. Another common factor is overt or covert marital discord.
- **c. Treatment** generally involves individual psychotherapy, marital therapy, or both.

3. Sexual arousal disorders. These disorders have been referred to as **inhibited sexual excitement** in recent years. In men, this condition has been termed **impotence**, and in women, it has been called **frigidity**. The negative connotation of these words in the description of sexual arousal disorder is not only unfortunate, it is inaccurate: Impotence implies weakness and powerlessness that goes beyond a sexual disorder; frigidity implies a coldness and reserve of personality. However, women with inhibited sexual excitement can be warm in other areas of their lives, and men with erectile failure may be aggressive and powerful in other areas of their lives.
- **a. Diagnosis** of a sexual arousal disorder cannot be made if the condition is caused by organic factors. Before diagnosing inhibited sexual excitement, the physician must determine that the sexual activity and stimulation level is adequate in focus, intensity, and duration.
  - **(1) In men**, there is:
    - **(a)** Recurrent and persistent partial or complete failure to attain or maintain an erection through completion of the sex act
    - **(b)** Recurrent or persistent lack of pleasure or excitement during sex
  - **(2) In women**, there is:
    - **(a)** Partial or complete failure to attain or maintain the lubrication and swelling response to sexual excitement until completion of the sex act
    - **(b)** Recurrent or persistent lack of pleasure or excitement during sex
- **b. Erectile dysfunction**
  - **(1) Primary erectile dysfunction** is a condition in which the man has never been able to have an erection sufficient to allow penetration of the vagina. It is not common and is usually associated with an overly rigid upbringing in which any expression of sexuality was punished. Occasionally, it is associated with homosexuality.
  - **(2) Secondary erectile dysfunction** involves the failure to achieve an erection for intercourse, having been successful on previous occasions. The failure must be a persistent event (i.e., it must occur in 20%–30% of all attempts). As is true in orgasmic dysfunction in women, the problem may be present in only certain situations or with certain partners. Approximately 10%–20% of all men have experienced secondary impotence. The incidence of erectile problems increases with age.
  - **(3) Etiology**
    - **(a) Psychological.** Anxiety from whatever source inhibits sexual arousal. The sympathetic nervous system is stimulated, thus inhibiting the parasympathetic nervous system, which is necessary for an erection. Anxiety about sexual performance is the most common psychological cause of inhibited sexual excitement.

(b) **Alcohol.** Overindulgence in alcohol often precipitates failure of erection. The patient subsequently becomes overly concerned and anxious about his sexual performance, and a vicious circle begins. Anxiety leads to failure, which increases the anxiety.

(c) **Organic causes.** Erectile failure that is chronic, invariable, and unrelated to situational factors is more likely to have an organic etiology. Failure of erection due to organic causes becomes increasingly common with age. In ruling out organic causes, it is important to inquire about the frequency of early morning erection, nocturnal emissions, and erection with self-stimulation and fantasy. Erections occur normally during rapid eye movement (REM) sleep. Plethysmography can be used to measure nocturnal tumescence: It measures the strength of an erection while the patient sleeps. The presence of erections at night indicates that the problem is less likely to be organic in origin. Medical illnesses thought to cause erectile failure include:

(i) Diabetes mellitus
(ii) Hyperthyroidism
(iii) Myxedema
(iv) Cirrhosis of the liver
(v) Mumps
(vi) Respiratory failure
(vii) Cardiac failure
(viii) Atherosclerosis
(ix) Leriche's syndrome (distal aortic obstruction)
(x) Multiple sclerosis
(xi) Amyotrophic lateral sclerosis
(xii) Parkinson's disease
(xiii) Syphilis
(xiv) Injuries to the spinal cord or peripheral nerves due to trauma or surgery
(xv) Hypopituitarism
(xvi) Urologic surgery, orchiectomy, or prostatectomy
(xvii) Drugs (see section VII D)

(4) **Treatment.** Management of contributing medical illness is necessary if the erectile dysfunction is related to such an illness. Psychological factors often respond to behavioral techniques. Marital therapy or sex therapy as described by Masters and Johnson may be necessary to deal with resistances to behavioral treatment approaches, which may be related to marital discord. Examples of behavioral techniques follow.

(a) **Sensate focus.** Couples are instructed to explore noncoital caressing, focusing on the discovery and enjoyment of sensual feelings. These exercises should have a pleasuring rather than demanding quality. This allows rediscovery of sensual feelings, which may have been suppressed by the sexual problem.

(b) **Managing anxiety.** Fear of failure and pressure to perform are common in erectile dysfunction. Prohibition of intercourse during sensate focus sessions removes this anxiety and allows the patient a feeling of success in enjoying arousal.

(c) **Regaining confidence.** As sensate focus exercises continue, the stop–start technique may be used. After the erection has occurred, the couple ceases the sexual stimulation and allows the erection to subside. They then continue the pleasurable activity, which allows recurrence of the erection. In this way, the man gains a sense of control of his own arousal level.

(d) **Gradual resumption of coitus.** As the man feels more confident, gradual approximation of coitus can occur. The man first achieves vaginal containment of the penis but then withdraws so that anxiety is managed and the sense of success can continue. As the man feels confident, active thrusting can be added with stopping and starting as needed to control anxiety.

c. **Female sexual arousal disorder.** The fact that the psychological form of this disorder is uncommon compared to hypoactive sexual desire disorder or inhibited orgasm suggests that conflicts in the female are more likely to be expressed as the latter disorders. Impaired sexual arousal in women is most likely due to a physical cause.

(1) **Etiology**

(a) **Estrogen deficiency** associated with menopause is the most common cause of failure to lubricate with normal sexual desire. Inadequate estrogen causes atrophic vulvovaginitis with drying of the vaginal epithelium.

(b) **Neurologic or endocrinologic causes or side effects from medications** occasionally cause female sexual arousal disorder.

(c) **Marital discord.** Psychogenic forms of this disorder are thought to be related to conflicts about intercourse and conflicts in the marriage.

(2) **Treatment**
  (a) **Estrogen replacement**, either orally or topically, readily reverses atrophic vulvovaginitis.
  (b) **Correction of any contributing medical or physical causes** is necessary.
  (c) **Psychotherapy and marital therapy** are indicated for psychological factors.

4. Orgasm disorders
  a. **Inhibited female orgasm** is defined in the *DSM-III-R* as recurrent and persistent inhibition of orgasm after a sexual excitement phase that ought to be adequate in focus, intensity, and duration. Some women experience difficulty in both the excitement and orgasm stages. Other women may be able to have an orgasm during noncoital clitoral stimulation but not during coitus, which, although probably a normal variation, concerns some patients.
  (1) **Primary orgasmic dysfunction.** Women who have never had an orgasm may have never learned what to expect physically. Primary orgasmic dysfunction may be easier to treat than secondary orgasmic dysfunction because the problem can be solved through education. Ninety percent of patients can be helped with behavioral therapy.
  (2) **Secondary orgasmic dysfunction** involves a history of successful achievement of orgasm with the subsequent failure to achieve orgasm in all or some situations, either with particular partners or in particular settings. This disorder is a common complaint. *DSM-III-R* lists the prevalence at 30% of the female population.
  (3) **Etiology.** Inhibited female orgasm is thought to be common but not indicative of psychopathology. Women with this problem may function quite well in all other areas of their lives.
    (a) **Cultural restrictions** of women's sexuality probably account for some inhibition.
    (b) **Financial concerns, alcohol abuse, and extramarital affairs** add tension to the relationship, making it more difficult to relax and achieve orgasm.
    (c) **Psychological issues** are the most common cause of secondary inhibition of orgasm. Problems of passivity versus assertiveness, issues of control, and guilt feelings can all interfere with sexual pleasure. **Lack of communication** of needs and desires between partners is common. The man may lack sensitivity to his partner's needs, and the woman may be unable to tell him because of perceived role expectations, anger, or guilt.
    (d) Inhibited female orgasm is rare secondary to organic illness (e.g., multiple sclerosis) or as a side effect to medications (e.g., antidepressants) but may occur.
  (4) **Symptoms.** Some women who do not have orgasms are nonsymptomatic and report satisfactory sex lives. Others may develop symptoms of pelvic pain, vaginal discharge, tiredness, and irritability.
  (5) **Treatment.** Behavioral techniques are helpful in 90% of cases. Therapy involves informing the patient about normal sexual response, giving the woman permission to experience sexual feelings and encouraging her to explore her sexual response by self-stimulation and then with a partner.
    (a) **Organic causes** should be corrected as necessary.
    (b) **Behavioral techniques**
      (i) **Sensate focus** exercises are initially used for the woman to explore her own sensuality. They start with the woman touching her skin, breasts, genitals, and noticing the pleasurable sensations. She then progresses to caressing the genitals while noting pleasurable sensations. She is then encouraged to explore clitoral and vaginal sensations and masturbation. A vibrator may be used to provide high level of stimulation and assist in the experience of orgasm.
      (ii) **Anxiety management.** Prohibiting orgasm during sensate focus exercises reduces performance anxiety. Relaxation techniques, hypnosis, and, occasionally, antianxiety agents may be used.
      (iii) **Strengthening pubococcygeal muscles** is associated with a high rate of orgasmic competence. This is accomplished by having the woman consciously tighten the pelvic floor muscles several times a day.
      (iv) **Experiencing orgasm with a partner.** After the woman has gained confidence in her ability to experience orgasm by herself, she then learns to experience it with a partner. The woman is then encouraged to educate her partner about activities that she finds stimulating. She is, thus, given permission to get pleasure for herself in the relationship.

(c) Group therapy for "preorgasmic women," which uses behavioral approaches, is effective; it allows the participants to learn from each other and gain the support of other group members.

(d) Individual psychotherapy is useful for those with conflicts not treatable by behavioral techniques.

(e) Marital therapy may be required when conflicts impede orgasmic function.

b. Inhibited male orgasm. In this uncommon condition, there is recurrent and persistent delay or absence of ejaculation, following an adequate phase of sexual excitement. The diagnosis is not made if the cause is organic.

(1) Etiology

 (a) Physical factors

  (i) The most common cause of delayed ejaculation is side effects of medications, particularly α-adrenergic blockers, such as antipsychotic drugs and antihypertensives.

  (ii) Neurologic disorders and surgical procedures rarely cause male orgasmic dysfunction without impairing erectile function as well.

 (b) Psychological factors are thought to be related to fear of trauma (external or intrapsychic), which becomes associated with ejaculation and then is reinforced. This disorder may be seen in men with obsessive–compulsive disorder.

(2) Treatment

 (a) Physical factors must be corrected when indicated.

 (b) Psychological factors must be identified and desensitized. This requires an understanding of the traumatic factors that initiated and maintain the inhibition. A series of exercises analogous to those used for the treatment of erectile dysfunction should be designed for individual needs [see section V C 3 b (4)].

c. Premature ejaculation is defined as recurrent ejaculation with minimal sexual stimulation before the man wishes it to occur. This condition is the most common sexual dysfunction of men, particularly young men. Previously, premature ejaculation was defined as the inability of the man to delay ejaculation during intercourse until his partner achieved orgasm in more than 50% of the attempts. This definition, however, did not take into account the possibility of sexual dysfunction in the partner. Some men complain if they cannot sustain intercourse for 30 minutes or more. Although this may be a problem to the patient, the diagnosis of premature ejaculation should not be made. More commonly, the man ejaculates one or two strokes after insertion or even before insertion.

(1) Etiology

 (a) Anxiety from any source can stimulate the sympathetic nervous system and lead to premature ejaculation as well as erectile failure.

 (b) Early sexual experiences. Learning theory suggests that the patient learned to ejaculate rapidly from early sexual experiences in which anxiety was high because of fear of getting caught by parents or other authorities. The disorder is more common in men who are highly educated. Ironically, these men may be more concerned about their partner's satisfaction and, thus, are more susceptible to performance anxiety.

 (c) Guilt about sex or hostility toward the partner are other causes of premature ejaculation.

(2) Treatment. Behavioral treatment is successful in over 90% of cases.

 (a) Behavioral approaches. Sensate focus and **anxiety reduction**, incorporating the **squeeze technique**, or **stop and go technique**, are similar to the treatment of erectile dysfunction [see section V C 3 b (4)]. In the sensate focus exercises, the man is stimulated just to the point of ejaculatory inevitability, at which point ejaculation is prevented by squeezing the penis at the frenulum and coronal ridge or simply by stopping stimulation. Using this technique, the man gains control of his arousal and the timing of ejaculation. As he gains confidence, his anxiety is reduced, which further improves performance. Eventually he learns to modulate arousal independent of the squeeze technique.

 (b) Psychotherapy

  (i) Couples therapy may be needed to address conflicts in the marriage.

  (ii) Individual psychotherapy may be needed for those with significant resistance to behavioral approaches.

5. Vaginismus is defined as involuntary tightening of the paravaginal muscles to prevent penile penetration, which can occur in all sexual encounters or only in specific situations. This problem is sometimes seen in the physician's office during a pelvic examination, preventing insertion of the speculum.

 a. Etiology

  (1) Rigid sexual upbringing. Patients often have backgrounds where sex was considered to be sinful and parents were overly controlling. Intercourse is experienced as painful and traumatic. The disorder is more common in women from high socioeconomic groups.

    (2) Traumatic sexual experiences. Some patients have had traumatic sexual experiences, such as incest and rape, which cause anxiety, tension, and pain in subsequent sexual experiences, that inadvertently reinforce the vaginal spasm.

    (3) Organic causes. Vaginismus can develop secondary to vaginal infections or painful conditions, such as vaginal repair after childbirth.

  b. Treatment involves correction of any painful physical condition and then behavior modification. The patient is taught to gradually desensitize herself by inserting graded sizes of catheters into her vagina. When she is able to tolerate a catheter the size of an erect penis, intercourse is attempted. This program is structured so that intercourse is under her control, and her partner is instructed to avoid active thrusting. As the woman is able to accept vaginal containment of the penis without anxiety or spasm, the couple then increases their sexual activity gradually until full active thrusting is possible.

6. Functional dyspareunia is defined as recurrent and persistent genital pain before or after intercourse, not due to lack of lubrication, vaginismus, or physical causes.

  a. Etiology

    (1) Organic causes. Forty percent of women presenting to sex therapy clinics with dyspareunia are found to have organic causes, such as infection or trauma. Dypareunia is rare in men and is usually secondary to an organic cause.

    (2) Learned dysfunctional patterns. Functional dyspareunia is thought to result from the patient having learned a dysfunctional sexual pattern, which leads to discomfort and avoidance that is reinforced each time the situation is repeated. Many of these women have histories of sexual abuse.

    (3) Psychopathology. Some reports suggest significant psychopathology in women with nonorganic dyspareunia. It is thought there is an unconscious fear of or aversion to the sex act.

  b. Treatment

    (1) Underlying physical conditions must be corrected.

    (2) Systematic desensitization by vaginal dilation as discussed in section V C 5 b.

    (3) Psychotherapy may be helpful in understanding the origin of the dysfunctional sexual pattern.

    (4) Couples therapy may be helpful in treating conflicts in the couple that perpetuate the dysfunction.

VI. TREATMENT OF SEXUAL DYSFUNCTION IN PRIMARY CARE MEDICINE. Most physicians can use the P-LI-SS-IT model developed by Annon in the treatment of sexual dysfunction.

  A. Permission (P). The physician's relaxed manner and interest facilitates the discussion of sexual concerns. Approval for enjoying sexual activity should be conveyed. The authority of the physician's role contributes to the effectiveness of this approach.

  B. Limited information (LI). Many cases of sexual dysfunction result from lack of information or misinformation about sex. The physician can reassure as well as educate the patient about "normality."

  C. Specific suggestion (SS). This type of intervention requires more skill on the part of the physician, and the level of interventions depends upon the complexity of the problem. Masters and Johnson, among others, have developed therapy programs for couples, which employ short-term behavior approaches. After an extensive history is taken and physical and laboratory examinations are conducted, the couple is taught **sensate focusing**. The couple learns to "pleasure" each other without the demand of intercourse. Further treatment depends upon the specific problem.

  D. Intensive therapy (IT). Patients who do not respond to the basic therapy described above may require psychotherapy and should be referred. In these cases, there are usually more complex problems in the relationship or associated psychopathology.

VII. SEX AND PHYSICAL ILLNESS

  A. General issues. Illness, whether medical or surgical, is a threat to self-esteem. The patient's physical appearance may be altered by either the illness or the treatment for the illness. The patient's self-image and sense of sexual attractiveness is also likely to be altered.

    Pain, malaise, and anxiety tend to decrease interest in sex markedly. Occasionally, however, as a compensatory reaction to the fear of loss of attractiveness, there is an increase in libido and sexual behavior. In acute illness, the disturbance in sexuality usually resolves with the illness. In chronic illness, however, the physician should explore the patient's adaptation with respect to sexual functioning as a part of ongoing medical care.

B. Specific conditions

1. **Cardiovascular disease**
   a. **Coronary artery disease.** Almost all patients with angina and those who have suffered a myocardial infarction are concerned that sex will affect their heart conditions. It is important to discuss the resumption of sex after a myocardial infarction with both partners since the spouse may also have concerns.
      (1) The patient may cease all sexual activity for fear of precipitating another myocardial infarction unless the physician intervenes. In general, if the patient can walk up two flights of stairs without symptoms, sexual intercourse should not present a problem. The position of the partners does not seem to make a difference in terms of cardiac stress.
      (2) The patient can be counseled to have sex in the morning after a good night's sleep rather than after a hard day's work or a party when he or she is tired and possibly intoxicated.
      (3) Occasionally, a patient may need to use nitroglycerine prophylactically prior to sex to prevent angina.
   b. **Hypertension.** The major sexual problems associated with hypertension are usually secondary to antihypertensive medication. These drugs can interfere with both erection and ejaculation. Reserpine and guanethidine cause the worst problems. Methyldopa is less likely to interfere, and propranolol and clonidine cause the fewest side effects.
   c. **Other cardiovascular diseases**, such as valvular disease of the heart, which interfere with cardiac output, may affect the patient's ability to sustain sexual activity.

2. **Neurologic illness**
   a. **Spinal cord lesions.** The support of the physician is crucial in facilitating a frank discussion of sexuality following injury to the spinal cord. Divorce rates increase following spinal cord injury in men. Exploration of alternative means of sexual expression, such as oral and manual stimulation, is necessary. Control of bowel and bladder function is an important aspect of sex. Avoiding stimulants, such as caffeine, may help prevent general muscle spasms.
      (1) The level of injury is crucial to whether the male patient is able to obtain an erection. Upper motor neuron lesions, especially those higher up in the spinal cord, may not affect reflexogenic erections, which occur either secondary to a full bladder or from direct stimulation of the penis. Loss of both ejaculation and the experience of orgasm occur if the upper motor neuron lesion is complete.
      (2) Female sexual responses, such as vaginal lubrication and orgasm, are also affected by the level of the injury, but the pathophysiology is less well understood.
   b. **Diabetes mellitus.** The possibility of adult-onset diabetes should always be considered in men over 50 years old who develop erectile failure. Approximately 50% of men with diabetes fail to have erections secondary to diabetic neuropathy. However, the sexual drive tends to remain strong in these men regardless of the success or failure in the treatment of the diabetes. Penile implants, which allow the patient to maintain an erection artificially, can be surgically inserted to allow continuation of an active sex life. The surgery usually involves removing some penile tissue, and thus, the patient can never again have a natural erection.
   c. **Multiple sclerosis** can also cause erectile failure, which can be treated by a penile implant.
   d. **Other illnesses** that cause neurologic impairment of sexual functioning include tumors, syphilis, and pernicious anemia.

C. Surgical procedures

1. **Prostatectomy.** Removal of the prostate gland secondary to benign hypertrophy is a relatively common procedure in elderly men. Impotence frequently occurs but is often due to the patient's expectation rather than to any surgical interruption of the sympathetic plexis of nerves around the abdominal aorta. Retrograde ejaculation into the bladder following surgery is also common.

2. **Orchiectomy.** Because of the risk of cancer, surgical removal of the testes may be necessary upon failure of one of the testicles to descend. Testicular carcinoma also requires removal of one or both testes. Erectile failure should not develop even with bilateral orchiectomy

in adult men, but it often occurs in boys when the testicles are removed. Reassurance and counseling are required to avoid unnecesary psychological and sexual dysfunction.

3. **Hysterectomy** is now the most common surgical procedure in the United States. The psychological associations of the uterus for the patient affect the psychological outcome of the surgery. Most women report no change in sexual functioning following hysterectomy. Because the fear of pregnancy is eliminated, some women derive more enjoyment from sex after surgery. When the surgery is performed for cancer, damage may be extensive, and the psychological stress is greater. This can lead both to increased organic and psychological impairment of sexual functioning.

4. **Mastectomy.** The breasts are an important aspect of a woman's sexual identity. Disfiguring loss of a breast due to mastectomy can have a major effect on a woman's self-image and, thus, her sexual functioning, even if there is no direct effect on sexual physiology.

   The patient may feel that she is no longer attractive to her husband and that he will shun her. The husband may feel guilty or may be afraid to touch or even look at his wife's body. He may think she wishes to be left alone. This withdrawal confirms the patient's fears that she is deformed and repulsive, leading to further isolation and a breakdown in the relationship. The physician must initiate open communication between the couple about the fears and misconceptions that both may have.

5. **Ostomy.** An ostomy usually causes concern about sex. Patients worry about pain, damage to the stoma, as well as about odors of elimination during sexual activity. A single patient who wants a sexual relationship is uncertain when and how a prospective sexual partner should be told about the ostomy. There are no simple or easy answers. It is crucial that the physician be willing and able to listen to the patient and offer support and understanding.

D. **Drugs and alcohol**

1. **Alcohol** is the most common cause of sexual dysfunction. It increases sexual desire but decreases performance. Chronic alcoholism also may affect sexual function because of liver disease. Cirrhotic livers are unable to detoxify estrogens in men, leading to testicular atrophy and decreased sexual performance.

2. **Narcotics and sedative-hypnotics** decrease libido. Drug abuse and addiction of any sort generally lead to decreased interest in sex.

3. **Medication-induced sexual dysfunction.** In one recent study of over 1,000 men in a medical outpatient clinic, at least one-third suffered from erectile failure. At least 25% of these cases were due to prescribed medications. The physicians in the clinic were unaware of the problem even though many of the patients discontinued their medications because of the sexual dysfunction.

   a. **Antihypertensives**
      (1) **Diuretics**
         (a) Thiazide-type diuretics cause erectile dysfunction probably secondary to their action in diminishing peripheral vascular resistance.
         (b) Spironolactone can also cause impotence, gynecomastia, and decreased libido due to its antiandrogen action.
      (2) **Adrenergic inhibitors (β-adrenergic blockers)**
         (a) Propranolol in doses over 320 mg/day is associated with erectile failure and decreased libido.
         (b) Cardiospecific agents, such as atenolol, metoprolol, nadolol, and pindolol, appear to have much less reported sexual dysfunction at usual dosages. High dosages may lead to problems because of loss of cardiospecificity.
      (3) **Central-acting adrenergic inhibitors**
         (a) Methyldopa causes erectile failure, ejaculation disturbances, and decreased libido at doses of 1–3 g/day.
         (b) Clonidine has also been implicated in impotence and reducing sexual drive at doses of 0.2–4.8 mg/day. The side effects of clonidine tend to occur early in treatment and decrease over time.
      (4) **Peripheral-acting adrenergic antagonists.** Guanadrel at dosages of 10–40 mg/day, guanethidine at dosages over 25 mg/day, and reserpine at 0.1 mg/day have all been implicated in decreased libido, ejaculatory difficulties, and impotence. The sexual problems are worse when these drugs are combined with diuretics.
      (5) **α-Adrenergic blockers**
         (a) Phenoxybenzamine has been associated with dry ejaculations in around 5% of men who take dosages up to 70 mg/day. The effect is dose-related.
         (b) Prazosin appears to have a very low incidence of sexual dysfunction.

(6) **Vasodilators.** Hydralazine and minoxidil have not been associated with sexual dysfunction unless used with hydrochlorothiazide or propranolol.

(7) **Slow channel calcium-entry blocking agents.** Verapamil has been implicated in erectile failure at doses of 240–480 mg/day. Libido is not affected.

b. **Psychiatric drugs**

(1) **Cyclic antidepressants.** Decreased libido is difficult to assess as a side effect of these medications because it is primarily a symptom of depression.

    (a) Amitriptyline, amoxapine, doxepin, nortriptyline, and protriptyline have all been associated with delayed or inhibited ejaculation.

    (b) Imipramine and maprotiline have been associated with impotence in men and anorgasmia in women as have the other cyclic antidepresssants.

    (c) Trazodone at doses of 100–300 mg/day, in addition to the side effects already noted, has been implicated in a few cases of priapism with irreversible damage.

    (d) Clomipramine, a new drug effective in the treatment of obsessive–compulsive disorder, has been reported to cause orgasms in both men and women as a result of yawning.

(2) **Monoamine oxidase inhibitors.** Phenelzine (30–90 mg/day), tranylcypromine (20–60 mg/day), and isocarboxazid (20–40 mg/day) have all been associated with impotence and delayed ejaculation in men and anorgasmia in women. Phenelzine has the highest incidence of side effects (20%).

(3) **Lithium.** Decreased libido and impotence have been reported with lithium. However, since hypersexuality is a symptom of mania, it is not clear how much any reported decrease in sex drive is a therapeutic effect and how much is dysfunctional. Many bipolar patients like the symptoms of hypomania, including the increased sex drive.

(4) **Antipsychotics**

    (a) Chlorpromazine-related dysfunction includes erectile failure, failure of ejaculation, and decreased libido. It appears to be dose-related at over 400 mg/day. Priapism has also been reported in a few cases.

    (b) Fluphenazine usage has been associated with the whole range of sexual dysfunction, including anorgasmia and dyspareunia in women.

    (c) Thioridazine is associated with fewer erectile problems, but is noted to interfere with ejaculation in as many as 50% of males on as little as 30 mg/day. Dry ejaculation is not necessarily due to retrograde ejaculation but to inhibition of emission. Painful ejaculation also occurs. Most problems with ejaculation using any of the antipsychotics occur in the first day of use.

(5) **Hormones**

    (a) Androgens other than testosterone and especially anabolic steriods cause decreased libido as well as testicular atrophy in men.

    (b) Estrogens have been reported to cause increased, decreased, and no change in sex drive in women and decreased libido in men.

    (c) The effect of corticosteroids on sexual functioning is unclear.

(6) **Other medications**

    (a) Antibiotics may suppress normal vaginal flora, leading to yeast infections and subsequent dyspareunia in women.

    (b) Cimetidine has been reported to cause erectile failure, gynecomastia, and decreased libido while ranitidine has not.

    (c) Digoxin and disopyramide, two cardiac drugs, have both been associated with impotence.

VIII. HOMOSEXUALITY

A. Overview

1. Homosexual behavior in itself does not imply homosexual orientation. Homosexuality is defined as strong preferential erotic attraction to members of the same sex.

2. Sexual behavior is highly variable, ranging from:
   a. Exclusive heterosexuality
   b. Sporadic homosexual encounters, usually in adolescence and early adulthood
   c. Bisexuality (attraction to partners of both sexes)
   d. Exclusive homosexuality

3. Kinsey's landmark studies showed that over 33% of men and over 10% of women have had an orgasm with a partner of the same sex at least once in their lives.

4. Homosexuality is no longer considered to be an illness; it is considered to be a normal variant of human behavior.

5. Psychopathology in homosexuals is as varied as it is in heterosexuals. The incidence and prevalence of mental illness in homosexuals are no higher than in heterosexuals. Disturbed individuals may have an impaired sense of self, affect regulation, reality testing, impulse control, and object relations (ability to have relationships). Healthy individuals, on the other hand, show high-level ego functions reflected in maturity, productivity, and sustained relationships.

6. Male homosexuals who have many sexual partners are at increased risk for medical illness, such as acquired immune deficiency syndrome (AIDS), hepatitis, and venereal disease. AIDS has profoundly modified the sexual practices in the homosexual community.

7. Female homosexuality carries less stigma than male homosexuality. Lesbians may have been married, and many have children. Lesbians are less likely to have multiple partners and more likely to have long-term relationships than homosexual men.

8. Homophobia refers to the irrational fear of homosexuality. Societal attitudes, including prejudice, discrimination, and harassment, are distressing for male and female homosexuals as they would be for any minority group. Internalizing such attitudes impedes the development of a positive identity for homosexual individuals.

9. Civil rights awareness and "homosexual activism" of the sixties and seventies raised the consciousness of the homosexual community and increased the support available for homosexual and lesbian individuals.

10. "Coming out" is the process whereby one's homosexual orientation is accepted and integrated with the sense of self and the external world. This can be viewed as a lifelong process.

B. **Etiology.** The causes of homosexuality are not well understood.

1. **Psychological factors.** Psychological theories of homosexuality have focused on disturbances in the family during early development.
   a. The stereotypical family constellation associated with male homosexuality is the overly close mother who devalues a distant or weak father. This is thought to result in failure of identification with the father and aversion to women. However, not all men from such a family constellation become homosexual, and many male homosexuals have different family backgrounds.
   b. Family backgrounds of female homosexuals are more diverse and less well understood.

2. **Biologic factors**
   a. Genetic factors are suggested by studies that show a higher concordance for male homosexual behavior in monozygotic than dizygotic twins. Other studies show an increased evidence of homosexuality in first-degree male relatives of male homosexuals.
   b. Fetal exposure to abnormal androgen levels has been postulated to affect differentiation of the brain and lead to changes in adult sexual orientation.

C. **Treatment** should deal with the issues with which the individual wishes assistance. It is inappropriate to try to force individuals to change their sexual preference unless they desire this. Techniques used include psychoanalysis, psychoanalytically oriented psychotherapy, group therapy, and conditioning techniques with adversive and reinforcing stimuli.

1. Homosexual individuals may seek treatment for a specific problem, such as depression, and not experience homosexuality as an issue that needs to be addressed. Such individuals require diagnosis and treatment of the presenting problem.

2. Some homosexual individuals seek treatment to come to terms with their homosexuality. Issues in such psychotherapy might include self-acceptance, self-esteem, dealing with guilt, dealing with the responses of others, and improving relationships.

3. A small number of homosexual individuals seek treatment to change their sexual object choice. This goal has a better prognosis if the patient:
   a. Is highly motivated
   b. Is under age 35
   c. Has a history of previous heterosexual behavior
   d. Has recent onset of homosexual behavior
   e. In males, has an aggressive personality pattern

IX. PREMENSTRUAL SYNDROME (PMS) OR LATE LUTEAL PHASE DYSPHORIC DISORDER (DSM-III-R)

A. Definition. PMS is defined as physical or psychological symptoms that begin the week prior to menstruation and resolve shortly after the onset of the menstrual flow. The symptoms must be of such severity as to impair functioning. In order to make this diagnosis, symptoms must be charted prospectively because retrospective reports have been shown to be invalid. As many as 80% of women who complain of premenstrual syndrome do not meet the criteria when prospective charting is used. Most women who complain of PMS but do not meet the charting criteria exhibit another *DSM-III-R* diagnosis, such as affective, anxiety or substance abuse disorders. Of the women whose cyclical symptoms are verified by prospective charting, a subgroup will meet the criteria for other *DSM-III-R* diagnoses and should receive treatment for these disorders. The diagnosis of premenstrual syndrome should be reserved for women with cyclic symptoms who do not meet other psychiatric diagnostic criteria. While a multitude of symptoms have been described for PMS, typical complaints include:

1. **Psychological complaints**
   a. Tension
   b. Irritability
   c. Depression
   d. Anxiety
   e. Lability
   f. Food craving

2. **Physical complaints**
   a. Breast tenderness
   b. Weight gain
   c. Bloating
   d. Fatigue

B. Etiology. The cause of PMS is not well established.

1. Theories about imbalance of estrogen and progesterone levels have not been validated.

2. There is an increasing interest in the effect of female gonadal hormones on central nervous system monoamine activity, particularly serotonin.

3. Thyroid abnormalities have been noted in some groups that meet the rigorous definition of PMS.

4. Endorphin activity may be altered by the menstrual cycle.

5. Aldosterone levels may be elevated, leading to water retention.

6. Prostaglandin levels may be elevated, leading to water retention, pain symptoms, and dysphoria.

7. When women expect to have PMS symptoms, they are more likely to report symptoms, whether or not they are actually premenstrual.

C. Treatment. Since the etiology of PMS is unclear, various empirical approaches are used.

1. **Education.** The patient can be taught to recognize her cyclic fluctuations and anticipate problems. The process of charting the symptoms is helpful in promoting self-awareness.

2. **Nonspecific approaches**
   a. Diet should consist of regular small meals low in sodium, sugar, sodium, and caffeine.
   b. Substance use, especially alcohol, should be avoided.
   c. Regular physical exercise will reduce tension and stress.

3. **Medications** have been shown to be helpful for some patients.
   a. Bromocriptine is useful in alleviating breast symptoms.
   b. Diuretics are useful for weight gain and edema.
   c. Prostaglandin inhibitors are useful for dysmenorrhea pain.
   d. Ovulation suppressants, such as oral contraceptives, are useful for some patients.
   e. Antianxiety medication is useful for tension and irritability symptoms.
   f. Progesterone suppositories have been a popular treatment for PMS, but numerous well-designed studies have shown them to be no better than placebo.
   g. Pyridoxine (vitamin B$_6$) and magnesium supplementation have also been popular, but their efficacy is unclear.

BIBLIOGRAPHY

Annon JS: *The Behavioral Treatment of Sexual Problems: Brief Therapy.* Harper and Row, New York, 1976

Kaplan HS: *The New Sex Therapy.* New York, New York Times Book Company, 1976

Kaplan HS: *The Evaluation of Sexual Disorders.* New York, Brunner Mazel, 1983

Kinsey, AC: *Sexual Behavior in the Human Male.* Philadelphia, Saunders, 1948

Kinsey AC, Pomeroy WB, Martin CE, et al: *Sexual Behavior in the Human Female.* Philadelphia, Saunders, 1953

Marmor J: Homosexuality and sexual orientation disturbances. In *Comprehensive Textbook of Psychiatry,* 2nd ed. Edited by Freedman AM, Kaplan HI, Sadach B. Baltimore, Williams and Wilkins, 1975

Masters WH, Johnson V: *Human Sexual Inadequacy.* Boston, Little, Brown, 1970

STUDY QUESTIONS

Directions: Each question below contains five suggested answers. Choose the **one best** response to each question.

1. All of the following statements about normal sexual response are true EXCEPT

(A) physical stimulation of the bladder may produce an involuntary sexual response
(B) erection and lubrication depend upon arousal of the parasympathetic nervous system
(C) arousal of the sympathetic nervous system inhibits sexual response
(D) stages of sexual response include excitement, plateau, and resolution
(E) psychic stimuli are mediated through the prefrontal cortex and the anterior spinal cord

2. Lubrication of the vagina is a prominent feature of which of the following stages of normal sexual response in women?

(A) Desire
(B) Excitement
(C) Plateau
(D) Orgasm
(E) Resolution

3. Transsexualism is best characterized by all of the following statements EXCEPT

(A) the disorder usually begins in childhood
(B) transsexual boys believe that they will lose their penises and testicles when they grow up
(C) transsexual girls usually have been dressed like boys by their mothers
(D) the etiology of transsexualism is not known for certain
(E) the transsexual wishes to live as a member of the opposite sex

4. Pedophilia is best characterized by all of the following statements EXCEPT

(A) it is often caused by an organic mental syndrome
(B) the adult perpetrator must be at least 6 years older than the victim
(C) the disorder involves prepubertal children of either sex
(D) the diagnosis can be made when sexual stimulation is achieved by fantasy
(E) sexual abuse of children may be more common than has been appreciated in the past

5. What it the most common reason that adequate sexual histories are not obtained from patients?

(A) The patient is embarrassed about the subject of sex
(B) The patient has religious or moral qualms about the subject of sex
(C) The physician does not think that sex is as important as other medical issues
(D) There is not enough time to cover the subject adequately in taking a routine history
(E) The physician is uncomfortable with the subject of sex

6. What is the most common reason for cessation of sexual activity in married couples?

(A) Aging
(B) Marital discord
(C) Physical illness
(D) Cultural prohibitions
(E) Depression

7. All of the following statements about secondary failure of erection are true EXCEPT

(A) it may be present in only certain situations
(B) it must occur in 20%–30% of attempts at intercourse for diagnosis
(C) it becomes increasingly common with age
(D) overindulgence in alcohol is often the precipitating factor
(E) it usually is associated with an overly rigid upbringing

8. What physical impairment is most responsible for sexual dysfunction in men?

(A) Spinal cord injury
(B) Diabetes mellitus
(C) Benign prostatic hypertrophy
(D) Testicular carcinoma
(E) Multiple sclerosis

Directions: Each question below contains four suggested answers of which **one or more** is correct. Choose the answer

    A if **1, 2, and 3** are correct
    B if **1 and 3** are correct
    C if **2 and 4** are correct
    D if **4** is correct
    E if **1, 2, 3, and 4** are correct

9. Correct statements concerning the sexual disorder of masochism include which of the following?

(1) fantasies of being bound or hurt that lead to sexual excitement are sufficient to make the diagnosis
(2) the patient takes on the martyr's role of suffering and sacrifice in interpersonal relationships
(3) the patient is not likely to achieve sexual gratification by inflicting pain on another, only by receiving it
(4) a single episode in which the patient was physically harmed in order to achieve sexual excitement is sufficient to make the diagnosis

10. Treatment for paraphilias can involve

(1) outpatient psychotherapy
(2) hormone treatment
(3) a high failure rate
(4) relaxation techniques

11. To obtain a thorough sexual history, it is necessary for the physician to inquire about

(1) familial attitudes about sex
(2) any history of sexual abuse
(3) the first sexual experience
(4) current sexual functioning

12. The psychosexual disorder of hypoactive sexual desire can be diagnosed in patients with which of the following findings?

(1) Little or no sexual desire lasting more than 6 months
(2) Lack of sexual desire following major surgery
(3) Distress reported by the sexual partner rather than by the patient
(4) Lack of sexual desire with the marriage partner but not with other partners

13. Sexual aversion disorder is characterized by which of the following statements?

(1) It is sometimes secondary to organic causes
(2) It is thought to be related to discord in the relationship
(3) It affects more than 20% of couples
(4) The diagnosis depends on cultural and lifestyle variables

14. True statements concerning inhibited female orgasm include

(1) inhibited female orgasm is common and usually does not indicate psychopathology
(2) primary orgasmic dysfunction is more difficult to treat than secondary orgasmic dysfunction
(3) associated symptoms include pelvic pain and vaginal discharge
(4) physiologic impairment is the most likely cause of secondary orgasmic dysfunction

15. Premature ejaculation has which of the following characteristics?

(1) It is uncommon in younger men
(2) It benefits from treatment of anxiety
(3) It is associated with major psychopathology
(4) Treatment benefits from assistance of the partner

16. Vaginismus involves tightening of the paravaginal muscles to prevent penile penetration. Characteristics of the disorder include

(1) occasional occurrence during pelvic examinations
(2) occasional development secondary to vaginal infections
(3) occurrence in all or only some sexual encounters
(4) a history of sexual abuse in childhood

SUMMARY OF DIRECTIONS

A	B	C	D	E
1, 2, 3 only	1, 3 only	2, 4 only	4 only	All are correct

---

17. Dyspareunia is defined by which of the following characteristics?

(1) Lack of lubrication
(2) Constriction of vaginal muscles
(3) Equal incidence among men and women
(4) Pain during intercourse

18. Spinal cord injuries in men can have which of the following effects?

(1) Increase the rate of divorce
(2) Impair orgasm
(3) Require careful management of bladder and bowel care
(4) Interrupt sexual responsiveness

19. Correct statements concerning women who complain of premenstrual syndrome include which of the following?

(1) The majority do not meet the diagnostic criteria on symptom charting
(2) Mood disorders are common
(3) Other psychiatric disorders must be ruled out
(4) Symptoms often include arthralgia, nausea, and vomiting

20. Treatment of PMS involves which of the following?

(1) Progesterone suppositories
(2) Avoidance of substance use, especially alcohol
(3) B_6 supplementation
(4) Dietary changes and exercise

Directions: The groups of questions below consist of lettered choices followed by several numbered items. For each numbered item select the **one** lettered choice with which it is **most** closely associated. Each lettered choice may be used once, more than once, or not at all.

Questions 21–24

For each phase of psychological development as described by Freud listed below, select the characteristic with which it is most closely associated.

(A) Undifferentiated gender
(B) Separation–individuation
(C) Interest in masturbation
(D) Identification with parent of same sex
(E) None of the above

21. Anal phase

22. Oedipal phase

23. Oral phase

24. Phallic phase

Questions 25–29

For each paraphilia listed below, select the object of desire or characteristic most commonly associated with it.

(A) Children
(B) Nonhuman object
(C) Hostility
(D) Requires suffering
(E) No physical contact

25. Fetishism

26. Pedophilia

27. Exhibitionism

28. Voyeurism

29. Masochism

ANSWERS AND EXPLANATIONS

1. The answer is E. (*I A 1, 2 a–c*) Psychic stimuli are mediated through the limbic system, the hypothalamus, and the lateral spinal cord. Physical stimulation of the bladder and the bowel as well as the genitals may produce an involuntary sexual response through the spinal cord. The parasympathetic nervous system is responsible for erection and lubrication; sympathetic arousal inhibits this response. The stages of sexual response are desire, excitement, plateau, orgasm, and resolution.

2. The answer is C. (*I C 2*)) During the plateau stage of normal sexual response in women, the clitoris becomes sensitive and retracts, the labia deepen in color, and the vagina becomes lubricated. During the excitement phase, breast size increases, nipples stand out, the clitoris lengthens, and the heart rate and blood pressure increase. During the orgasm stage, there is a rhythmic contraction of the orgasmic platform. During resolution, vasocongestion is lost.

3. The answer is C. (*III A 1–3, B*)) Although the etiology of transsexualism is not known for certain, boys have histories of being crossdressed by their mothers as well as having overly close physical and emotional ties to them; their fathers generally have been absent. Girls tend to have distant relationships with their mothers, who are seen as unavailable physically or emotionally during the formative years. The disorder begins in childhood, and boys believe that they will lose their penises and testicles when they grow up. This is not a homosexual condition; patients wish to live as members of the opposite sex.

4. The answer is A. (*IV C 4*)) When an individual with an organic mental syndrome engages in sexual activity with a child, pedophilia is not diagnosed; inappropriate sexual activity can be characteristic of brain damage. By definition, an adult with pedophilia must be at least 6 years older than the victim. When the perpetrator is a late adolescent, the age difference is less clear and clinical judgment must be used. The disorder involves prepubertal children of either sex, and the diagnosis can be made when the sexual stimulation is achieved by fantasy alone. The incidence of sexual abuse of children appears to be much higher than had been previously thought, and statistics are changing as the general population becomes more aware of the problem.

5. The answer is E. (*V B 1*) The most common reason that physicians do not ask adequate questions concerning sexuality is their own anxiety about the subject. Patients are certainly embarrassed as well, but, if there is a problem, they usually hope that their physicians will take the lead in discussing it. Religious and moral objections to talking about sex are not very common. Physicians' impressions that sex is not as important as other medical issues is usually only a cover for their anxiety. It takes only a moment to ask screening questions about sexuality, and, if there are difficulties, the subject can be dealt with later when there is adequate time.

6. The answer is B. (*V C 1 a, b*) Many factors can affect the sexual activity of couples, including aging, physical illness, and psychiatric illness, such as depression. However, more commonly than not, the reason that sexual activity ceases is discord in the marital relationship. Cultural prohibitions may play a role but usually not as frequently as discord.

7. The answer is E. [*V C 3 b (1)–(3)*] Primary erectile dysfunction is usually associated with an overly rigid upbringing in which any expression of sexuality was punished. Secondary erectile dysfunction usually results from anxiety about sexual performance. It may be present in only certain situations or with certain partners. Diagnosis is not made when it is a rare or occasional event but when it occurs in about 25% or more of attempts at intercourse. It becomes increasingly common with age and is often precipitated by a bout of drinking, which leads to increased anxiety about performance.

8. The answer is B. (*VII B 2 b*) Diabetes mellitus is a very common cause of sexual impairment in men, and it should always be considered as a possible cause of erectile failure in men over 50 years of age. Approximately one-half of men with adult-onset diabetes develop erectile failure secondary to diabetic neuropathy. Spinal cord injury is a far less common cause of sexual impairment, but certainly issues of sexuality need to be discussed with these patients. Benign prostatic hypertrophy should not cause sexual impairment, but occasionally, the surgery for the condition does. In comparison to diabetes, testicular carcinoma and multiple sclerosis are rare causes of dysfunction.

9. The answer is D (4). (*IV C 7*) If the patient even once allows him- or herself to be harmed in order to achieve sexual excitement, the diagnosis of the sexual disorder of masochism can be made. Fantasies about being bound or hurt by themselves are not sufficient to make the diagnosis. The martyr's role of suffering and sacrifice in an interpersonal relationship is moral masochism; it is not the sexual disorder of masochism. Whereas the other paraphilias are almost exclusively seen in men, masochism is also seen in women, although not commonly. Sadism, the achievement of sexual gratification by inflicting pain on others, is often seen in conjunction with masochism, hence the disorder, sadomasochism.

10. The answer is A (1, 2, 3). (*IV D 1, 2*) Despite limited effectiveness, outpatient therapy is commonly used for paraphilias. Antiandrogen drugs have been effective in reducing sexual drive in some paraphilias. Overall, the treatment of paraphilias has been discouraging with a high failure rate. This is thought to be due to the fact that paraphilias involve sexual gratification, and it is difficult for anyone to give up sexual pleasure, even if the legal risk is high. Relaxation techniques have no role in the treatment of this disorder.

11. The answer is E (all). (*V B 3 b*) A discussion led by the physician with the patient concerning the attitudes of the patient's family about sex is important in obtaining a thorough sexual history. Was sex seen as dirty and was discussion prohibited, or was there an openness about sexuality? In addition, it is increasingly important that discussion with the patient include any history of sexual abuse; this is particularly important with women patients. Questioning the patient about his or her first sexual experience is also important, particularly whether it was a pleasant or frightening event. Even the most basic screening questions should evaluate the patient's current sexual functioning.

12. The answer is B (1, 3). (*V C 1*) The diagnostic criterion of hypoactive sexual desire is persistent and pervasive inhibition of sexual desire or fantasies about sex. The clinician must take into account factors that affect sexual desire, such as health. Generally, the disorder is not diagnosed if the patient has a normal lack of sexual desire immediately following major surgery or if there are marital problems, such that one partner lacks sexual desire for the spouse but not for other partners. If the patient's sexual desire has been inhibited for more than 6 months, the diagnosis can be made. A diagnosis is also valid upon report of distress from the partner rather than the patient.

13. The answer is C (2, 4). (*V C 2*) Sexual aversion disorder in which patients suffer from a persistent or recurrent extreme aversion to genital sex with a sex partner is often associated with discord in the relationship. The diagnosis of sexual aversion disorder requires an evaluation of cultural and lifestyle variables, which may affect sexual expression; it is not an appropriate diagnosis if the cause is organic. There is little information about the prevalence of this disorder, but clinical experience suggests that it is less than 20% of couples.

14. The answer is B (1, 3). (*V C 4 a*) While some women who do not have orgasms are nonsymptomatic, others may develop symptoms of pelvic pain, vaginal discharge, and feelings of tiredness and irritability. The disorder is common, but its presence does not always indicate psychopathology because there are often cultural restrictions regarding women's sexuality. These women have a normal excitement phase, but it does not lead to orgasm. Primary orgasmic dysfunction may be more easily treated because women may not have "learned" to have an orgasm and can be taught once inhibitions about sexuality have resolved. When secondary orgasmic dysfunction develops, it is almost always as a result of psychological issues in the sexual relationship.

15. The answer is C (2, 4). (*V C 4 c*) Premature ejaculation is defined as recurrent ejaculation with minimal stimulation before the man wishes it to occur. It is the most common sexual dysfunction of men, particularly young men, and it is not associated with major psychopathology. Behavioral techniques, which require a cooperative partner, are successful in reducing performance anxiety in most cases.

16. The answer is E (all). (*V C 5 a*) Patients with vaginismus often come from backgrounds in which sex was considered sinful and behavior by the parents was overcontrolling; some patients have had traumatic sexual experiences, such as incest and rape, which cause anxiety, tension, and pain in subsequent sexual experiences that inadvertently reinforces the vaginal spasm. The paravaginal muscles are tightened involuntarily, thus preventing penile penetration. Occasionally, this condition occurs in the physician's office during a pelvic examination; sometimes it develops secondary to vaginal infections and irritation. By definition, it can occur in all sexual encounters or only in some.

17. The answer is D (4). (*V C 6*) Dyspareunia refers to pain during intercourse. Lubrication may or may not be normal. While some cases may involve constriction of vaginal muscles, such symptoms usually indicate vaginismus, not dyspareunia. Dyspareunia is rare in men.

18. The answer is A (1, 2, 3). (*VII B 2*) Divorce rates increase following spinal cord injuries in men as adjustment to these injuries is difficult. Physicians must facilitate frank discussions of sexuality following spinal cord injury, including alternative means of sexual expression and control of bowel and bladder function. Contrary to popular belief, spinal cord injuries do not commonly stop sexual responsiveness or impair orgasmic abilities; however, loss of ejaculation and the experience of orgasm do occur if upper motor neuron lesions are complete.

19. The answer is A (1, 2, 3). (*IX A*) Most women who complain of the premenstrual syndrome (PMS) do not meet the diagnostic criteria after prospective charting of symptoms. Of these women, many exhibit another *DSM-III-R* diagnosis, such as affective, anxiety, or substance abuse disorders. Arthralgia, nausea, and vomiting are not usually associated with PMS.

20. The answer is C (2, 4). (*IX C*) The treatment of premenstrual syndrome is largely empirical and commonly involves dietary changes, including the avoidance of substance use, and increased exercise. Some medications have been shown to be useful, including bromocriptine, diuretics, prostaglandin inhibitors, ovulation suppressants, and antianxiety medication. Despite considerable popularity, recent studies have shown progesterone suppositories and vitamin B_6 supplementation to be no better than a placebo.

21–24. The answers are: 21-B, 22-D, 23-A, 24-C. (*II B 1 b–d*) Freud's concept of the anal phase, which refers to issues of control over bodily function, was applied to children age 1½–3 years. Other developmental tasks associated with this period are separation–individuation, wherein the child gradually becomes a separate entity from the mother, gender identification, the beginning of socialization, and language readiness.

In the fourth and fifth years, strong sexual feelings about the opposite sex parent are common (oedipal phase). In normal development, if the same sex parent does not overreact and remains accepting to the child, the child will accept the reality of his or her position in the family and develop a healthy identification with the same sex parent.

Freud's concept of the oral phase was applied to children in the first year of life. The infant initially shows no evidence of gender differentiation, and only with maturation and interaction with the parents does the child gain a sense of gender differentiation. Also during this period, the child experiences the regular satisfaction of his or her needs and, thus, develops a sense of basic trust.

In normal development, the child experiences pride in his or her genitalia and self in the preschool years, which Freud labeled the phallic phase. Masturbation becomes more obviously pleasurable, and fear of bodily injury is common in this period (fear of castration in boys and fear of genital penetration and mutilation in girls).

25–29. The answers are: 25-B, 26-A, 27-C, 28-E, 29-D. (*IV C 1, 4–7*) Fetishism involves sexual excitement from a nonliving object, such as women's clothing. This disorder does not include objects designed for sexual stimulation, such as vibrators. Pedophilia involves sexual interest, either activity or fantasy, in prepubertal children. Exhibitionism is associated with a conscious wish to shock the observer. Affected individuals expose their genitals in order to obtain sexual gratification. Hostility is usually present. Voyeurism involves sexual excitement from observing unsuspecting people naked or in the act of disrobing. The voyeur does not seek contact with the observed person and achieves orgasm by masturbating while looking. Masochism involves the achievement of sexual pleasure only through physical pain or suffering.

9
Eating Disorders
Donald W. Bechtold

I. ANOREXIA NERVOSA is an eating disorder exemplified by obsessional weight loss without an identifiable organic cause.

A. Diagnostic and associated findings

1. **Diagnostic findings***
   a. The age of onset is before 25 years except in unusual cases.
   b. Weight loss is at least 15% of the original body weight or of the ideal body weight.
   c. Fear of becoming obese (and of eating) is paramount in the clinical picture.
   d. The body image of the patient is disturbed (i.e., the patient feels fat despite emaciation). This perception may not be limited to anorectics, however, and is sometimes found in normal-sized adolescents.
   e. The patient refuses to maintain a normal weight and becomes preoccupied with weight-losing activities.
   f. Amenorrhea (absence of three consecutive menstrual cycles) is a classic presentation. It may occur before, during, or after weight loss; menses do not necessarily resume with weight gain in contrast to amenorrhea secondary to simple malnutrition. The reason that menstruation is not necessarily tied to weight in anorexia nervosa is unknown.

2. **Associated findings**, which may precede or accompany the onset of illness
   a. Lanugo hair development
   b. Heightened activity level
   c. Vomiting and purging
   d. Laxative, cathartic, and diuretic abuse
   e. Lowered metabolic rate manifested by bradycardia, hypotension, and hypothermia
   f. Normal thyroid-stimulating hormone levels; possible low triiodothyronine (T_3) levels
   g. Normal or overstimulated adrenal axis; a possible loss of normal diurnal variation in cortisol secretion
   h. Characteristically normal protein and albumin concentrations
   i. Increased serum carotene, which is rare in other causes of weight loss
   j. Partial development of diabetes insipidus
   k. Possible increase in growth hormone levels
   l. Dehydration and serious electrolyte abnormalities
   m. Abdominal pain
   n. Three personality styles, which are classically cited as preceding the onset of anorexia nervosa:
      (1) **Obsessive–compulsive (perfectionistic).** A girl who is perfectionistic about other areas of her life may focus her compulsivity on eating.
      (2) **Hysterical.** An hysteric overly sexualizes his or her relationships because of conflicts about sexuality. Such conflicts may also play a role in the etiology of anorexia nervosa.
      (3) **Schizoid (schizotypal).** Because a schizoid individual is prone to odd behavior, he or she is more likely to have unusual eating behavior.

B. Epidemiology

1. **The prevalence** of anorexia nervosa is approximately 1 in 200 girls at puberty. The disorder

---

*This information is taken from the American Psychiatric Association's *Diagnostic and Statistical Manual of Mental Disorders*, 3rd ed., revised. Washington, D.C., American Psychiatric Association, 1987.

occurs in girls much more commonly than in boys at a ratio of between 10 and 20 to 1.

2. **The incidence** of the disorder is increasing, probably due to altered social attitudes and changing roles for women (e.g., the high value placed on thinness in Western societies).

3. **Race and socioeconomic status.** Anorexia nervosa appears to be more common in Western civilization, and Caucasians have the highest rate of this disorder, particularly girls of Jewish and Italian families. Middle- and upper-class families are at the greatest risk.

4. **Age.** The average age of onset of the illness is 13–14 years; the onset often is preceded by a period of mild obesity or mild dieting. It is interesting to note that a relatively high percentage of anorectics lose a parent within the year preceding the onset of the illness.

5. **Genetic predisposition.** Anorexia nervosa has a higher incidence among patients with Turner's syndrome, which is characterized by the absence of the second X chromosome (45,XO) than in the population at large. The genetic implications of this association are not presently understood.

6. **Mental illness**
   a. There may be a slightly increased risk of anorexia nervosa developing in mentally retarded children, although many anorectic individuals are high achievers with above-average intelligence.
   b. Anorectic patients are at greater risk than the general population of developing either unipolar or bipolar mood disorders. These disturbances tend to occur later in life and probably are not the underlying cause of anorexia nervosa.
   c. The risk for suicide is increased in anorectic patients.

C. **Etiology**

1. **One psychological theory** holds that anorectic patients have a deep fear of impregnation and an accompanying fantasy that impregnation occurs through the oral route. They defend themselves against pregnancy by not eating. A corollary to this theory is that affected adolescents fear sexuality, menarche, and pregnancy and starve themselves to remain prepubertal. In this theory, anorexia nervosa is understood as an attempt to avoid developmental, phase-specific conflicts.

2. **The transactional theory** considers the interactions between parent and child. A series of particular interactions may cause slight changes in the family system, which, in turn, may lead to a new and more deviated set of interactions. The child's request not to eat or refusal to eat is overridden by the parent's need to feed the child. Eventually, the child loses the ability to regulate her own eating and becomes dependent on her environment in a pervasive way for cues concerning this and other areas of self-regulation. For example, anorectic girls are unable to maintain weight at a norm. Lacking the ability to follow internal cues (e.g., satiety and hunger), such girls rely on strict diet, observations of parents, and careful calorie counts to guide eating behavior. They may depend on parental approval to guide social activity rather than feeling a sense of who *they* are and what *they* want to do with themselves.

3. **Family system models** also consider the interactions between parents and children. An underlying assumption of this model is that family systems seek to maintain a dynamic equilibrium. Changes in any part of the system result in a disequilibrium and require compensatory changes in other parts of the system to establish a new equilibrium. Attempts of adolescent children to begin the developmental process of separation and emancipation in overinvolved families or to exert developmentally appropriate autonomy and self-control in rigid, autocratic families are seen as disequilibrating factors in the family system. To the extent that the parental component of the family system resists change, the regression of the child from normal adolescent strivings to a preadolescent developmental posture through the symptoms of anorexia nervosa represents an accommodation within the family system, resulting in a new equilibrium. Thus, the active involvement of parents in the treatment of children with anorexia nervosa is mandatory.
   a. **The mother-daughter relationship** could play a role in the etiology. Mothers of anorectic girls are often controlling, allowing their daughters little autonomy. The child's developing and maintaining control over eating and weight could be a method of counteracting such maternal effects. Mothers of anorectic girls may also be fragile in terms of feminine identity and self-esteem, perceiving their pubescent daughters as competitive and threatening. Regression of the child to a prepubertal body morphology may serve to relieve this disequilibrating force in the family system.

b. The fathers of anorectics are often obsessive–compulsive. They may participate in quasi weight-control activities, such as distance running, and may transmit their attitudes about weight to their daughters. ("Obligate running" among males has been considered by some to be a male equivalent to anorexia nervosa.) Fathers of anorectic girls may also be fearful of their own sexual impulses toward their daughters, which are heightened by their pubertal development. Again, the regression to a prepubertal body morphology may relieve this disequilibrating force in the family system.

4. Endocrine disorders

    a. An increase in catecholamine activity at various central nervous system sites could account for some of the stigmata of this illness.

    b. A variety of endocrine abnormalities (listed in section I A 2 f, g), which may signify some alteration in normal hypothalamic–pituitary function, occur in this disease.

D. Differential diagnosis

1. Medical conditions

    a. Addison's disease may present with weight loss, anorexia, vomiting, and electrolyte abnormalities. It differs from anorexia nervosa in that listlessness and depression are frequent concomitants (in contrast to the hyperactivity of anorexia nervosa). Sodium concentration is low, potassium concentration is high, and serum cortisol levels should be suppressed in Addison's disease.

    b. Hypothyroidism may present with cold intolerance, constipation, bradycardia, low blood pressure, and skin changes similar to those seen in anorexia nervosa (i.e., dry, scaling skin). Obsessional food handling, weight loss (and accompanying fear of weight gain), and hyperactivity are not usual, however.

    c. Hyperthyroidism presents with elevated vital signs, hyperactivity, and, sometimes, weight loss. However, hyperthyroid patients usually are not obsessive about food.

    d. Any chronic illness (e.g., Crohn's disease, ulcerative colitis, rheumatoid arthritis, collagen-vascular disease, and tuberculosis) can cause progressive weight loss but should be readily identifiable as a physical disorder.

    e. Neoplasms, especially central nervous system tumors, can cause endocrine malfunction (e.g., tumors of the hypothalamus or third ventricle). Visual disturbances or panhypopituitarism secondary to the tumor should be evident.

    f. Superior mesenteric artery syndrome can cause vomiting and anorexia. The mechanism is thought to involve compression of the duodenum by the superior mesenteric artery, particularly when the patient is supine and especially in individuals who are thin. When found concomitantly with anorexia nervosa, it is often difficult to ascertain whether it is primary and etiologic or secondary to the weight loss of anorexia nervosa.

2. Psychiatric conditions

    a. Schizophrenia. Although schizophrenics may be delusional about food, the delusions are much more bizarre than those seen in anorectics (e.g., "there's poison in this" versus "this will make me fat"). Other stigmata of schizophrenia should be present.

    b. Bulimia nervosa involves binge eating followed by some form of purging in a patient who otherwise maintains her weight.

    c. Depression is often accompanied by anorexia. In this case, the anorexia is a so-called vegetative sign of depression, and a depressed mood is usually pronounced.

    d. Hysterical noneating is distinguishable by the absence of a morbid concern with weight and calories.

3. Anorexia nervosa as a syndrome. Recent research suggests that anorexia nervosa is a syndrome that can be subclassified. Such subclassification is useful both prognostically and (perhaps) in treatment.

    a. Patients with anorexia accompanied by bulimia may form a distinct subgroup. As such, these patients seem to be more extroverted, present with the disorder later in life, and have a worse prognosis than patients who indulge only in persistent self-starvation.

    b. The anorexia nervosa subgroup is characterized by strict self-starvation.

    c. Vomiters may form another subgroup; they tend to herald a more chronic course with a poorer prognosis.

    d. Male anorectics may form yet another distinct subgroup.

E. Treatment

1. Medical management

    a. The anorectic patient must be protected from the potentially lethal complications of starvation, metabolic disturbances and cardiac dysrhythmias. It is important to determine how much weight has been lost and within what time period so that a medical emergency is not missed. In severe cases, medical intervention may be lifesaving.

    b. It is also important to understand the propensity of anorectics to deny and conceal the severity of their conditions. Careful attention should be paid to accuracy of weight measurements. Serial weights should be obtained at the same time of day, on the same scale, in the same garb (preferably a hospital gown only), and after voiding. Attempts to artificially pad weight by drinking large quantities of water or concealing objects on the body are typical of anorectics.

2. Medications

    a. Antidepressant drugs are not of universal value, but they may be useful in certain individual cases. Responsivity to antidepressant medications may suggest a co-existent mood disorder.

    b. Cyproheptadine may be of some value because it has appetite-stimulating properties.

    c. Antipsychotic medication should be used only when the patient suffers from pre-schizophrenic illness.

3. Psychotherapy is nearly always a useful adjunct to other treatment modalities, but it is rarely effective alone. Psychoanalysis is usually particularly ineffective in anorexia nervosa if it is the only treatment intervention. Both can foster a regression in patients, which, in treatment, is useful only when the patient has the ability and strength to pull out of the regression at the end of the session. Neither of these treatments provides enough structure for the patient (e.g., anorectics may need to be watched and instructed most of the day).

    a. Mechanism and approach

        (1) Initially, the therapeutic work should be aimed at forming an alliance with the patient to work on particular problems.

        (2) Gaps in the patient's ego should be clarified (e.g., when the patient is obviously angry about something but is unaware of this, her affect can be pointed out to her).

        (3) Transference reactions should be interpreted if and when they interfere with the patient's ability to work on and talk about her problems.

        (4) An empathic stance should be maintained with the patient.

    b. Contraindications

        (1) The patient steadfastly refuses to work with the therapist.

        (2) If the patient suffers from a severe borderline personality disorder, psychotherapy may worsen her condition because anorectics may be intolerant of regression. This is usually not predictable, however, until a trial of psychotherapy has been instituted.

4. Family therapy. Some form of **family intervention is nearly always indicated**, especially for adolescents.

    a. Approach. Styles of family interaction should be clarified, and projections and vicarious pleasures that family members derive from the patient's symptoms should be interpreted. The family should be allied with the staff, working toward the patient's betterment, and not with the patient to her detriment.

    b. Contraindications. There are none.

5. Hospitalization

    a. Indications

        (1) The patient loses weight despite outpatient intervention.

        (2) The patient is suicidal.

        (3) Vomiting and purging are causing acid–base or electrolyte problems.

        (4) The family cannot tolerate having the child at home any longer and adequate, less restrictive alternatives are not available.

    b. Treatment approach

        (1) Medical management should include:

            (a) Monitoring the electrolyte and hydration status of the patient. Thyroid stimulation is usually unnecessary.

            (b) Weighing the patient every other day

            (c) Providing alimentation by a nasogastric tube if the patient steadfastly refuses to eat

            (d) Readministering food if the food is vomited

            (e) Providing hyperalimentation through a central intravenous line if all of the above measures fail

        (2) Behavior modification is usually necessary. The patient's privileges (e.g., confinement in a locked unit versus freedom to leave the ward) should be tied to the behavioral approach and be commensurate with the patient's ability to regulate her own activity and eating. Splitting (pitting one staff member against another) and manipulations concerning eating are common and should be discussed at staff meetings and with the patient. Flexibility is important. These patients can be extraordinarily manipulative. Peer interaction and feedback should be sought and emphasized since adolescents often pay more attention to their peers than to adults.

- (a) **Indications for behavior modification**
    - (i) If psychotherapy fails
    - (ii) If there is no time to wait for the results of psychotherapy
- (b) **Approach**
    - (i) The patient's weight should be the target symptom, not the eating behavior, amount of exercise, or vomiting, and reinforcers should be tied to weight fluctuation.
    - (ii) Once the patient is stable medically and has some weight reserve, urine can be monitored for ketones before each meal. This checks starvation states, provides the patient with immediate feedback, and offers her the opportunity to alter her starvation state immediately.
    - (iii) If the patient is spilling ketones, her activities and privileges should be completely restricted until her urine reverts to normal.

  c. **Contraindications.** There are no contraindications. If the patient refuses hospitalization and is in danger either medically or psychiatrically (if she is suicidal), she should be held against her will.

F. Prognosis

1. The earlier the onset of the disease, the better the prognosis, and the longer the disease course, the worse the prognosis. Decreased denial of a problem and admitting to feeling hungry are good prognostic signs, as is gainful employment. A schizoid personality disorder bodes a bad prognosis, as does recurrent bulimia, vomiting, and laxative abuse.

2. On the average, 30%–40% of patients have a relatively complete recovery; 30% or more may undergo a period of obesity; and 40% continue to demonstrate bizarre eating habits, weight loss, and a severe disease course.

3. The mortality rates are reported to be 5%–15%. Death, when it occurs, is due to electrolyte abnormalities, suicide, cardiac dysrhythmias, or possibly a too rapid rehydration and weight gain.

II. BULIMIA NERVOSA

A. **Definition.** As a distinct diagnostic entity, bulimia nervosa consists of ravenous overeating followed by guilt, depression, and anger at oneself for doing so. Although there usually is some accompanying feeling of loss of control of eating, there is no significant loss of weight below the normal for age and size. Other findings include the following:

1. High-calorie food is usually ingested.

2. Individuals with bulimia usually hide their eating.

3. There are wide fluctuations in weight.

4. There is a persistent overconcern with weight and body shape.

5. There may be attempts to lose weight (e.g., dieting, exercise, and use of cathartics, diuretics, and enemas).

6. Eating episodes may be terminated by sleep, abdominal pain, social interruption, or self-induced vomiting.

7. There may be lengthy phases of normal eating.

B. **Epidemiology.** Primarily a disorder of adolescent girls, the disorder is probably very common, existing in gradations from mild (perhaps a variant of normal) to severe.

C. **Etiology.** Very little is known about the cause of the disorder; the following etiologies remain tentative.

1. **Psychological**
   a. Bulimia could be caused by a need to take in something orally—perhaps as a substitution for some degree of maternal deprivation.

    b. Some children of short stature fantasize that eating ravenously can help them grow.

    c. Bulimia has been described in children with psychogenic dwarfism (retarded growth due to emotional neglect).

    d. Bulimia could be a disorder of self-regulation. There are high rates of co-existent substance abuse and stealing. Stealing may be due in part to the cost of maintaining a very expensive food habit.

  2. Medical. A lesion of the satiety center in the hypothalamus could contribute to bulimia, but such a lesion has not been defined or discovered.

D. Medical complications

  1. Metabolic abnormalities (e.g., hypokalemia and hypochloremic alkalosis)

  2. Parotid gland swelling

  3. Dental erosion and caries

  4. Menstrual irregularities

  5. Gastric dilatation and rupture

  6. Chronic sore throats and esophagitis

  7. Anemia

E. Differential diagnosis

  1. Prader-Willi syndrome is characterized by continuous overeating, obesity, mental retardation, hypogonadism, hypotonia, and diabetes mellitus. While apparently a genetic syndrome, the mode of transmission is unknown. It is thought to be due to a hypothalamic lesion.

  2. Klüver-Bucy syndrome. Objects are examined by mouth, and hypersexuality and hyperphagia are characteristic. Visual agnosia, compulsive licking and biting, and hypersensitivity to stimuli are common as well. The condition may result from temporal lobe dysfunction.

  3. Kleine-Levin syndrome manifests as hyperphagia and hypersomnia, both of which occur in spurts of 2–3 weeks at a frequency of 2 or 3 cycles per year. Loss of sexual inhibitions may occur as part of the syndrome. This disorder is more common in boys and appears to represent a limbic or hypothalamic dysfunction.

  4. Hypothalamic lesions should be considered.

  5. Anorexia nervosa. A component of anorexia nervosa may be binge eating, but simple bulimia does not include significant weight loss.

  6. Binge eating in obesity. In obesity, binging represents a pattern of overeating, is not terminated by purging, and is not accompanied by a preoccupation with body shape.

  7. Epileptic seizures

  8. Central nervous system tumors

F. Treatment. Long-term efficacy of any one treatment modality has not been established. Bulimia has traditionally been viewed largely as a treatment-resistant condition. However, mixed modality treatment appears to offer promising results.

  1. Individual psychotherapies of psychodynamic, behavioral, and cognitive orientations have been variably helpful. Individual therapy that combines elements of the various therapeutic orientations in conjunction with supportive group psychotherapy offers promising results.

  2. Medications are not universally indicated; however, the following drugs have been reported to be useful.

    a. Tricyclic antidepressants

    b. Monoamine oxidase inhibitors

    c. Lithium

    d. Carbamazepine

    e. Phenytoin

  3. Hospitalization is indicated for the management of serious medical complications, relentless binging and purging (several times daily), and for the severely depressed or suicidal bulimic patient.

III. RUMINATION

A. Definition. This is a rare disorder of infancy that is potentially fatal, consisting of purposive expulsion of previously ingested food, followed by rechewing the food. This usually occurs while the infant is alone.

B. Epidemiology. The disorder is very rare and may be decreasing in incidence.

C. Etiology. Although theories abound, the disorder often occurs in families where the parents are psychosexually immature and distant. Food and chewing may take on a transitional quality for the child and soothe the infant when alone, much in the way of a special doll or blanket.

D. Treatment

1. Dyad (mother–child) interactions should be observed. Cues that the parent gives the child that encourage regurgitation should be interpreted and eradicated.

2. In-depth psychotherapy of one or both parents is often needed.

3. The infant's nutritional status should be followed closely.

IV. PICA

A. Definition. Pica is a disorder involving the persistent eating of nonfood products, such as dirt, clay, paper, or plaster. Mouthing inanimate objects is normal between 6 and 12 months of age.

B. Epidemiology. This problem may be more common in lower socioeconomic groups.

C. Etiology

1. Mentally retarded children mouth objects more than normal children.

2. Iron deficiency can cause a craving for ice and nonfood items.

3. Mother–child problems (especially where repeated, traumatic separations are involved) are etiologic in some cases.

4. A variety of rare neurologic conditions can cause children to mouth nonfood items (e.g., Klüver-Bucy syndrome).

D. Complications

1. Bezoars

2. Lead poisoning, which can present with a variety of neurologic and psychiatric manifestations. It is extremely dangerous, more common in areas of older homes with lead-based paint, and should be suspected in any child with an encephalopathy or unusual behavior.

E. Treatment

1. Dangerous objects should be removed from the child's environment.

2. Increasing the amount of stimulation to a child can be helpful. (Most cities offer infant-stimulation programs.)

3. Psychotherapy for the child and parents may be needed.

V. FAILURE TO THRIVE

A. Definition. Failure to thrive is diagnosed when a child fails to maintain weight above the third percentile for his or her age-group. Failure to grow in height sometimes accompanies this, but failure of head circumference growth occurs only in severe cases.

B. Etiology

1. Failure to thrive as a **psychiatric condition** (nonorganic failure to thrive) has protean causes and manifestations. The following list divides these causes by developmental phase, but it is not meant to be complete.
   a. **Early infancy.** Prior to 8 or 9 months of life, a child is inactive and relies on parental feeding. Failure to thrive in this age range may mean poor parenting or troubled parent-child interactions.

    b. Late infancy. After 8 months, failure to thrive may be secondary to anaclitic depression, poor parenting, or childhood psychosis.

    c. Toddler stage. The negativism associated with the terrible twos can also apply to eating. Children may refuse to eat in the service of autonomy. Sometimes this negativism may develop earlier, as when parents frantically force food on a 1-year-old child.

  2. A variety of medical conditions can cause failure to thrive and should be evaluated. These include juvenile-onset diabetes mellitus, other endocrine disorders, and malabsorption syndromes.

C. Treatment. Any organic cause must be ruled out, and parent–child interactions should be evaluated carefully. The child should be hospitalized in some cases to observe if he or she can gain weight in a new environment. Underlying disorders should be treated.

BIBLIOGRAPHY

American Psychiatric Association: *Diagnostic and Statistical Manual of Mental Disorders,* 3rd ed, revised. Washington DC, American Psychiatric Association, 1987

Halmi KA, Falk JR: Anorexia nervosa; a study of outcome discriminators in exclusive dieters and bulimics. *J Am Acad Child Psychiatry* 21:369, 1982

Lesser LI, Ashenden BJ, Debuskey M, et al: Anorexia nervosa in children. *Am J Orthopsychiatry* 30:572, 1960

Sameroff AJ, Chandler M: Reproductive risk and the continuum of caretaking causality. In *Review of Child Development Research,* vol 4. Edited by Horowitz F. Chicago, University of Chicago Press, pp 187–244, 1975

STUDY QUESTIONS

Directions: Each question below contains five suggested answers. Choose the **one best** response to each question.

1. The mortality rate associated with anorexia nervosa is

(A) less than 1%
(B) 5%–15%
(C) 20%–30%
(D) 35%
(E) 50%

2. The differential diagnosis of anorexia nervosa includes all of the following conditions EXCEPT

(A) neoplasms
(B) depression
(C) Addison's disease
(D) Cushing's disease
(E) ulcerative colitis

3. A 15-year-old girl presents to the emergency room with severe weight loss. On physical examination, she is cachectic with a weight of 68 lb; her heart rate is 36, and her blood pressure is 72/50. The first intervention should be to

(A) evaluate the family to determine the family dynamics
(B) immediately administer a high-protein and carbohydrate diet via a nasogastric tube
(C) draw blood for a serum electrolyte determination and then start intravenous feeding
(D) arrange to have the patient admitted to the psychiatric service
(E) arrange for electroconvulsive therapy

4. Mortality associated with anorexia nervosa may result from all of the following EXCEPT

(A) cardiac dysrhythmias
(B) metabolic disturbances
(C) myocardial infarction
(D) starvation
(E) suicide

5. Psychotherapy is contraindicated in the treatment of anorexia nervosa in which of the following circumstances?

(A) When the patient gets angry at the therapist
(B) When the patient's weight drops below 80 lb
(C) When the patient starts abusing laxatives
(D) When the patient says she no longer wants to be in psychotherapy
(E) In none of the above circumstances

6. Which of the following statements concerning the use of a nasogastric tube in the treatment of anorexia nervosa is true?

(A) It is contraindicated because the tube may remind the patient of a penis; therefore, hyperalimentation through a central intravenous catheter should be used
(B) It is contraindicated because of the pain involved in passing the tube
(C) It is contraindicated because not enough calories can be provided to the patient by a nasogastric tube
(D) It is indicated in cases where the patient is at risk of starving to death
(E) It is indicated as a form of punishment when the patient refuses to eat

7. Characteristics of patients with bulimia nervosa include all of the following EXCEPT

(A) cathartic abuse
(B) diuretic abuse
(C) intermittent dieting
(D) severe weight loss
(E) persistent concern about weight

8. The differential diagnosis of bulimia nervosa includes all of the following conditions EXCEPT

(A) anorexia nervosa
(B) Holt-Oram syndrome
(C) Klüver-Bucy syndrome
(D) Kleine-Levin syndrome
(E) Prader-Willi syndrome

9. The Prader-Willi syndrome is characterized by which constellation of symptoms?

(A) Overeating, mental retardation, and stealing food
(B) Hypersexuality, overeating, and mouthing objects
(C) Wide fluctuations of weight with lengthy phases of normal eating
(D) Overeating and hypersomnia
(E) None of the above

10. Eating disorders of early childhood include all of the following EXCEPT

(A) failure to thrive
(B) colic
(C) obesity
(D) pica
(E) rumination

11. A child presents with an encephalopathy, bizarre behavior, and a history of pica. The diagnostic test most likely to reveal the etiology of this child's problem is

(A) electroencephalogram
(B) computed tomography scan of the head
(C) serum lead levels
(D) serum arsenic levels
(E) none of the above

12. Failure to thrive usually presents with

(A) weight loss
(B) reduced height or length
(C) reduced head circumference
(D) vomiting
(E) regurgitation

Directions: Each question below contains four suggested answers of which **one or more** is correct. Choose the answer

> A   if **1, 2, and 3** are correct
> B   if **1 and 3** are correct
> C   if **2 and 4** are correct
> D   if **4** is correct
> E   if **1, 2, 3, and 4** are correct

13. Rumination disorder is characterized by which of the following statements?

(1) The incidence is fairly common and appears to be increasing
(2) The disorder usually poses no medical risk to the child
(3) Pathogenic family interactions are not prominent
(4) Symptoms appear to be under voluntary control

14. Which of the following factors may be etiologic in the development of anorexia nervosa?

(1) Cultural influences
(2) Hypothalamic–pituitary abnormalities
(3) Controlling parents
(4) Schizophrenia

15. True statements concerning the presentation of anorexia nervosa include

(1) age of onset is 13–14 years
(2) boys are affected at an older age than girls
(3) onset is often preceded by a period of normal dieting
(4) a suicide attempt is a frequent indication of onset

16. Factors associated with anorexia nervosa include which of the following?

(1) Mental retardation
(2) Turner's syndrome
(3) Above-average intelligence
(4) High socioeconomic status

17. Personality types that have been described as common among anorectic individuals include

(1) hysterical
(2) schizoid/schizotypal
(3) obsessive–compulsive
(4) avoidant

18. Behavioral disturbances that may occur concomitantly with bulimia nervosa include

(1) aggression
(2) stealing
(3) promiscuity
(4) substance abuse

19. The Klüver-Bucy syndrome is characterized by which of the following signs or symptoms?

(1) Visual agnosia
(2) Hypersexuality
(3) Compulsive licking and biting
(4) Electroencephalogram abnormalities

20. The Kleine-Levin syndrome is characterized by

(1) hyperphagia
(2) male predominance
(3) hypersomnia
(4) examination of objects by mouth

21. Pica is characterized by which of the following statements?

(1) Infant-stimulation programs may be therapeutically helpful
(2) Mouthing inanimate objects is not considered developmentally abnormal until after 36 months of age
(3) The etiology may be either environmental (interactional) or physiologic
(4) Poisoning via ingestion of toxins is the only physical complication

22. Correct statements concerning failure to thrive include which of the following?

(1) Diagnosis is established when weight falls beneath the tenth percentile for age
(2) It may represent an interactional problem between a parent and the child
(3) Weight, height, and head circumference all tend to be low for age
(4) Hospitalization is sometimes indicated; however, even then some children continue to fail to gain weight

Directions: The group of questions below consists of lettered choices followed by several numbered items. For each numbered item select the **one** lettered choice with which it is **most** closely associated. Each lettered choice may be used once, more than once, or not at all.

Questions 23–26

For each disorder listed below, select a typical complication that is likely to be associated with it.

(A) Bezoars
(B) Hypercarotenemia
(C) Cyclic hypersomnia
(D) Extreme guilt
(E) Urticaria

23. Pica
24. Anorexia nervosa
25. Kleine-Levin syndrome
26. Bulimia

ANSWERS AND EXPLANATIONS

1. The answer is B. (*I B 6 c, F 3*) The usual causes of death in anorexia nervosa are serum electrolyte abnormalities and suicide. The workup of a patient with anorexia nervosa should include the following: careful physical examination, determination of the serum electrolyte count, electrocardiogram (ECG), and a blood chemistry profile (i.e., serum protein and liver and renal function studies). A mental status examination should be performed. This screens for suicidal ideation and other psychiatric conditions that cause weight loss (e.g., depression and schizophrenia).

2. The answer is D. (*I D 1 a–f*) The differential diagnosis of anorexia nervosa includes all of the causes of weight loss in adolescence, including neoplasms, depression, Addison's disease, and ulcerative colitis. Cushing's disease is not typically characterized by weight loss.

3. The answer is C. (*I E 1 a, b, 5 a–c, F 3*) Anorexia nervosa may be a life-threatening illness. There is a significant mortality that accompanies this condition, most commonly due to the metabolic or cardiac complications secondary to starvation. The first intervention with anorectic patients is always an assessment of the medical state by drawing blood for serum electrolyte determination, followed by supportive or emergency medical intervention, such as starting intravenous feeding. A too rapid hydration or weight gain should be avoided as it may lead to further complications and even death. A high-protein and carbohydrate diet by nasogastric tube would not correct fluid and electrolyte problems quickly. Evaluation and treatment of the individual and family dynamics are always secondary to the emergency medical management.

4. The answer is C. (*I E 1 a, F 3*) Mortality among anorectics is significant, ranging from 5%–15%, depending on the study. When death occurs, it is most commonly due to either suicide or the effects of starvation with its concomitant cardiac dysrhythmias and metabolic disturbances. While cardiac death caused by disturbances in the conduction system is common among anorectics, cardiac death caused by myocardial infarction is not.

5. The answer is E. (*I E 3 b*) Anger is common in the course of treatment of anorectic patients as are issues surrounding individual choices and control. When expressed in the course of treatment, these become therapeutic issues to be considered, not contraindications to continued treatment. Persistent weight loss and laxative abuse may indicate the necessity for more stringent behavioral controls or additional medical management, but they do not preclude ongoing psychotherapy. In fact, they are issues that should be considered in psychotherapy.

6. The answer is D. (*I E 5 b*) In most cases, a nasogastric tube is the treatment of choice when an anorectic patient suffers from severe inanition. Its use is simple and safe and can provide the patient with sufficient calories. Although there may be negative connotations in association with the use of a nasogastric tube, these should not prevent appropriate medical management of the patient. Some pain is associated with the use of the tube, but it is much safer than a central intravenous catheter. Nasogastric tubes are used appropriately to reverse starvation, not as a form of punishment.

7. The answer is D. (*II A 1–7*) Bulimia nervosa is characterized by alternating episodes of binging and purging. Methods of purging include self-induced vomiting, cathartic abuse, and diuretic abuse. Bulimics are persistently concerned about weight, and intermittent dieting is common. Severe weight loss, however, is more likely to represent a subset of anorectic patients who have concomitant bulimia. Bulimics tend to demonstrate no significant weight loss below the normal for age and size.

8. The answer is B. (*II E 1–3, 5*) The symptoms of bulimia nervosa may mimic those of anorexia nervosa with the exception that severe weight loss is not prominent among bulimics. The Klüver-Bucy syndrome, Kleine-Levin syndrome, and Prader-Willi syndrome are all characterized by hyperphagia among a variety of other behavioral manifestations. The Holt-Oram syndrome is a congenital heart condition unrelated to eating disorders.

9. The answer is A. (*II E 1–3*) The Prader-Willi syndrome is characterized by ravenous overeating and is accompanied by obesity, mental retardation, and hypotonia. It is probably due to a hypothalamic lesion. Examining objects by mouth, hypersexuality, and hyperphagia are attributed to the Klüver-Bucy syndrome, and overeating and hypersomnia are associated with the Kleine-Levin syndrome. Wide fluctuations in weight with lengthy phases of normal eating may be seen in bulimia nervosa.

10. The answer is B. (*III–V*) Failure to thrive is diagnosed when a child fails to maintain weight above the third percentile for his or her age-group. Obesity describes an increase in body weight as a result of excessive overeating. Pica is a disorder that involves the persistent eating of nonfood products, such as dirt, clay, paper, or plaster. Rumination describes a rare disorder of infancy, consisting of purposive expulsion of previously ingested food, followed by rechewing the food. All of these disorders occur as a result of problems in parent–child relationships. Colic describes abdominal pain, usually of infancy. It is not considered an eating disorder.

11. The answer is C. (*IV D 2*) Lead toxicity can present with a variety of neurologic and psychiatric manifestations and should be suspected in patients presenting with acute encephalopathy or unusual behavior. It is relatively more common in areas of older homes and among lower socioeconomic groups.

12. The answer is A. (*V A*) Weight loss, or failure to gain weight, is usually the first symptom of failure to thrive, followed by a reduction in growth rate relative to length, and late in the course, a reduction in growth rate relative to head circumference. Most commonly, failure to thrive derives from nonorganic etiologies. Typically, these relate to disturbances in the parent–child relationship. Organic etiologies do occur and must be considered. In some cases, repeated vomiting may occur, but by definition, the diagnosis of failure to thrive is established on the basis of inadequate weight gain, rather than on those factors that contribute to inadequate weight gain.

13. The answer is D (4). (*III A–D*) Rumination disorder is a rare disorder of infancy that is potentially fatal, consisting of purposive expulsion of previously ingested food, followed by rechewing or ejection of the food. The incidence appears to be decreasing. Failure to thrive may be a severe complication of this disorder. It most often occurs in the presence of an overtly dysfunctional parent–child relationship. The purposive symptoms seem to represent a self-soothing quality.

14. The answer is A (1, 2, 3). (*I B 2, C 3, 4, D 2*) In Western societies in which thinness is associated with beauty, a higher incidence of anorexia nervosa is observed. A variety of endocrine abnormalities are also observed, which may signify some alteration in the normal hypothalamic–pituitary functioning. Parental overcontrol may cause the child to fight for autonomy by controlling her eating. An eating disorder that occurs in schizophrenia is usually the result of the psychotic thinking of the individual (i.e., this food has been poisoned) in contrast to the likely etiologies of anorexia nervosa (i.e., this food will make me fat).

15. The answer is B (1, 3). (*I B 1, 4*) The average age of onset of anorexia is 13½ years, and the onset is usually preceded by a period of normal dieting. The disease rarely occurs in boys. Suicide attempts, although increased in incidence, are infrequent.

16. The answer is E (all). (*I B 2, 3, 5, 6*) Anorexia nervosa is associated with mental retardation, Turner's syndrome, above-average intelligence, and high socioeconomic status; however, these are associations only and do not imply cause or effect. Anorexia nervosa is more common in Caucasians, especially girls from Jewish or Italian families, and in Western civilizations. The incidence of the disease is increasing, probably due to cultural factors (i.e., thin is beautiful).

17. The answer is A (1, 2, 3). (*I A 2 n*) An hysterical personality style may be recognized among those anorectic individuals with major conflicts regarding sexuality. A schizoid (or schizotypal) character style may be recognized among those anorectics with qualitative oddities in their thinking. An obsessive–compulsive personality style may be recognized among anorectics who are overtly perfectionistic in most areas of their lives. An avoidant personality style is one characterized by social shyness and awkwardness; it is not commonly associated with anorexia nervosa.

18. The answer is C (2, 4). (*II C 1 d*) Bulimia nervosa may represent a disorder of self-regulation. Stealing behavior and substance abuse commonly occur concomitantly in bulimic patients. While aggression or promiscuity may be character traits of certain bulimic patients, they are not part of a characteristic profile of bulimia nervosa.

19. The answer is A (1, 2, 3). (*II E 2*) The Klüver-Bucy syndrome is characterized by the examination of objects by mouth. Additional symptoms include visual agnosia, hypersexuality, compulsive licking and biting, hyperphagia, and hypersensitivity to stimuli. Electroencephalogram abnormalities are not common, although the condition may result from temporal lobe dysfunction.

20. The answer is A (1, 2, 3). (*II E 3*) The Kleine-Levin syndrome is a disorder more common in boys, apparently secondary to a limbic or hypothalamic dysfunction. It is characterized by intermittent cycles of hyperphagia and hypersomnia, which occur in 2–3-week intervals. Examination of objects by mouth is characteristic of the Klüver-Bucy syndrome.

21. The answer is B (1, 3). (*IV A–E*) Pica is a disorder involving the eating of nonfood products, especially after 12 months of age at which time normal developmental mouthing of inanimate objects begins to wane. Problems with the parent–child relationship may be etiologic in some cases, as may physiologic problems, such as iron deficiency anemia. The development of bezoars and poisoning are common complications.

22. The answer is C (2, 4). (*V A–C*) Failure-to-thrive is diagnosed when a child fails to maintain weight above the third percentile. Failure to maintain weight is necessary for the diagnosis; failure to maintain height is an infrequent finding, and failure to maintain head circumference occurs only in severe cases. There may be either an organic or a nonorganic etiology. Dysfunction in the parent–child relationship is common in nonorganic failure-to-thrive. Hospitalization is sometimes indicated. When a child is hospitalized and continues to fail to gain weight, an organic etiology should be considered likely.

23–26. The answers are: 23-A, 24-B, 25-C, 26-D. (*I A 2 i; II A, E 3; IV D 1*) Pica is the eating of nonfood substances, and bezoars can form as the result of ingesting nondigestible material. Trichobezoars, hair balls in the stomach, and phytobezoars, masses of vegetable matter, can cause intestinal obstruction, necessitating surgery.

Hypercarotenemia may be seen in anorexia nervosa and is uncommon in other causes of weight loss. The resultant orange skin discoloration is characteristic. Otherwise, hypercarotenemia is clinically insignificant.

Kleine-Levin syndrome causes overeating and hypersomnia. These symptoms are periodic, lasting several weeks. The disorder begins in adolescence and is more common in boys.

Binge episodes in bulimia nervosa are followed by guilt. Guilt is relieved by subsequent purging. Purging usually is by vomiting.

10
Child Psychiatry
Donald W. Bechtold

I. INTRODUCTION. Child psychiatry is the study and treatment of the mental and behavioral problems of childhood. As such, it overlaps with a variety of pediatric subspecialties. An understanding of standard childhood development is essential to the understanding of childhood psychopathology, since seemingly major difficulties may be normal at certain ages (e.g., negativism is usual at 2 years of age and again at adolescence, but it is problematic during the latency period and in adulthood).

A. Developmental concepts

1. **Epigenesis.** There is a natural and unalterable sequence in which development must occur (e.g., in Freudian psychology, the anal period must follow the oral stage and cannot be reversed).

2. **Developmental continuities.** Some childhood personality traits and experiences are continuous with and have ramifications for adulthood; others do not; for example, children who are abandoned at 3 years of age by their parents may feel depressed every time someone leaves them later in life. Thus, this early childhood experience is *continuous* with later experiences.

3. **Critical phases.** It was previously accepted that particular phases of development must occur at certain ages. For example, if a child suffered a severe psychological trauma at 4 years of age, causing a developmental arrest, he or she would not experience a normal oedipal period, even though the trauma is overcome, and development recommences at 7 years of age. This distorted oedipal phase might result in irrational fears of physical or psychological harm in competitive situations, a fear that could persist into adulthood. This example is hypothetical; very little is actually known about which developmental phases are critical. In fact, the concept of critical phases has been largely replaced by that of "sensitive" phases in which development is most efficient, but not limited to that phase of development.

4. **Invulnerability.** Certain children are able to negotiate seemingly overwhelming psychological trauma with no apparent effect on their subsequent personality development; however, what makes certain children invulnerable is unknown. The match or fit between a child's needs and the ability of his or her caregivers to meet those needs and the innate temperamental differences of children have been postulated as causative factors.

B. Overview of childhood psychopathology

1. **Most disorders are more common in boys** than in girls. This probably reflects an inherent increased vulnerability of the male to stress and trauma.

2. **Psychopathology is usually the result of chronic, maladaptive interactions** between the child and the environment, often combined with some biologic propensity towards developing a mental illness. Isolated traumatic events (e.g., one episode of sexual abuse by a nonfamily member) can cause transient anxiety, anger, and depression; however, they generally do not cause psychopathology unless they generate long-lasting changes in the child's interactions with his or her environment.

3. **Misbehavior may be the result of the parents' conscious or unconscious prompting.** Children usually behave in a way that is consistent with the parents' desires.

C. Approach to the child patient

1. **The physician must be an advocate for the child,** not for the parents. To do otherwise is to subject the child to the parents' wishes, which may or may not be realistic or appropriate. Nevertheless, the child psychiatrist must develop a working relationship with the child's parents; they often represent a limitation in terms of the child's psychological growth.
    a. Parents should be seen frequently, especially at the beginning of psychotherapy.
    b. Preadolescents should be seen alone but usually after the parents have been seen. An attempt to communicate with the child patient by talking should be made. If this is difficult, a small assortment of toys, including a dollhouse, paper and crayons, puppets, checkers, and blocks, can help a child communicate through play.
    c. Adolescents should be seen alone and before the parents are seen. Use of unnatural slang to bridge the generation gap should be avoided. An attitude of concern for the adolescent suffices, usually establishing rapport with the patient.

2. **The patient interview should reveal:**
    a. The child's reaction to separation from the parents
    b. The child's behavior towards the interviewer (e.g., anxious, very open, or shy)
    c. The child's perception of people in general (e.g., trustworthy or dangerous, reliable or neglectful, kind or hostile)
    d. The choice of verbal versus play communication
    e. The clarity of the child's thought processes
    f. The level of development (i.e., social, language, motor, or cognitive) of the child and its appropriateness to the child's age
    g. The ability of the child to identify different affective states and to discharge these states in an age-appropriate manner
    h. The ability of the child to tolerate frustration and to control his or her impulses
    i. The child's perception of him- or herself (e.g., competent or ineffectual, master or victim) and the relative strength of his or her self-esteem
    j. The child's reaction to rejoining the parents after the interview

3. **Gathering information from the child** can be facilitated by requesting the child to:
    a. Make three wishes and elaborate on each wish.
    b. Make drawings of anything, and elaborate on each drawing. Drawings of people and families are especially helpful.
    c. Describe the family.
    d. Describe important nonfamily members.
    e. Describe favorite television shows, movies, and musicians, noting with whom the child identifies.
    f. Describe the problem that initiated therapy and how the family told him or her of the appointment.

II. BONDING AND ATTACHMENT

A. Definitions

1. **A bond** is defined as an affective relationship of the parent with the child. Bonding develops over time; there appears to be no critical phase of bonding as is described in animal studies. It is likely that bonding commences long before the birth of the child and is apparent in the parents' attitudes, fantasies, and wishes for the child.

2. **Attachment** describes the child's affective relationship with the parent. Attachment, like bonding, develops over time.

B. Assessment of bonding

1. Ask the parents when and how a name was chosen for the child, which indicates when they began planning for the new arrival. The name can have special meaning; it may indicate how the family perceives the child.

2. Determine what sort of dreams the parents had about the child during pregnancy.

3. Determine how the parents' relationship towards each other changed during the pregnancy. The husband often assumes a maternal role towards his wife; however, if he begins abusing her, has affairs, or grows uninvolved, a poor relationship between the parents and the new baby is likely.

4. Determine whether or not the parents visited the nursery following delivery.

5. Determine the mental health of the parents. Depression, psychosis, and drug abuse are problems that can distort the way the parent perceives the child.

6. Special problems are posed if the newborn has to spend extra time in the nursery due to illness. A family with a child in the critical care unit nursery should be evaluated prior to discharge to assure adequate care for the child.

7. Determine of whom the child reminds the parents. This question determines transferences and preconceived attitudes about the infant.

C. Disorders of bonding and attachment

1. **Hospitalism** is an extreme example of failure of any affective relationship to develop. Affected infants suffer from:
   a. Susceptibility to infection
   b. Apathy
   c. Retarded development
   d. Failure to thrive

2. **Anaclitic depression** results when an attachment relationship is disrupted during a sensitive phase of development (see section IV A 1).

3. **Child abuse** may occur if parents have not adequately bonded with the child. This is especially prevalent with premature infants.

4. **Vulnerable child syndrome** was originally described by Green and Solnit. Parents may continue to treat a child who has been ill and recovered as though he or she is still vulnerable. Such children may later show a variety of psychological traits, including:
   a. Those resulting from parental overprotectiveness
   b. Hypochondriasis
   c. Hyperactivity
   d. Separation anxiety
   e. Learning difficulties

5. **Separation from parents** in infancy probably also induces a range of reactions later in life.

D. Treatment

1. Parents should be counseled to spend time with the newborn. In situations in which the parents have not visited a sick infant or have been reluctant to see a newborn, a structured plan to facilitate parent–child interactions should be implemented.
   a. There should be a mandatory visitation of at least 24 consecutive hours.
   b. Nursing support should be available when parents' questions arise.
   c. Grief over a child's prematurity and illness may require psychiatric intervention when the grief is thought to contribute to the lack of parental involvement.
   d. Follow-up in a special clinic for premature infants is indicated.

2. When parents cannot demonstrate a bond to their child and an understanding of the child's needs and when these problems may contribute to the development of either hospitalism or child abuse, the child should be placed in a foster home.

3. Psychopathology in either parent should be evaluated and treated.

4. Vulnerable child syndrome is managed by informing the parents that the child has recovered and is doing well. Surprisingly, parents may not realize this, and their attitude towards the child may change with this reassurance. However, if reassurance fails, psychotherapy for the parents is indicated. Psychotherapy for the child is also indicated if he or she has internalized this sense of fragility and vulnerability into his or her personal identity.

III. CHILDHOOD PSYCHOSES

A. Autistic disorder

1. **Clinical data.** Autistic disorder is an illness most commonly commencing early in childhood (before the age of 36 months) in which the child is relatively unresponsive to other human beings, demonstrates bizarre responses to his or her environment, and has unusual language development.
   a. Autistic children treat other individuals indifferently, almost as though they are inanimate objects.
   b. Language abnormalities include echolalia, pronoun reversals (e.g., use of the pronoun "you" when "I" is correct), mutism, and delays.
   c. Autistic children have a great need for consistency in their environment and may de-

compensate if, for example, furniture is rearranged. The etiology of this need for sameness is unknown.
  d. Social development is usually abnormal
2. **Epidemiology.** Although the disorder has an even socioeconomic distribution, it occurs more commonly in boys.
3. **Etiology**
   a. **A cold, distant mother figure** was thought to be responsible for the development of coldness and aloofness in the child (i.e., growing up in an emotional vacuum leads to unrelatedness in the child). However, this theory has been replaced by the abnormal sensory integration theory.
   b. **Abnormal sensory integration theory.** An increased threshold to sensory stimuli or delayed integration of communicative stimuli may place the child out of synchrony with the environment.
4. **Associated findings**
   a. Abnormal auditory evoked potentials, which are tracings of the transmission of sound stimuli from the brain stem to the cerebral cortex
   b. Decreased nystagmus in reponse to vestibular stimulation
   c. Developmental distortions (i.e., qualitative abnormalities in development) above and beyond mere delays
5. **Differential diagnosis**
   a. Hearing deficits
   b. Mental retardation accompanied by global developmental delays, not simply social and language delays as in autism
   c. Organic mental disorders, such as hepatic encephalopathy and congenital cytomegalovirus, which can mimic autism
6. **Treatment**
   a. A highly structured classroom setting is important to help autistic children focus their attention on learning and communication tasks. Precautions should be taken to insure that the environment remains stable.
   b. Psychotherapy for both the child and parents may be of value in cases in which parental factors are considered to be partly etiologic. It may also be indicated when the family is having trouble coping with the stress of having an autistic child.
   c. Medication is rarely of value unless agitation is pronounced, in which case thioridazine at an oral dose of 0.5–1.0 mg/kg daily or haloperidol at an oral dose of 0.5–5.0 mg daily may be necessary. Alternatively, some hyperactive autistic children may benefit from stimulant medication (e.g., fenfluramine).
7. **Prognosis.** Many autistic children develop grand mal seizures prior to adolescence. However, the prognosis for autistic disorder is better if the child has:
   a. A high IQ
   b. Reasonable language development

B. **Childhood schizophrenia**

1. **Clinical data.** The symptom profile of childhood schizophrenia may include:
   a. Preoccupation with gory or grotesque fantasies
   b. Hallucinations (usually not prominent and not a criterion in the *DSM-III-R*)
   c. Propensity to digress with poor attention span
   d. Responsiveness to individuals in the environment without consistent demonstration of sociability, reciprocity, or empathy
   e. Possible abnormal motor movements
   f. Unusual mannerisms
2. **Etiology**
   a. A genetic cause for childhood schizophrenia has not been well delineated as it has for adult schizophrenia.
   b. A **grossly chaotic upbringing** with constant exposure to aggressive and sexual themes (e.g., chronic violence in the family) could be causative.
   c. A failure of repression is also considered to be active in the disorder. For example, a child who is repeatedly exposed to violence may be unable to repress sexual and aggressive fantasies, which normally occur by the age of 6 years.
3. **Treatment**
   a. Psychotherapy is very helpful. Family therapy may be indicated when disruption of the

family is evident. When aggression and sexualized stimulation cannot be minimized within the home, out-of-home placement should be considered.

> **b.** Antipsychotic medication, especially thioridazine at an orally administered dose of 1 mg/kg daily or haloperidol at an orally administered dose of 1–5 mg daily may be necessary.

4. Prognosis. The prognosis for childhood schizophrenia is generally favorable provided adequate treatment and remediation of environmental deficits occur. A family history of schizophrenia worsens the prognosis.

C. Symbiotic psychosis

1. Clinical data. Symbiotic psychosis is a disorder in which parents misperceive themselves as their child. The reciprocal is usually true also. Although this disorder usually occurs in mothers and their children, fathers occasionally are affected.

> **a.** A loss of ego boundaries (i.e., the inability to distinguish oneself from others) is apparent.
>
> **b.** Great anxiety at the threat of separation of the child from the parent is seen in both. Upon reuniting, the anxiety clears.
>
> **c.** The overlap between parent and child can be manifested in almost any area (e.g., if parents diet, they assume that the child needs to diet too).

2. Etiology. Parents who have poor object relations may see their child as an extension of themselves. Borderline psychopathology may predispose to the disorder. Although the parent is the cause of the problem, the child usually manifests the symptoms (e.g., severe separation anxiety).

3. Treatment. Psychotherapy aimed at separating the child from the parent is needed. Sometimes parents may require support to help them permit the separation and development of autonomy in the child. In certain refractory cases, an actual separation through out-of-home placement may be necessary.

4. Prognosis is good; symbiotic psychosis carries the best prognosis of all the childhood psychoses.

IV. CHILDHOOD DEPRESSION. Biologic markers are even less valuable in identifying childhood depressive disorders than in identifying adult disorders. They remain under investigation.

A. Clinical data. Depressive illness presents at all stages of development.

1. Children between the ages of 7 and 30 months demonstrate **anaclitic depression.** The cause is a lengthy separation (more than 1 week) from caregivers. Symptoms include listlessness, anorexia, psychomotor retardation, and sad facial expressions. The treatment is restitution of the relationship.

2. Preschool children who are depressed often demonstrate more behavioral difficulties, such as hyperactivity and aggressiveness, than older children. These symptoms are called **depressive equivalents.** Separation from caregivers or a sense of poor mastery over developmental tasks (e.g., toilet training) may be etiologic. Treatment should be aimed at changing the child's environment. Psychotherapy may help.

3. Schoolchildren may manifest the usual signs and symptoms of depression (e.g., vegetative signs and a depressed mood). Biologic vulnerabilities and a sense of helplessness or incompetence may play an etiologic role at this age. Treatment is psychotherapy aimed at helping the child feel a sense of competence vis-à-vis his or her environment.

4. Adolescents also demonstrate the usual signs of depression, especially a pervasive sense of boredom and lack of future orientation. The incidence of depressive disorders increases in adolescence with girls affected more frequently than boys.

B. Treatment. Antidepressant medication may be a useful adjunct in the treatment of depression in certain children and adolescents. It should never be used without individual or family psychotherapy. Parents must take the responsibility for administering the medication and for safeguarding siblings from inadvertent overdosage.

C. Associated mood disorders

1. Manic–depressive illness may present in childhood but does so uncommonly. Hyperactivity can be mistaken for mania.

2. **Childhood suicide** may be a complication of a mood disorder. The incidence of suicide is probably increasing in preadolescence and in adolescence. Depressed children should be carefully evaluated for suicidal ideation.

V. TOURETTE'S SYNDROME

A. **Clinical data.** Tourette's syndrome consists of recurrent, involuntary, purposeless motor movements accompanied by vocal tics (e.g., coprolalia and involuntary swearing). Motor tics may precede or follow the development of vocal tics. Psychological stress exacerbates the symptoms, but the cause, although unknown, is probably organic.

B. **Epidemiology**

1. The disorder is more common in boys, and onset is prior to the age of 21, often in early childhood.

2. There may be a familial pattern.

3. It occurs in all socioeconomic classes.

C. **Treatment**

1. **Psychotherapy** is indicated when the tics are causing psychological problems.

2. **Medical treatment** includes the use of:
   a. Haloperidol, which suppresses the tics.
   b. Pimozide, a relatively new drug, which appears to be effective. However, pimozide can cause cardiac arrhythmias.
   c. Cloridine, which has also proven to be effective in some cases of haloperidol-resistant Tourette's syndrome.

VI. SLEEP DISORDERS

A. **Parasomnias** are sleep disorders that usually affect stages 3 and 4 of sleep, which predominate early in the sleep cycle. Thus, these disorders usually occur early in the night. Examples include the following:

1. **Somnambulism (sleep walking)** is exacerbated by psychological stress in some cases. It is normal much of the time. Alcoholism unmasks somnambulism in adults.

2. **Night terrors** are very common between the ages of 2½ and 5 years, affecting 30% of children in this age bracket. Terrors are sometimes exacerbated by stress. Night terrors should be distinguished from nightmares, which occur during rapid eye movement (REM) sleep and whose content is remembered as a bad dream, by:
   a. The inconsolability of the child during the event.
   b. The absence of recall of the content of the dream
   c. The absence of recall of the event the following morning

3. **Nocturnal enuresis** (see section VII A 1) is due generally to stress or slow central nervous system maturation. The disorder dissipates with increasing age and is, therefore, self-limited.

B. **Narcolepsy** is a sleep disorder that is characterized by REM-onset sleep. REM sleep normally occurs after sleep stages 1–4.

1. **Manifestations**
   a. The entire sleep cycle is affected, resulting in **excessive daytime drowsiness.**
   b. **Cataplexy** is the loss of motor tone in response to an emotion (e.g., anger and excitement).
   c. On awakening, the patient may be transiently completely **paralyzed.**
   d. **Hypnagogic hallucinations** are vivid hallucinations occurring at sleep onset.

2. **Treatment.** Administration of amphetamines and tricyclic antidepressants helps.

VII. ENURESIS

A. **Clinical data.** The child with enuresis continues to urinate at inappropriate times and places after the time when he or she normally should have been toilet trained (i.e., between the ages of 2 and 4 years). The disorder is much more common in boys.

1. **Primary enuresis** is that which has never been interrupted by a period of good bladder control.
   a. **Nocturnal enuresis** is a parasomnia, occurring during stages 3 and 4 of sleep.
   b. **Diurnal enuresis** occurs during the waking hours.
2. **Secondary enuresis** is that which develops after a period of at least 1 year of good bladder control. As in primary enuresis, the disorder may occur both during the sleeping and waking hours.

B. Etiology

1. **Organic disorders** may cause enuresis. These include:
   a. **Systemic illnesses**
      (1) Juvenile-onset diabetes mellitus
      (2) Sickle cell anemia or sickle cell trait
      (3) Diabetes insipidus
   b. **Central nervous system disorders**
      (1) Frontal lobe tumor
      (2) Spinal cord lesion (e.g., spina bifida or spina bifida occulta)
      (3) Peripheral nerve damage
   c. **Anatomic disorders**
      (1) Posterior urethral valvular dysfunction
      (2) Proximal genitourinary malformations
   d. **Urinary tract infections**
   e. **Delayed central nervous system maturation** (after the age of 4½ years, as many as 10% of boys remain enuretic, frequently due to delayed maturation)
2. **Psychological factors** account for the majority of cases of secondary enuresis.
   a. Acute stress can cause enuresis (e.g., the birth of a sibling or starting kindergarten).
   b. Enuresis sometimes occurs in very ambitious boys. Strength and quality of the urine stream may become equated with physical prowess. Micturition can then become conflicted, resulting in urination at inappropriate times.
   c. Hostility can be expressed through the symptom of enuresis. Such an expression of hostility is nearly always unconscious; the child does not deliberately void at inappropriate times.
   d. Family reaction to the enuresis sometimes causes more psychopathology than the psychological causes of the enuresis per se.
   e. The family may encourage enuresis unconsciously. A possible vicarious pleasure for the parents in the child's enuresis may exist.
   f. Some children wet their pants because they are too busy or preoccupied to use the bathroom.

C. Treatment may be only sporadically helpful. Since enuresis is a self-limited disorder, sometimes no treatment is the best.

1. Probing diagnostic procedures to search for an organic etiology, unless the preponderance of evidence points to such, should be avoided.
2. The parents should be assured that the child is not purposefully wetting (enuresis is usually beyond the child's control). Remedial measures include:
   a. Reduction of fluid intake after dinner
   b. Awakening the child to urinate after 1–2 hours of sleep
   c. Bladder exercises (having the child hold urine during the daytime)
   d. Use of special feedback devices that set off an alarm upon urination in bed
3. Tricyclic antidepressant therapy can be effective. Imipramine should be administered in a 10–25 mg dose after school. The medicine should be kept out of reach in a child-proof bottle since overdoses can cause serious problems. Enuresis is a self-limited condition; therefore, the use of antidepressants is discouraged except in refractory or unusual cases (e.g., the parents are completely intolerant of the condition). Though initial symptom response to imipramine is common, breakthrough on that same dose may occur, resulting in the recurrence of enuresis.
4. The child should be treated for any psychological stress. In refractory cases, long-term psychotherapy may be indicated.

VIII. ENCOPRESIS

A. Clinical data. Encopresis is fecal incontinence beyond the period when bowel control should normally have developed. Most encopresis is unconscious and involuntary; only occasionally does it occur deliberately.

1. **Primary encopresis** is that which has occurred continuously throughout the child's life.

2. **Secondary encopresis** develops following a period of at least 1 year of good bowel control.

B. Etiology

1. **Organic disorders.** Hirschsprung's disease rarely presents in older children as encopresis.

2. **Psychological factors**
   a. Unresolved anger at a parent sometimes is expressed unconsciously through fecal incontinence. The child consciously and unconsciously perceives that his or her stool has a negative impact on the family.
   b. Fecal smearing may be a psychotic symptom, especially if the child is older than 4 or 5 years of age.
   c. As is true with enuresis, parents can get vicarious pleasure from their child's symptoms.
   d. When autonomy and control battles focus on toilet training at the age of 2–3 years and when parents are too punitive and unyielding in their approach to the toilet training, conflicts over bowel evacuation develop in the child.

C. Treatment

1. **Correcting fecal impaction** is necessary. Some pediatricians recommend a bowel regimen that consists of periodic cathartic administration to insure that no impaction develops and to help regulate bowel control [e.g., administration of a bisacodyl (Dulcolax) suppository daily at the same time, immediately followed by placing the child on the toilet].

2. **Behavior modification** that reinforces continence is effective in some children (e.g., rewarding a child after a day of good bowel control or after evacuation in the toilet).

3. **Long-term psychotherapy** is indicated in refractory cases. Occasionally, encopresis is a symptom of psychosis. The underlying disease should then be treated.

IX. MASTURBATION

A. Definition. Childhood masturbation involves genital manipulation and fondling. It definitely is not a disease, but many parents complain to the physician about this behavior in their children. An open attitude on the part of the physician is important in allowing the parents to express concern. Any notions that masturbation may cause growth retardation or mental retardation should be dispelled.

B. Incidence. Masturbation occurs in 100% of children. It can develop before the age of 1 year. During the oedipal period (i.e., between the ages of 3½ and 6 years), there is heightened focus on the genitalia.

C. Etiology. Continuous masturbation may be a sign of severe understimulation, environmental deprivation, or of excessive sexual stimulation.

1. Other signs of self-stimulation (e.g., rocking, head banging, and hair pulling) should be sought. The child should be enrolled in a stimulation program, and the situation should be followed up.

2. Signs of child abuse should also be sought. A careful history of the child's exposure to sexual stimulation should be elicited.

X. THUMB SUCKING

A. Incidence. Thumb sucking is more common in girls and is normal at transitional periods in the child's life (e.g., at bedtime and at times of separation from the parents). Approximately 30% of children around 12 years old still suck their thumbs.

B. Treatment is not usually needed. If thumb sucking is chronic and occurs after the age of 3½ years, it can cause changes in dentition. An in-depth exploration of the child's relationship with the parents is indicated as is, usually, psychotherapy. Thumb sucking in the older child can be a sign that the child is insecure or withdrawn. Behavior modification can be useful.

XI. SCHOOL PHOBIAS

A. **Definition.** School phobias are a phobic attitude towards and avoidance of school. In adolescence, they can herald schizophrenia.

B. **Incidence.** School phobias most commonly occur when a child is first introduced to school (at age 4 or 5 years) and in early adolescence when children are required to shower at school after gym. They occur throughout childhood, however.

C. **Etiology.** School phobia is best considered as a symptom. It is caused by a variety of conditions, including:

1. Separation anxiety suffered by the child

2. Extreme separation anxiety suffered by the parent (as opposed to that suffered by the child)

3. Malingering (e.g., the child has not completed a homework assignment)

4. A legitimate cause of fear to the child at school (e.g., gangs or a cruel teacher)

5. Vulnerable child syndrome

6. Homosexual panic in an older child

D. **Treatment**

1. Legitimate causes of fear should be eliminated, and the child should usually be sent back to school immediately. Thus, school avoidance is not reinforced by staying home.

2. Psychotherapy to treat the underlying disorder may be needed.

3. Some cases are exceedingly refractory to treatment interventions and may even require psychiatric hospitalization.

XII. ATTENTION-DEFICIT HYPERACTIVITY DISORDER

A. **Definition.** Hyperactivity is defined subjectively as an increase in motor activity to a level that interferes with the child's functioning either at school or at home. It is important to note, however, that symptoms of attention-deficit disorder may exist with or without the symptom of hyperactivity. Key symptoms of an attention deficit include:

1. Short attention span

2. Difficulty concentrating

3. Impulsivity

4. Distractibility

5. Excitability

B. **Etiology**

1. Medication (e.g., sedative-hypnotics paradoxically cause hyperactivity in children)

2. Depression (e.g., depression is poorly tolerated by some children, who express their sad feelings by means of increased activity)

3. Anxiety

4. Vulnerable child syndrome

5. Severe central nervous system disease (e.g., a grossly abnormal central nervous system or a history of significant head trauma)

6. Constitutional hyperactivity (e.g., some children have a hyperactive temperament, which is present from birth)

7. An intolerant parent, teacher, or supervisor (e.g., factitious hyperactivity—the child is not truly suffering from increased motor activity)

8. Specific learning disabilities, which may be associated with hyperactivity

C. Treatment

1. Any underlying disorder should be treated (e.g., depression should be treated by means of psychotherapy, possibly in conjunction with antidepressant medication).

2. **Medications**
   a. Stimulant medications are effective (e.g., methylphenidate administered in a divided dose of 5–50 mg/day; alternate choices include dextroamphetamine. Growth curves should be followed on all children on stimulant medication as appetite and growth suppression are the most common side effects.
   b. Tricyclic antidepressants, phenytoin, and thioridazine have all proved to be valuable in certain refractory cases.

3. An alteration in the child's diet may be helpful, presumably because the emphasis on food alters a parent's relationship with a child in some meaningful way, although studies have not proven any beneficial dietary effects as yet. Many parents of hyperactive children report that reducing the child's sugar intake reduces the hyperactivity. These parents may pay more attention to their child, feel more in control of the problem, and spend more time with the child at mealtime as a result of changing the child's diet. All of the secondary effects can be beneficial.

XIII. LEARNING DISORDERS

A. **Definition.** There are a wide range of disorders that interfere with the child's ability to perform certain intellectual functions. Children may suffer from specific reading, processing, writing, mathematical, and language disabilities (e.g., developmental dyslexia). Diagnosis is established by documenting a mismatch between the child's performance on standardized measures of the skill in question and his or her intellectual capacity as measured by IQ testing.

B. **Differential diagnosis** of learning problems includes a variety of psychiatric conditions.

1. **Depression** develops in childhood and manifests differently at varying ages.
   a. In infancy, anaclitic depression occurs between 7 and 30 months of age in response to prolonged separation from the primary caretaker.
   b. In toddlers, depression may present as heightened aggression or clinging.
   c. Latency-aged children may be hyperactive, aggressive, frankly depressed, or withdrawn.
   d. Adolescents may act out as a depressive equivalent.

2. **Hyperactivity** can be either primary or secondary to the learning disorder. This distinction is important since treatment differs with the etiology of the hyperactivity.

3. **School phobias** of any etiology can lead to learning disorders.

4. **An interaction problem with the teacher** (specific transference reactions) can prove causative.

5. **Homosexual panic** (in older children) may interfere with learning.

6. **Childhood psychosis**, with its attendant developmental delays, may be at the root of a learning disability.

C. **Treatment** is aimed at the underlying disorder when present. Educational remediation is always necessary.

XIV. PROBLEMS OF ADOLESCENTS. A variety of disorders increase in incidence during adolescence (e.g., anorexia nervosa, adult schizophrenia, and depression). Discussion of these disorders may be found elsewhere. Specific problems of adolescent development are discussed below.

A. **Identity disturbances.** Adolescents struggle to achieve a stable identity. Certain problems result when this aspect of development breaks down.

1. **Identity diffusion.** An adolescent has a poor sense of him- or herself and is easily swayed by the opinions of others.

2. **Peer-related disorders.** Some adolescents can be persuaded to do dangerous things (e.g., take drugs and drive recklessly) to meet the identity of their peer groups.

B. **Adult sexual development.** In adolescence, adult sexual functioning is achieved and sexual preferences are solidified.

1. **Homosexuality** is found commonly in early adolescence, but when it occurs, consistently throughout adolescence, it usually represents a true homosexual preference.

2. **Sexual perversions.** Transvestism, voyeurism, and exhibitionism usually become full-blown in adolescence.

3. **Pregnancy** may be the outcome of increased sexual promiscuity or may manifest as emancipation difficulties. For example, an adolescent who is struggling with separating from her family may become pregnant and turn the infant over to the parents for care. The infant, thus, replaces her and makes her emancipation easier.

C. **Separation.** In adolescence, the individual negotiates leaving his or her family.

1. Difficulty with emancipation can be etiologic in a variety of clinical disorders. For example, psychosis becomes evident in many schizophrenics when they first leave home. The battle over food is really a struggle for autonomy and independence in anorectics. Separation and loss can trigger depressive feelings.

2. Difficult emancipation can lead to **mobilization of aggression** on the part of the adolescent, and intrafamily fighting ensues.

3. **Incest** can develop to prevent a child from emancipating, and inappropriate sexual contact within a family sometimes signifies separation problems.

D. **Treatment.** Special problems develop in the psychotherapy of adolescents.

1. **Labile allegiances.** Adolescents love the therapist one day and hate him or her the next day.

2. **Labile moods.** Because adolescents are in great endocrine and psychological turbulence, unstable moods frequently result.

3. **Communication difficulties.** Adolescents may not be comfortable with verbal communication but are too old for communication through play. Some adolescents communicate by means of their behavior (e.g., reckless driving may signify anger or depression). Obstinancy may signify an emancipation problem because the child refuses to take responsibility for him- or herself.

4. **Overprotective parents** may meddle in an adolescent's treatment. An adolescent should be seen by a physician for evaluation even if he or she asks that the parents not be made aware of the request for treatment. However, parents should be notified if the patient is:
   a. A danger to him- or herself
   b. A danger to others
   c. Gravely disabled

XV. **CHILD ABUSE** occurs when the individuals in a child's environment retard his or her development by hurting the child.

A. **Epidemiology**

1. Child abuse may be physical, sexual, or emotional. Significant neglect should be considered equivalent to abuse.

2. Approximately 15% of children who come to the emergency room with obvious trauma have been physically abused.

3. Parents who were abused as children are at greater risk for abusing their own children.

4. Parents who are not overtly abusive may be silently participating in the abuse by failing to protect the child from the abusive parent.

5. Premature infants are abused more often than full-gestation infants, which is probably due to poor bonding.

6. Reasons for the abuse of infants probably differ from those for the abuse of older children. Abuse of the latter is often associated with psychosexual development (e.g., a 3-year-old soils her pants and is beaten). The former are abused because their parents are emotionally needy and feel that the infant is taking attention away from them. Problems with feeding may result in abuse of infants. It is unusual for child abuse to begin after the age of 6 years with the exception of sexual abuse.

7. Abuse occurs in all socioeconomic groups.

B. Effects on the child

1. Occasionally, development may be precocious. The expectation that a child function as "a parent" causes some children to develop quickly. Fear of being abused for mistakes can also lead to precocious development. The precocity, however, tends to be superficial and defensive. The underlying desire to be validated as a child for age-appropriate attributes is usually also apparent.

2. Development may be retarded if the abuse is severe.

3. There may be a role reversal with the parents. Abusive parents may expect their children to function as adults and care for them.

4. Physical injuries are constantly a risk.

5. There is a risk of abusing future offspring when the abused child grows up and identifies with his or her parents.

6. Exposure to chronic violence can increase aggression and antisocial behavior in the abused child.

C. Treatment

1. Suspected abuse must be reported to the county protective services. If the child's health or life is in jeopardy, he or she should be removed from the abusive environment. If there is no improvement at 1–2 years postdiagnosis, severance of parental rights should be considered.

2. Most abused children need psychotherapy.

3. Parents almost always need long-term psychotherapy and often parenting classes.

BIBLIOGRAPHY

American Psychiatric Association: *Diagnostic and Statistical Manual of Mental Disorders,* 3rd ed, revised. Washington DC, American Psychiatric Association, 1987

Emde RN, Harmon RJ, Good WV: Depressive feelings in children: a transactional model for research. In *Depression in Childhood: Developmental Perspectives.* Edited by Rutter M, Izard D, Reed P. New York, Gilford Press, 1986

Green M, Solnit AJ: Reactions to the threatened loss of a child. A vulnerable child syndrome. *Pediatrics* 34:58–65, 1964

Klaus MH, Kendall JH: *Parent-Infant Bonding.* St. Louis, CV Mosby, 1982

Spitz RA: Hospitalism: an inquiry into the genesis of psychiatric conditions in early childhood. *Psychoanal Study Child* 1:53–74, 1945

Steele BF, Pollock CB: A psychiatric study of parents who abuse infants and small children. In *The Battered Child.* Edited by Helfer RE, Kempe CH. Chicago, University of Chicago Press, 1968, pp 103–145

STUDY QUESTIONS

Directions: Each question below contains five suggested answers. Choose the **one best** response to each question.

1. The view that there is a natural and unalterable sequence in which development must occur is referred to as

(A) critical phases of development
(B) developmental lines
(C) developmental continuity
(D) epigenesis
(E) none of the above

2. The sequence of the oral-anal-genital psychosexual stages has which of the following characteristics?

(A) It starts when a child is 2 years old
(B) It must be negotiated in this order
(C) It does not really exist
(D) It is based on Jungian theory
(E) None of the above

3. True statements concerning the use of play in a child psychiatric evaluation include all of the following EXCEPT

(A) play materials may diminish the child's anxiety, facilitating communication
(B) play materials allow the child a vehicle through which to communicate in metaphor
(C) play materials should be used in the evaluation of all preschool and latency-aged children
(D) play materials may at times interfere with, rather than facilitate, communciation
(E) play materials should be carefully selected and limited in number

4. Childhood psychopathology is best described by which of the following statements?

(A) Childhood psychiatric disorders are more common in boys than in girls
(B) Childhood disorders are more common in latency-aged children (i.e., those 6–12 years of age)
(C) Childhood psychopathology is always transient
(D) It is impossible to evaluate psychiatric disorders in children alone; their families must also be evaluated
(E) None of the above

5. Physician advocacy for the child patient is complicated by the issue of confidentiality. Which of the following statements accurately describes situations in which patient confidentiality is applicable?

(A) It does not apply because parents have a right to know what their children are thinking and talking about
(B) It does not apply because children think that their parents know and understand most things
(C) It applies in all situations except when a child is a danger to him- or herself or others
(D) It applies to children over the age of 15 years
(E) None of the above

6. A 22-year-old woman has just delivered a healthy boy by cesarean section under general anesthesia. When she awakens she is frantic because she has not bonded to her child. The physician should

(A) reassure the patient that bonding is a lengthy process
(B) suggest that the mother breast-feed to offset the effects of poor postnatal bonding
(C) return in 1 day to see if the patient's concerns have dissipated
(D) recommend psychiatric counseling aimed at helping the patient attach to her child
(E) none of the above

7. True statements concerning bonding and attachment include all of the following EXCEPT

(A) both terms refer to an affective relationship
(B) bonding describes the parent's feelings toward the child
(C) attachment describes the child's feelings toward the parent
(D) attachment relationships may be formed throughout the life cycle
(E) bonding and attachment relationships begin with the birth of the child

8. The prognosis of autistic disorder is most accurately described by which of the following statements?

(A) The prognosis is good if the onset of the illness is at birth
(B) The prognosis is good if the child has normal auditory evoked potentials
(C) The prognosis is determined by language development
(D) The prognosis is bad if either of the child's parents has manic–depressive illness
(E) None of the above

9. Which of the following statements about childhood schizophrenia is most accurate?

(A) A genetic linkage with the adult syndrome of schizophrenia has been established
(B) A failure of repression has been suggested etiologically
(C) Auditory hallucinations are prominent
(D) Antipsychotic medication is seldom indicated due to the age of the child
(E) None of the above

10. Night terrors are most likely to occur at what time during the night?

(A) Between 9:00 P.M. and 1:00 A.M.
(B) Between 1:00 A.M. and 3:00 A.M.
(C) Between 2:00 A.M. and 5:00 A.M.
(D) Between 5:00 A.M. and 6:30 A.M.
(E) At any time

11. True statements concerning primary nocturnal enuresis include all of the following EXCEPT

(A) most often, it is not based in psychological conflict
(B) invasive urologic procedures are seldom indicated
(C) some children never outgrow the condition, which persists into adolescence
(D) seldom is medication a first-line treatment
(E) at times, no treatment may be the best treatment

12. True statements concerning the epidemiology of child abuse include all of the following EXCEPT

(A) parents who were abused will likely abuse their own children
(B) parents who fail to protect their children from abuse within the home may be considered silent partners in the abuse
(C) abuse may derive in part from problems in bonding
(D) most abusive parents do not overtly desire to hurt their children
(E) abuse cuts across all socioeconomic strata

Directions: Each question below contains four suggested answers of which **one or more** is correct. Choose the answer

A	if **1, 2, and 3** are correct
B	if **1 and 3** are correct
C	if **2 and 4** are correct
D	if **4** is correct
E	if **1, 2, 3, and 4** are correct

13. In child psychiatry, toys are used for which of the following reasons?

(1) For the child's enjoyment
(2) To facilitate communication between the child and the therapist
(3) To avoid discussion of upsetting issues in therapy
(4) Symbolically by the age of 3 years

14. Phases of the life cycle during which the bonding process occurs include

(1) the mother's childhood
(2) pregnancy
(3) the immediate postnatal period
(4) the toddler stage

15. Findings that support a neurologic etiology of autistic disorder include

(1) high incidence of grand mal seizures
(2) abnormal auditory evoked potentials
(3) decreased responsivity to vestibular stimulation
(4) enlarged ventricles on computerized tomography

16. Anaclitic depression can be described as occurring

(1) after 4 months of life
(2) after 7 months of life
(3) anytime in the life span
(4) prior to 30 months of life

17. Symptoms that are necessary to establish the diagnosis of Tourette's syndrome include

(1) vocal tics
(2) multiple motor tics
(3) onset before age 21
(4) coprolalia

18. Symptoms of narcolepsy include

(1) hypnagogic hallucinations
(2) cataplexy
(3) sleep attacks
(4) sleep paralysis

19. Correct statements concerning encopresis include

(1) soiling is rarely deliberate
(2) the symptom may signify severe psychopathology
(3) the illness is usually self-limited
(4) soiling is an expression of ambition

20. Etiologically, encopresis may represent

(1) parent–child struggles around normal tasks of development
(2) childhood psychosis
(3) parental psychopathology
(4) fecal impaction

21. Correct statements concerning thumb sucking in children include which of the following?

(1) It is usually a benign and self-limited condition
(2) It may be a normal means of self-soothing for young children
(3) If it persists beyond ages 3½–4, changes in dentition can develop
(4) It is more common in boys than in girls

22. Etiologies of school phobia include

(1) homosexual panic
(2) separation anxiety
(3) malingering
(4) cruel teacher

23. The pharmacotherapy of attention-deficit disorder is described by which of the following statements?

(1) Antidepressants are generally considered first-line medications for this disorder
(2) Appetite and growth suppression may occur in children on medication for this disorder
(3) In most cases, medication alone provides adequate management for this disorder
(4) Administration of dextroamphetamine tends not to induce behavioral stimulation in children as it does in adults

24. Symptoms that are necessary for the diagnosis of an attention-deficit disorder include

(1) short attention span
(2) impulsivity
(3) distractibility
(4) hyperactivity

25. Accurate statements concerning learning disorders include which of the following?

(1) Learning disorders may involve reading, writing, or arithmetic skills
(2) Learning disorders usually occur in mentally retarded children
(3) Diagnosis is established as a mismatch between cognitive ability and actual performance of the skill in question
(4) Learning disorders are also known as pervasive developmental disorders

ANSWERS AND EXPLANATIONS

1. The answer is D. (*I A 1*) The view that development progresses according to a fixed sequence, which cannot be reversed, is referred to as epigenesis. The concept of critical phases of development, while largely outdated, held that certain developmental tasks could be accomplished only at certain ages. The concept of developmental lines relates to a view of longitudinal development within certain domains, such as eating, toileting, and relationships. Developmental continuities are those personality traits beginning in childhood with later relevance for adulthood.

2. The answer is B. (*I A 1–3*) Epigenesis is a principle that states that development must occur in a sequential fashion. Although some children may become arrested at certain points of development, they still progress through these psychosexual stages in the correct order. When a child is psychologically traumatized at one of these levels, he or she may continue to show characteristics of that level. These psychosexual stages begin at birth. They were first conceptualized by Freud.

3. The answer is C. (*I C b*) The psychiatrist must facilitate communication and expression on the part of a child during a child psychiatric evaluation. Some children are able to do this directly without the use of play materials. If the child is sufficiently verbal, play materials may be unnecessary. However, play materials may diminish the child's anxiety as well as provide the child with a vehicle through which to communicate in metaphor. When used, however, play materials should be carefully selected and limited in number so as not to distract or impede the child's communication.

4. The answer is A. (*I B 1, C 1, 2*) The incidence of almost all childhood psychiatric conditions is higher in boys; only anorexia nervosa and thumb sucking occur more frequently in girls. Boys are more vulnerable for a number of reasons. They may be raised differently, and they probably have a genetic vulnerability. The incidence of many psychiatric conditions, such as anorexia nervosa, depression, and schizophrenia, increases at puberty. Childhood psychopathology is more likely to be transient when it follows a clear psychological stressor. When a child has been raised in a chronically damaging way, he or she may have lasting psychological problems. Although family history and evaluation are helpful, a child can be evaluated independently of either.

5. The answer is C. (*I C 1; XIV D 4*) A child should be assured that the information that he or she provides the psychiatrist is confidential. When a child is at risk of harming him- or herself or others, it is appropriate and necessary to inform the family. Although children assume that parents know a great deal, the ability to understand and keep a secret probably develops by 3 years of age. While the principle of confidentiality is typically of more concern to teenagers than to young children, it is applicable to all.

6. The answer is A. (*II A, B*) Bonding and attachment are processes that occur over a lengthy period of time. Although many parents worry that a cesarean section interferes with this process, simple reassurance usually is helpful to them. Breast-feeding would not necessarily offset any sort of aberration in bonding and attachment. At first, many new mothers feel that their infants do not belong to them. This feeling can last several days. Returning to see the patient is a good idea but should be done 3–4 days later; however, conditions can warrant returning sooner. When the mother is severely depressed, anxious, or psychotic, she should be evaluated for psychiatric treatment and follow-up.

7. The answer is E. (*II A*) Bonding and attachment refer to an affective relationship between parent and child. Bonding refers to the parent's relationship with the child, and attachment refers to the child's relationship with the parent. Attachment relationships may be formed throughout the life cycle as is demonstrated by adopted children and their families. The process of parent-child bonding has its roots during preconception and relates to the parent's own experience with attachment relationships. The process of bonding is greatly accelerated in utero as the parents fantasize about and begin to relate to the developing fetus.

8. The answer is C. (*III A 7*) Although the prognosis of autistic disorder relates to the level of language development and intelligence, in general, the prognosis for the syndrome is very guarded. The condition cannot be diagnosed at birth. Delays and distortions in development must be documented over time. While there are associated neurologic findings (e.g., grand mal seizures, vestibular dysfunction, and abnormal auditory evoked potentials), these do not affect prognosis. A manic–depressive parent would not affect prognosis, and there is no association of manic–depressive illness (bipolar disorder) with autistic disorder.

9. The answer is B. (*III B 2*) Childhood schizophrenia is a regression to a psychotic state after previous attainment of better mental functioning. Suggested etiologies include a grossly chaotic upbringing with constant exposure to aggressive and sexual themes with a subsequent failure of repression. A genetic cause is possible as well; however, it has not been as well delineated as it has for adult schizophrenia. Auditory hallucinations may be present but are seldom prominent. Antipsychotic medications may be helpful to the child, though children tend to respond less completely to antipsychotic medications than do adults.

10. The answer is A. (*VI A 2*) Night terrors occur during the deep stages (stages 3 and 4) of sleep, which are early in the sleep cycle. Therefore, night terrors would be most likely to occur between 9:00 P.M. and 1:00 A.M. The physiology of night terrors is only partly understood. Apparently, arousal from these deep stages of sleep triggers night terrors in some children. Since so many children (30%) experience night terrors, delayed central nervous system maturation is hypothesized as a cause.

11. The answer is C. (*VII A, C*) Primary nocturnal enuresis is bed wetting that occurs only during deep sleep and that has never been interrupted by a period of good nocturnal bladder control. Most commonly, it derives from a benign delay in central nervous system maturation. Consequently, invasive urologic procedures are seldom indicated. Insofar as it is a generally benign condition, and all medications carry attendant risks, seldom is medication indicated as a first-line of treatment. Since enuresis is a self-limited disorder, which all children outgrow, sometimes no treatment is the best. Unlike secondary enuresis, which commonly derives from psychological conflict, this conflict is seldom etiologic in primary nocturnal enuresis.

12. The answer is A. (*XV A*) Child abuse is a condition that cuts across all socioeconomic strata. While abusive parents are a heterogeneous population, it is true that most abusive parents do not consciously desire to hurt their children. Abusive parents tend to control their own impulses poorly. Abusive parents may have failed to bond adequately with their children for a variety of reasons. Parents who are not overtly abusive may be silently participating in abuse by failing to protect a child from an abusive parent. Although a high percentage of abusive parents were themselves abused as children, it does not follow that a high percentage of abused children will become abusive parents.

13. The answer is E (all). (*I C 1 b, 3*) As with all forms of communication, play and the use of toys inform the therapist of conflict and can be used defensively. For example, a child may insist on playing checkers for the entire session to avoid talking or playing out his or her problems. Consequently, special attention should be paid so that toys facilitate communication between the child and the therapist rather than providing a source of interference or impediment to communication. Symbolic play, that is, using toys to express an idea, develops very early in childhood, usually before 3 years of age.

14. The answer is E (all). (*II A*) A bond is defined as an affective relationship of the parent with the child. Bonding occurs throughout an individual's life span. There is no critical phase. The process of bonding begins even before conception. For example, a young girl plays with dolls and imagines her attitudes towards her future children. When she is pregnant, these vague attitudes about children become focused on the fetus and child-to-be. After the child is born, the affective relationship grows and changes. It probably persists throughout the child's life span and is passed on to the next generation.

15. The answer is A (1, 2, 3). (*III A 4*) Autistic disorder is an illness that commences in early childhood (before the age of 36 months) in which the child demonstrates disturbed relatedness to other human beings, bizarre responses to his or her environment, and delays and oddities in language development. Findings that support the neurologic etiology of this condition include abnormal auditory evoked potentials in most autistic children, a high incidence of grand mal seizures during childhood, and decreased nystagmus in response to vestibular stimulation. Enlarged ventricles on computerized tomography have not been consistent findings in this condition.

16. The answer is C (2, 4). (*IV A 1*) Anaclitic depression occurs after 7 months of life and before 30 months of life. During this phase of development, children are aware of who their primary caretaker is but do not yet have object constancy; that is, they lack the ability to maintain an image of their caretaker in the caretaker's absence. Therefore, they are vulnerable to lengthy separations (i.e., more than 1 week). Such separations from caretakers can result in a depressive syndrome that includes sad facial expressions, anorexia, apathy, and withdrawal from other individuals. The best treatment is to avoid prolonged separations. If that is not possible, a familiar individual or surrogate caretaker should be available to the child.

17. The answer is A (1, 2, 3). (*V*) Tourette's syndrome consists of recurrent, involuntary, purposeless movements (i.e., motor tics) accompanied by vocal tics. The onset occurs before the age of 21.

DSM-III-R criteria for the diagnosis of Tourette's syndrome include the occurrence of motor and vocal tics for at least 1 year. While coprolalia is a particular type of vocal tic, it is not necessary to establish the diagnosis of Tourette's syndrome.

18. The answer is E (all). (*VI B 1*) Narcolepsy is a sleep disorder that is characterized by rapid eye movement (REM)–onset sleep. Associated manifestations include hypnagogic hallucinations (visual and auditory), occurring at sleep onset, cataplexy (loss of motor tone) in response to an emotion, sleep paralysis, and daytime sleep attacks. Treatment is aimed at the suppression of REM sleep and consists of the administration of amphetamines and tricyclic antidepressants.

19. The answer is A (1, 2, 3). (*VIII A, B 2*) Soiling is rarely deliberate and is usually self-limited. Sometimes encopresis does signify severe psychopathology, but not necessarily. The symptom may be associated with harsh or punitive toilet training. It is often an expression of anger but not ambition. With no treatment, an encopretic child could be expected to stop soiling by adolescence. Underlying psychopathology would probably remain, however.

20. The answer is E (all). (*VIII B*) Encopresis is characterized by fecal incontinence. Parental coercion around issues of autonomy and control during toilet training may result in conflict, which is subsequently expressed as encopresis. Encopresis may also represent a symptom of childhood psychosis, particularly in the older child and when fecal smearing is present. In certain cases, the symptom of encopresis may be unconsciously generated and propagated as an expression of the parent's own conflict. A significant number of children with encopresis have an impaction, which must be treated.

21. The answer is A (1, 2, 3). (*X A, B*) Thumb sucking is usually a benign and self-limited condition. It is both common and normal at transitional periods in the child's life (bedtime and times of separation from parents) in which it becomes a means of self-soothing. Changes in dentition can develop when thumb sucking persists beyond the ages of 3½–4. It is one of the few conditions that is more common in girls than in boys.

22. The answer is E (all). (*XI A, C*) School phobias are a fear and avoidance of school. They occur throughout childhood but are most common when a child is first introduced to school. School phobia is best considered as a symptom. It may be caused by a variety of conditions, including homosexual panic (e.g., in an older child), separation anxiety (e.g., suffered either by the parent, child, or both), malingering (e.g., to avoid a consequence, such as incompletion of homework), and a legitimate cause of fear at school (e.g., threatening children or a cruel teacher). Legitimate causes of fear should be eliminated, and in most cases, the child should be returned to school immediately.

23. The answer is C (2, 4). (*XII C*) Stimulant medications are generally considered the pharmacologic agents of choice for attention-deficit disorder. Stimulants may cause appetite and subsequent growth suppression in children, so growth curves should be followed on all children on stimulant medication. Children tend not to experience the behavioral stimulation from these medications as do adults. Tricyclic antidepressants, phenytoin, and thioridazine may be valuable as second-line medications in certain refractory cases. In addition to medication management, underlying conditions should be treated, and children should be taught compensatory means to deal with their attention deficit.

24. The answer is A (1, 2, 3). (*XII A*) Key symptoms of attention-deficit disorder include short attention span, difficulty concentrating, impulsivity, distractibility, and excitability. Hyperactivity, which is defined subjectively as an increase in motor activity to a level that interferes with the child's functioning, may be present; however, it is not necessary to establish the diagnosis.

25. The answer is B (1, 3). (*XIII A*) Specific developmental disorders (i.e., learning disorders) may involve a number of skills, including reading, writing, and arithmetic. Diagnosis is established by documenting a mismatch between the child's performance on standardized measures of the skill in question and his or her intellectual capacity as measured by IQ testing. Typically, learning disorders occur in children of normal intelligence. Pervasive developmental disorders, by contrast, involve significant distortions in the development of social relatedness, language, and responsivity to the environment, rather than a circumscribed deficit in a specific academic skill.

11
Personality Disorders
James H. Scully

I. INTRODUCTION. Each of us has a repertoire of coping devices or defenses that allows us to maintain an equilibrium between our internal drives and the world around us. This repertoire is **personality—the set of characteristics that defines the behavior, thoughts, and emotions of an individual**. The characteristics become ingrained and dictate our life-styles.

A. **Personality traits** are generally viewed as a result of development that has been influenced by culture and society as well as by the child-rearing practices of the individual family. In addition, recent studies in child development suggest that there may be genetically determined temperamental factors involved in the course of personality development. Certain genetic characteristics may make a specific behavioral response more likely to occur, thus leading to a specific personality style. When this stable pattern of response leads to problems, a personality disorder may be present. The *Diagnostic and Statistical Manual of Mental Disorders*, 3rd ed., revised (*DSM-III-R*) defines a personality disorder as present when personality traits are inflexible and maladaptive, causing either significant impairment in social or occupational functioning or subjective distress. Manifestations of a personality disorder are generally recognized early, usually by adolescence, and continue into adulthood; however, symptoms may become less obvious in later years.

B. **Expression of symptoms.** Personality disorders are the most common emotional disorders seen in psychiatric practice, particularly in the outpatient clinic. The patient's perception of the problem and the expression of symptoms, however, are different from those demonstrated in other psychiatric illnesses, making treatment difficult. Patients with personality disorders may complain of mood disturbances, particularly depression or anxiety. They may exhibit:

1. **Ego-syntonic symptoms**, whereby patients do not recognize that anything is wrong with them that needs to be changed. They view existing disturbances as being the result of the world being out of step with them.

2. **Ego-dystonic symptoms**, whereby patients may be experiencing internally distressing symptoms, which are self-induced, but they are still unable to alter their behavior.

C. **Clinical picture.** Symptoms of personality disorders almost always effect other individuals. The symptoms involve work and play and all relationships.

1. Individuals with personality disorders have trouble in their work settings; they have often had many jobs and work below their capacities.

2. Social relationships are disrupted or absent altogether. Because individuals with personality disorders can be irritating and infuriating to those involved with them, the reactions to personality disorders by these involved individuals are often more pronounced than the disorder itself in the affected person.

3. These patients may seek help as a result of a concurrent medical or surgical problem or because of a primary emotional distress; in any case, these patients may elicit strong negative reactions in the physicians and other health care personnel who take care of them.

4. In general, patients with personality disorders tolerate stress poorly, and they do not seek help to change their characters but to alleviate the outside stress. If stress is great, as it can be in physical illness, patients may regress even more and can develop transient psychotic

reactions in which they lose touch with reality and become unable to function for brief periods of time.

D. Diagnosis

1. It is sometimes difficult to diagnose a specific personality disorder when a patient has a mix of traits; however the *DSM-III-R* allows for the diagnosis of more than one personality disorder if the patient meets the diagnostic criteria for several disorders.

2. Diagnosis of a personality disorder should be made with care in someone who is reacting to a major environmental or social stress; for example, some young men develop maladaptive coping mechanisms in the military that they do not otherwise employ.

3. Some environments are compatible with certain personality traits and even reward them; for example, the histrionic and narcissistic personality types may function well in the entertainment field, while schizoid and avoidant types might do better in an isolated environment, such as a laboratory.

II. CLUSTERS OF PERSONALITY DISORDERS. Eleven specific personality disorders are described in the *DSM-III-R*. Because of the similarities in symptoms or traits they are grouped into three clusters: A, B, and C.

A. Cluster A. The odd or eccentric group includes the **paranoid, schizoid, and schizotypal personality disorders**.

1. Affected individuals use the defense mechanisms of projection and fantasy and may have a tendency towards psychotic thinking.
   a. **Projection** involves attributing to another person thoughts or feelings of one's own that are unacceptable, such as prejudice, excessive fault-finding, and paranoia.
   b. **Fantasy** is the creation of an imaginary life with which the patient deals with loneliness. A fantasy can be quite elaborate and extensive.
   c. **Paranoia** is a feeling of being persecuted or treated unfairly by others. Paranoid patients may feel that others are talking about or making fun of them.

2. Biologically, patients with cluster A personality disorders may have a vulnerability to cognitive disorganization when stressed.

3. Schizotypal patients have been found to have some of the same biologic markers seen in schizophrenic individuals, including low levels of monoamine oxidase (MAO) activity in platelets and disorders of smooth pursuit eye movements.
   a. It has been speculated that not everyone who has a genetic vulnerability to schizophrenia becomes psychotic, but some of these individuals may be diagnosed as having a schizotypal personality disorder.
   b. In families where there is a history of schizophrenia, there is also an increased number of relatives with schizotypal personality disorder. This is not true of paranoid or schizoid personality disorders.

B. Cluster B. The dramatic, emotional, and erratic group includes **histrionic, narcissistic, antisocial, and borderline personality disorders**. These are the most problematic personality disorders to treat because of the reactions that they stir up in the therapist.

1. Affected individuals tend to use certain defense mechanisms, such as dissociation, denial, splitting, and acting out.
   a. **Dissociation** involves the "forgetting" of unpleasant feelings and associations. It is the unconscious splitting off of some mental processes and behavior from the normal or conscious awareness of the individual. When extreme, this can lead to multiple personalities.
   b. **Denial** is closely associated with dissociation. In denial, the patient disavows a thought, feeling, or wish but is unaware of doing so.
   c. **Splitting**, often seen in borderline personalities, occurs when the patient divides individuals into all good and all bad and cannot experience an ambivalent relationship. The patient cannot even be ambivalent in regard to his or her own self-image.
   d. **Acting out** involves the actual motor expression of a thought or feeling that is intolerable to the patient; this can involve both aggressive and sexual behavior. Patients with these types of personality disorders may be biologically vulnerable to stress because of a tendency to low cortical arousal and a wide variation of autonomic and motor activities. Thus, a psychobiologic pattern may develop, which increases the potential for acting out and which is not associated with any particular anxiety.

2. Mood disorders are more common in cluster B and may be the chief complaint.

3. Somatization disorder is associated with histrionic personality disorder.

C. Cluster C. The anxious and fearful group includes **avoidant, dependent, compulsive, and passive–aggressive personality disorders**.

1. Affected individuals use defenses of isolation, passive aggression, and hypochondriasis.

  a. Isolation occurs when an unacceptable feeling, act, or idea is separated from the associated emotion. Patients are orderly and controlled and can speak of events of their lives without feeling.

  b. Passive aggression occurs when resistance is indirect and often turned against the self. Thus, failing examinations, clownish conduct, and procrastinating are aspects of passive–aggressive behavior.

  c. Hypochondriasis is often present in patients with personality disorders, particularly in dependent, passive–aggressive patients. Biologically, these patients may have a tendency towards higher levels of cortical arousal and an increase in motor inhibition. Thus, stressful stimuli may lead to high anxiety or affective arousal.

2. Twin studies have demonstrated some genetic factors in the development of cluster C personality disorders; for example, obsessive–compulsive traits are more common in monozygotic twins than in dizygotic twins.

III. SPECIFIC CLUSTER A PERSONALITY DISORDERS

A. Schizoid personality disorder

1. Definition and symptoms (*DSM-III-R*). Schizoid individuals have defects in their capacity to form social relationships. Close friends are limited to no more than one or two people, including family members.

  a. They lack warm, tender feelings and often are characterized by emotional coldness and aloofness. They are indifferent to praise, criticism, and the feelings of others.

  b. They are not psychotic, and they do not have the eccentric thoughts, speech, and behavior seen in individuals with schizotypal personality disorder.

  c. These individuals are loners; they almost always choose activities that are solitary. Certain work situations that require social isolation may allow them to perform well.

  d. These individuals tend to be humorless and dull. They are self-absorbed and absent-minded and seem to be unrelated to their surroundings.

  e. They have little or no interest in sex.

  (1) Men with this disorder are unlikely to marry because they lack social skills.

  (2) Women may passively accept a relationship and marriage.

2. The prevalence of schizoid personality disorder is unknown as these patients rarely come to treatment.

3. Medical–surgical setting. Illness brings these patients into close contact with caregivers, which is often seen as a threat to their equilibrium. Patients may intensify their aloofness and are likely to leave the hospital against medical advice if intruded upon too much. Physicians should respect the patients' distance and intrude as little as possible. They should expect the development of trust to take a long time and not demand emotional reactions from their patients.

4. Treatment. Individuals with schizoid, paranoid, and schizotypal personality disorders do not usually seek treatment. If treatment is sought, the physician should be respectful but scrupulously honest in dealing with the patient. Individual psychotherapy is usually the only possible way to begin, but, if the patient can tolerate it, **group therapy** can be more successful.

B. Paranoid personality disorder

1. Definition (*DSM-III-R*). The central features of paranoid personality disorder are a pervasive and unwarranted suspicion and mistrust of people, hypersensitivity to others, and an inability to deal with feelings. Individuals with this disorder are neither psychotic nor schizophrenic. While many paranoid individuals are careful observers and often energetic and capable, they routinely misinterpret the actions of others as deliberately demeaning or threatening.

2. Symptoms

  a. Paranoid individuals are hypervigilant and:

  (1) Continually scan the environment for signs of a threat

  (2) Expect to be tricked or harmed

  (3) Are guarded and secretive

      (4) Avoid accepting blame when it is deserved
      (5) Question the loyalty of others
      (6) Search continuously and intensely for confirmation of their biases with loss of appreciation of the larger context
      (7) Exhibit overconcern for hidden motives and special meanings
      (8) Exhibit pathologic jealousy
      (9) Have difficulty relaxing and are ready to counterattack when any threat is perceived
     (10) Exaggerate their problems
     (11) Are quick to take offense
  b. Paranoid individuals are often litigious and:
      (1) React to perceived insults with anger and counterattack
      (2) Bear grudges
      (3) Do not forgive insults or slights
      (4) Are very aware of the power and rank in others
  c. Paranoid individuals have a restricted ability to feel and:
      (1) Appear cold and aloof
      (2) Have no sense of humor
      (3) Lack passive, soft, tender, and sentimental feelings
      (4) Pride themselves on being objective and rational
      (5) Favor mechanical or electronic devices, not art

3. The prevalence of paranoid personality disorder is unknown. They tend to group themselves in esoteric religions and pseudoscientific and quasipolitical groups. Groups of paranoid individuals who set themselves apart and see others as "the enemy" tend to provoke negative reactions from the outside, thus reinforcing their paranoid views.

4. Medical–surgical setting. Illness tends to exacerbate the personality style of paranoid patients. They tend to become more guarded, suspicious, and quarrelsome. They are frequently overly sensitive to slights and project their concerns onto others. They complain and are suspicious. Physicians should be courteous, honest, and respect the defenses of paranoid patients. There is a need to be straightforward and explain everything. Physicians should not expect to be trusted and should not impose closeness upon these patients but remain professional and even a little aloof.

5. Treatment. Individuals with paranoid personality disorders, like those with schizoid and schizotypal personalities, rarely seek treatment. If treatment is sought, the physician needs to be respectful, but scrupulously honest. For example, if the patient finds something amiss, such as lateness for an appointment, the therapist should admit fault and apologize immediately.
  a. Individual therapy is usually the only possible way to begin.
  b. Occasionally, a patient can tolerate group therapy, but great care must be taken in the selection of patients.
  c. The therapist needs to avoid getting too close to the patient too quickly. Some patients may become agitated or threatening. Limits then must be set.
  d. Antipsychotic medications can be used in small doses for short periods of time to manage agitation. However, the physician must be sure to explain the side effects.

C. Schizotypal personality disorder

1. Definition. The central features of this disorder are pervasive patterns of "strange" or "odd" behavior, appearance, or thinking. These peculiarities are not so severe that they can be termed schizophrenic, and there is no history of psychotic episodes.

2. Symptoms. At least five of the following symptoms should be present in one context or another.
  a. Undue anxiety about social situations, especially situations involving unfamiliar people
  b. Ideas of reference
  c. Magical thinking and odd beliefs (e.g., superstitions, clairvoyance, and telepathy)
  d. Eccentric and strange appearance or behavior
  e. Recurrent perceptual experiences of an unusual nature (e.g., sensing a force or individual not actually present)
  f. Peculiar speech without loosening of associations or incoherence (i.e., speech that is digressive, overelaborate, circumstantial, and metaphoric)
  g. Social isolation (no close friends or confidants other than first-degree relatives)
  h. Inadequate rapport in face-to-face interactions due to inappropriate or constricted affect
  i. Paranoia or suspicion

3. **Prevalence.** Some studies indicate that 3% of the population have this disorder.

4. **Medical–surgical setting.** The problems in treating schizotypal personality with medical or surgical illness are similar to those encountered with schizoid patients. Schizotypal individuals tend to put off caregivers. Illness threatens their isolation.

5. **Treatment.** If treatment is sought, the physician should be very honest in dealing with the patient. The odd behavior of these patients can cause uneasiness in the physician who must avoid all ridicule. There is more of a chance of success with group therapy than individual psychotherapy; however, only select patients can tolerate this.

IV. SPECIFIC CLUSTER B PERSONALITY DISORDERS

A. Antisocial personality disorder

1. **Definition** (*DSM-III-R*). Individuals with this disorder have a history of continuous and chronic antisocial behavior by which the rights of others are violated. The essential defect is one of character structure in which affected individuals are seemingly unable to control their impulses and postpone immediate gratification. Antisocial personalities lack sensitivity to the feelings of others; they are egocentric, selfish, and excessively demanding and are usually free of anxiety, remorse, and guilt. Antisocial personalities have been termed sociopathic and psychopathic. They persist in lifelong habits of violating the laws and customs of the communities in which they live.

2. **Symptoms**
   a. In order to diagnose antisocial personality disorders in adults, there should be evidence of a conduct disorder in childhood, manifested by at least three of the following:
      (1) Truancy
      (2) Running away from home at least twice
      (3) Initiating physical fights
      (4) Physical cruelty to other people
      (5) Physical cruelty to animals
      (6) Use of a weapon in more than one fight
      (7) Deliberate destruction of property
      (8) Fire setting
      (9) Lying
      (10) Forcing someone into sexual activity
      (11) Frequent thievery without confronting the victim
      (12) Stealing with confrontation of the victim (e.g., mugging or extortion)
   b. Problem behavior, both antisocial and irresponsible, since age 15 should be manifested in at least four of the following areas:
      (1) Frequent job changes, significant unemployment, serious absenteeism, and walking off the job
      (2) Inability to function as a responsible parent as indicated by malnutrition of a child, poor hygiene, lack of medical care, or failure to arrange for a caretaker when away
      (3) Failure to accept social norms with respect to lawful behavior as indicated by repeated thefts, an illegal occupation (e.g., pimping, prostitution, or drug dealing), multiple arrests, or felony convictions)
      (4) Inability to sustain a monogamous relationship for more than 1 year
      (5) Irritability and aggressiveness as indicated by repeated physical fights or assaults, including spouse and child abuse
      (6) Failure to honor financial obligations and debts, failure to provide child support, and failure to support other dependents on a regular basis
      (7) Failure to plan ahead or impulsiveness as indicated by moving about without a prearranged job or clear goal or the lack of a fixed address for 1 month or more
      (8) Disregard for the truth as indicated by repeated lying or conning others for personal profit
      (9) Recklessness as indicated by driving while intoxicated or recurrent speeding
      (10) Lack of remorse or guilt for behavior that hurts others

3. **Prevalence.** It is estimated that 3% of American men and 1% of American women have an antisocial personality disorder. The disorder is more common among individuals of lower socioeconomic groups, and individuals with this disorder tend to do poorly economically and leave their families destitute. Illiteracy and substance use disorders are frequent complications.

4. **Etiology.** The etiology is not clear.
   a. There is often a history of antisocial personality disorder in both men and women in

the family. In fact, a sociopathic or alcoholic father is a powerful predictor of an antisocial personality whether or not the child is reared in the presence of the father.
   b. Some antisocial behavior is precipitated by brain damage secondary to closed head trauma or encephalitis. In these cases, the proper diagnosis is **organic personality syndrome** rather than antisocial personality disorder. The causative factors are generally felt to be psychosocial.
   c. Other studies show that inconsistent and impulsive parenting are more damaging than the loss of a parent.

5. **Medical–surgical setting.** Patients with antisocial personality disorder may be superficially charming when under stress and not cause any particular problems initially. However, they tend to be manipulative if given a chance and will chafe against the rules of the hospital. Young patients with antisocial personality have particular difficulty with the authority of physicians and tend to be noncompliant with treatment. They are likely to leave the hospital against medical advice when threatened and generally disrupt the hospital setting.

6. **Treatment**
   a. Setting of firm limits is crucial, and, in general, inpatient settings are the only places where behavior can be controlled.
   b. Group therapy is more helpful than individual therapy because the patient sees it as less authoritative. Inpatient groups can confront antisocial behavior since the group is made up of experts at recognizing this behavior. Group treatment may involve therapeutic communities as well.
   c. Outpatient treatment usually is totally unsatisfactory because the patient flees treatment as soon as unpleasant affects are elicited.

B. Borderline personality disorder

1. **Definition.** The term borderline originated with the concept that this disorder was on the border between neurosis and psychosis. The disorder has also been called borderline schizophrenia, pseudoneurotic schizophrenia, or ambulatory schizophrenia, but it is now thought to be distinct from schizophrenia. The most important features of the disorder are instability of self-image, interpersonal relationships, and mood. An identity disturbance is usually present and is manifested by an uncertainty about sexual orientation, goals, types of friends, and self-image.

2. **Symptoms.** The disorder begins in early adulthood and involves the following symptoms.
   a. Impulsive and unpredictable behavior, which is potentially self-damaging, such as suicidal gestures, self-mutilation, recurrent accidents, fighting, substance abuse, binge eating, shoplifting, or reckless driving
   b. Mood instability, shifting from depression to anxiety or irritability over the course of hours to days
   c. Intense, inappropriate outbursts of anger
   d. Symptoms of a profound identity disturbance, including uncertainty about self-image, gender, and long-term goals
   e. An inability to tolerate being alone, which produces frantic behavior when faced with the prospect

3. **Prevalence.** The disorder may be present in 1%–2% percent of the population. The diagnosis is made twice as frequently in women. Of the individuals with this diagnosis, 90% also have one other *DSM-III-R* diagnosis, and 40% have two other diagnoses.

4. **Etiology.** Almost all theories related to the cause of the borderline personality have postulated problems in early development. It is speculated that there is failure of the child to separate and individuate, and, therefore, a symbiotic relationship with the parental figures persists.

5. **Medical–surgical setting.** When an individual with a borderline personality becomes ill, there is an increase of stress and the potential for an exacerbation of symptoms related to the personality. The illness can mean a threat to any emotional homeostasis that the patient has developed. **Splitting** is seen. The hospital staff may unconsciously take sides and, with the patient, see things as all good or all bad. This split often occurs between the physicians and the nurses. The intensity of the feelings stirred up by the patient may make medical treatment difficult.

6. **Treatment**
   a. Psychological. There are two general approaches to the psychological treatment of the borderline patient.

(1) The psychodynamic approach aims to understand the underlying psychopathology. In general, standard long-term psychotherapy is difficult because the patient tends to regress, and the reactions of therapists are intense.

(2) Treatment oriented towards supportive reality is confrontational rather than interpretational. The therapist helps the patient recognize the feelings that are being stirred up and their connection with behavior. The therapist sets limits and provides structure. This approach is more appropriate in the general hospital setting.

  b. Pharmacologic treatment. Clinically important, although modest improvement in patient mood and behavior can be obtained with pharmacotherapy.

    (1) Antidepressants, particularly monoamine oxidase (MAO) inhibitors (e.g., tranylcypromine) have been effective in improving mood but not in effecting behavioral changes.

    (2) Carbamazepine, an anticonvulsant, has been shown to decrease behavioral dyscontrol.

    (3) Antipsychotic medications in low doses for brief periods are also effective.

    (4) Benzodiazepines are contraindicated for most patients because they make symptoms worse.

C. Narcissistic personality disorder

1. Definition. Individuals with narcissistic personality disorder have a grandiose sense of their own importance, but they are also extremely sensitive to criticism. They have little ability to empathize with others. They are more concerned about appearance than substance.

2. Symptoms (*DSM-III-R*). The narcissistic individual demonstrates at least five of the following symptoms by early adulthood:

  a. Reacts to criticism with anger, shame, or humiliation

  b. Takes advantage of others either for self-aggrandizement or to indulge personal desires

  c. Has grandiose sense of self-importance or uniqueness and expects to be acknowledged as "special"

  d. Has excessive and unrealistic fantasies, involving unlimited success, ability, power, wealth, brilliance, and ideal love

  e. Exudes a sense of entitlement with the expectation of special favors without the assumption of reciprocal responsibilities

  f. Forms relationships with others that lack empathy

  g. May overidealize others but also devalues them

  h. Needs constant attention from others and may exploit others to get this

  i. Is preoccupied with feelings of envy

3. Prevalence. The prevalence of this disorder is unknown. Although the diagnosis has been made more often in recent years, this is likely to be due to a greater interest in this disorder rather than to an increased prevalence.

4. Associated features. Depression or a depressed mood is common with this disorder. Painful preoccupation with appearance occurs. Features of other cluster B disorders are often present.

5. Medical–surgical setting. An individual with a narcissistic personality reacts to illness as a threat to his or her sense of grandiosity and self-perfection. There is usually intensification of characteristic behavior and either overidealization or devaluation of the physician. The patient expects special treatment.

6. Treatment. Individual psychotherapy is the treatment of choice with an attempt at understanding the pain suffered by the patient with this disorder. The therapist must deal with transitions from being overidealized to being devalued. These transitions can be stormy, and they occur when the therapist has misunderstood the patient or has not been perfectly empathic. It is important that the therapist is not defensive about his or her mistakes.

D. Histrionic personality disorder

1. Definition (*DSM-III-R*) People with this disorder are flamboyant, seek attention, and demonstrate an excessive emotionality. Their emotions are shallow and shift rapidly. Typically, they are attractive and seductive and, like the narcissistic personality, are overly concerned with their appearance. This disorder was formerly called "hysterical personality," but that term has been dropped because of the many meanings of "hysterical." Over the years, the word hysterical has been used to describe a personality type, a conversion reaction, and a psychoneurotic disorder characterized by phobias and anxiety; generally speaking, it has been used pejoratively when applied to women.

2. **Symptoms.** The individual with histrionic personality disorder has at least four of the following:
   a. Constantly seeks praise, reassurance, or approval
   b. Is sexually seductive in inappropriate ways
   c. Is vain and overly concerned with appearance
   d. Self-dramatizes and exaggerates emotions
   e. Is egocentric and inconsiderate of others
   f. Is intolerant of delayed gratification
   g. Has shallow emotions that shift quickly
   h. Exhibits bored or irritated behavior if not the center of attention
   i. Has excessively overgeneralized and impressionistic speech

3. **Prevalence.** The prevalence of histrionic personality disorder is not known with certainty. It is thought to be common. The disorder is diagnosed in women much more frequently than men.

4. **Associated features.** As with all of the cluster B disorders, mood and somatization disorders are common, especially depression.

5. **Medical–surgical setting**
   a. Patients may be seen as charming and fascinating by the physician, especially when they are of the opposite sex.
   b. The illness is often seen as a threat by patients to their physical attractiveness. It may be seen as a punishment for their thoughts or feelings, and in men it may be seen as a threat of castration.
   c. Men may behave in an inappropriate sexual manner with nurses and physicians who are women. The sexual behavior may be a cover for deeper concerns about dependency. These patients learn that they can be taken care of by being cute or sexually attractive, and this behavior is accentuated under the stress of illness. The physician should approach the patient as a professional and remind him or her that the roles are set; at the same time, it is important to remain warm and noncritical.

6. **Treatment**
   a. Psychotherapy, either individual or group, is generally the treatment of choice for histrionic personality disorder. In general, the therapist helps the patient become aware of the real feelings underneath the histrionic behavior.
   b. Antidepressant medications, especially MAO inhibitors, have been useful in treating mood disorders associated with this personality type.

V. SPECIFIC CLUSTER C PERSONALITY DISORDERS

A. Avoidant personality disorder

1. **Definition** (*DSM-III-R*). Individuals with this disorder are timid and shy but do wish to have friends. They are so uncomfortable and afraid of rejection or criticism that they avoid social contact. If given strong guarantees of uncritical acceptance, they will make friends. They are very self-critical with poor self-esteem.

2. **Symptoms.** An individual with this disorder should demonstrate by early adulthood a pervasive pattern, including at least four of the following:
   a. Is easily hurt by disapproval or criticism
   b. Has no (or almost no) close friends except close relatives
   c. Avoids involvement with anyone unless there is a guarantee of acceptance
   d. Avoids social or work activities that require social interaction
   e. Holds back and is shy in social situations for fear of saying something stupid or embarrassing
   f. Expects and fears embarrassment, such as blushing or crying when in the presence of others
   g. Avoids new activities because of inappropriate worry about potential difficulties or risks associated with anything outside the usual routine

3. **Prevalence.** The prevalence is unknown, but it is probably common.

4. **Associated features.** Social phobias and agoraphobia may be present, but they are also separate disorders that need to be ruled out.

5. **Medical–surgical setting.** Unlike schizoid patients, patients who are avoidant may do well in the hospital. These patients are undemanding and generally cooperative; their illness can allow them to be taken care of and establish relationships with the staff. They are sensitive

to criticism and may misinterpret equivocal statements as being derogatory or ridiculing and withdraw emotionally.

  6. Treatment
  a. Psychotherapy, either individual or group, can be useful. These patients respond to genuine caring and support.
  b. Assertiveness training may give these patients new social skills and be very useful.

B. Dependent personality disorder

  1. Definition (*DSM-III-R*). Individuals with dependent personality disorder are **passive**. They allow others to direct their lives because they are unable to do so themselves. Other people, such as a spouse or parents, make all of the major decisions of their lives, including where to live and what type of employment to obtain. Their own needs are placed secondary to those of the people upon whom they depend to avoid any possibility of having to be self-reliant. They lack self-confidence and see themselves as helpless or stupid. Some authorities believe that the presence of this disorder depends to a large extent upon cultural roles (i.e., certain groups are expected to assume dependent roles on the basis of certain criteria, such as gender or ethnic background).

  2. Symptoms. This disorder begins no later than early adulthood and is characterized by at least five of the following:
  a. Unable to make everyday decisions without excessive reassurance. Important decisions, such as where to live, are made by others.
  b. Is overly agreeable with the opinions of others, even when he or she believes they are wrong
  c. Cannot initiate things by him- or herself
  d. Will agree to do unpleasant or demeaning tasks just to be liked
  e. Cannot tolerate being alone and will go to great lengths to avoid it
  f. Exhibits extreme reactions to ending relationships; feels helpless and devastated
  g. Worries about being abandoned
  h. Is easily hurt by criticism or disapproval

  3. Prevalence. The prevalence is unknown, but the disorder is apparently common. The diagnosis is more frequent in women.

  4. Associated features. Children who have had a chronic physical illness or who have had separation anxiety may be at risk for this disorder in adulthood. Depression is common.

  5. Medical–surgical setting
  a. Being sick usually means being taken care of, and one might expect that dependent individuals would be good patients. However, illness may stir up intolerable feelings of fear of abandonment and helplessness for these patients. There is a pull to regress to an earlier state of dependency, which may frighten the patients because of its intensity. Feelings of dependency increase. Generally these patients become demanding and complaining when sick.
  b. Physicians need to set limits. It is important for the physicians, nurses, and other staff to get together to plan with the patient what kind of care is going to be given. For instance, it should be clear to the patient how often the nurse will come by to check on him or her. If this is not done early, the negative reactions that these patients stir up can lead to punitive behavior on the part of the caregivers.

  6. Treatment
  a. Psychotherapy can be very useful in the treatment of dependent patients. The focus is on the current behavior and its consequences. The therapist should be careful when there is a challenge to a pathologic but dependent relationship. The patient may leave therapy rather than give up such a relationship.
  b. Behavioral therapies, including assertiveness training, can be helpful.

C. Obsessive–compulsive personality disorder

  1. Definition. Individuals with this disorder are perfectionistic, inflexible, and unable to express warm and tender feelings. They are preoccupied with trivial details and rules and do not appreciate changes in routine. **Obsessive–compulsive disorder** is an anxiety disorder, which involves time obsessions and compulsions and should be distinguished from obsessive–compulsive *personality* disorder. Individuals with obsessive–compulsive disorder may not have the personality disorder, and individuals with the personality disorder may not have the anxiety disorder.

2. **Symptoms.** This disorder begins by early adulthood. The individual with this disorder demonstrates at least five of the following:
   a. Is a perfectionist to the point at which it gets in the way of completing a task
   b. Is preoccupied with rules, lists, and details so that the point of the activity is lost
   c. Insists that things be done his or her way and displays an unreasonable reluctance to delegate work because of fear others will not do it correctly
   d. Devotes time and energy to work to the exclusion of social life
   e. Gets lost in the rules and details and, thus, cannot make decisions
   f. Is inflexible and scrupulous about issues of ethics or morality
   g. Is stingy with both compliments and gifts
   h. Is unable to discard worn out or useless objects despite lack of sentimental value

3. **Prevalence.** This disorder is more common in men, although the prevalence is not known with certainty.

4. **Associated features.** People with this disorder have few friends. Hypochondriasis in later life may develop. Increased risk for myocardial infarction has been suggested for people with "type A" personality traits, which are similar to this disorder.

5. **Medical–surgical setting**
   a. Illness may be perceived by compulsive individuals as a threat to their control over impulses. Generally, stress increases compulsive behavior with an intensification of self-restraint and obstinacy. Patients become more inflexible than before, which may lead to complaints about the sloppiness of the hospital and imprecision of the care being given. When these patients are critical of failure to meet their standards, physicians should avoid defensive, authoritarian rebuttal. There is a fear of losing control of a situation on the part of these patients, and this may lead to a struggle for control with their physicians.
   b. Control should be shared with the patient in as many ways as possible. The patient should be allowed active participation in the decisions and details of his or her actual medical care. This may include charting medication times, carefully calculating caloric intake, and monitoring fluid intake and output.

6. **Treatment.** In general, individuals with compulsive personalities recognize that they have problems, unlike those with the other personality disorders. These patients know that they suffer from their inability to be flexible and realize that they do not permit themselves to have good feelings. Individual psychotherapy can be helpful, but treatment is difficult because these patients use the defense of isolation of affect. Group therapy may be more useful. Therapy should focus on current feelings and situations, and excessive time should not be spent on examining the psychological etiology of the condition. Struggles for control should be avoided. Depression, when present, should be treated.

D. Passive–aggressive personality disorder

1. **Definition** (*DSM-III-R*). Individuals with this disorder refuse to perform adequately at work or in social situations, but their refusal is indirect and passive. This social and occupational ineffectiveness is a hidden expression of aggression and anger.

2. **Symptoms.** Beginning in early adulthood, the individual with passive–aggressive personality disorder demonstrates at least five of the following:
   a. "Forgets" duties and obligations
   b. Makes unjustified protests that others are making unreasonable demands
   c. Makes mistakes or dawdles on jobs that he or she does not want to do
   d. Sulks or argues when asked to do something
   e. Procrastinates beyond deadlines
   f. Has an unrealistically positive assessment of own performance
   g. Resents any suggestion for improving performance
   h. Obstructs efforts of others by poor performance
   i. Resents and scorns authority figures

3. **Prevalence** is unknown.

4. **Associated features.** People with this disorder have poor self-esteem. Alcoholism and depression are seen.

5. **Medical–surgical setting**
   a. Some illnesses require patients to take an active role in the treatment. When this situation occurs with passive–aggressive patients, they tend to be noncompliant and develop new symptoms when discharge is pending. Staff reactions generally are anger

and frustration in dealing with these patients. This may be the first clue to the personality diagnosis.
   b. The physician should support the positive aspects of the behavior (e.g., encouraging the patient to walk rather than be pushed in a wheelchair). Early confrontation of the passive–aggressive behavior is preferable before angry feelings become too strong and the wish to punish the patient interferes with care. It is sometimes important for physicians to recognize that these patients cannot be cured and that it is not the physician's responsibility if the patient continues to smoke or abuse alcohol in the face of multiple warnings.

   6. **Treatment.** In general, supportive psychotherapy is indicated for those patients who seek therapy. The therapist should calmly confront the patient's behavior and its consequences. The goal is to help the patient see that his or her behavior causes certain reactions in the environment, which, in turn, cause pain in the patient.

VI. PERSONALITY DISORDERS UNDER EVALUATION.
Many clinicians believe that the following disorders exist, but in order for them to be properly studied and treated, they must first be diagnosed.

A. **Self-defeating personality disorder**

   1. **Definition.** Individuals with this disorder are repeatedly involved in relationships or situations that are self-defeating. They avoid or sabotage pleasurable experiences. This disorder has also been called masochistic personality disorder, but because masochism also refers to an outmoded theory of normal female sexual development, this term is no longer used. The diagnosis of self-defeating personality disorder should not be made if the behavior occurs in a setting of physical or psychological abuse, if the patient is depressed, or if the behavior is limited to sexual masochism.

   2. **Symptoms.** The individual with self-defeating personality disorder has a pervasive pattern of behavior, including at least five of the following:
      a. Chooses situations or people that inevitably lead to disappointment or mistreatment despite other choices
      b. Rejects attempts by others to help
      c. "Undoes" positive experiences by feeling depressed and guilty or by behavior (i.e., an accident)
      d. Provokes rejection from others and then feels bad
      e. Avoids pleasure or denies feeling good when enjoying himself or herself
      f. Fails to take care of tasks needed to accomplish personal objectives despite obvious abilities
      g. Not interested in relationships with people who are caring and concerned
      h. Martyrdom and excessive self-sacrifice, even when it is not requested by others

   3. **Prevalence.** The prevalence is unknown, but many clinicians believe it is common. Women are diagnosed twice as frequently as men.

   4. **Associated features.** Other personality disorders, such as dependent, borderline, and passive–aggressive personalities, are common. Children who have been abused physically, sexually, or psychologically are at risk for developing this disorder. Depression can be a complication.

   5. **Medical–surgical setting.** Patients with this disorder are uncomfortable with others caring for them and may covertly alienate the nursing staff. They are also likely to be noncompliant in cooperating with treatment.

   6. **Treatment**
      a. Individual psychotherapy that addresses the condition of impaired self-esteem is crucial. Cognitive therapy as well as psychodynamic therapy may be successful.
      b. Antidepressants may be indicated when there are features of depression.
      c. Self-help groups that focus on changing roles are also useful.

B. **Sadistic personality disorder**

   1. **Definition.** Individuals with this disorder are cruel, aggressive, and demeaning. When the purpose of the behavior is solely for sexual arousal or is only directed at one person (e.g., spouse or child), the diagnosis is not made. Individuals with sadistic personality lack empathy and respect for others.

2. **Symptoms.** The individual who is sadistic demonstrates repeated occurrences of at least four of the following:
   a. Dominates a relationship with cruelty or violence
   b. Humiliates and demeans others in public
   c. Treats others under his or her control unusually harshly (e.g., students, patients, or prisoners)
   d. Takes pleasure in the suffering of others, including animals
   e. Lies for the purpose of causing suffering or pain in others
   f. Intimidates others to do his or her bidding
   g. Limits autonomy of significant others (e.g., will not allow spouse to leave the house)
   h. Is fascinated by weapons, torture, or violence

3. **Prevalence.** In medical settings, this disorder is rare. In the military, it is less rare, and in prison populations, it is common. The disorder is far more common in men than in women.

4. **Associated features.** Other personality disorders, such as antisocial and narcissistic personalities, may be present. Spouse and child abuse are common. Substance use disorders are also common complications.

5. **Medical–surgical setting.** People with this disorder avoid medical institutions. They may try to threaten the staff, but generally, they leave against medical advice when anxious. Illness is a major threat to their ability to intimidate. They are generally noncompliant.

6. **Treatment.** As with antisocial personality disorder, individuals with sadistic personality disorder are difficult to treat. Often treatment is possible only when they are in an institutional setting, such as prison. If they can be engaged in psychotherapy, the central issue of cruelty in their lives must be addressed.

STUDY QUESTIONS

Directions: Each question below contains five suggested answers. Choose the **one best** response to each question.

1.   When individuals with personality disorders are unable to see their role in the disturbances in their lives, the symptoms that develop are considered

(A) self-induced
(B) ego-syntonic
(C) ego-dystonic
(D) internal
(E) characterologic

2.   The defense mechanism whereby an individual attributes to another individual thoughts or feelings of his or her own that are unacceptable is called

(A) fantasy
(B) splitting
(C) regression
(D) projection
(E) identification

3.   Somatization disorder is associated most commonly with

(A) paranoid personality
(B) histrionic personality
(C) narcissistic personality
(D) dependent personality
(E) passive–aggressive personality

4.   Chronic lateness, clowning around, and missed appointments are examples of

(A) splitting
(B) projection
(C) regression
(D) acting out
(E) passive aggression

5.   Factors thought to be involved in the etiology of an antisocial personality disorder include

(A) closed head injury
(B) encephalitis
(C) an alcoholic father
(D) loss of a parent
(E) low socioeconomic status

6.   In which disorder listed below do 90% of cases have another *DSM-III-R* diagnosis and 40% of cases have at least two other *DSM-III-R* diagnoses?

(A) Borderline personality
(B) Paranoid personality
(C) Antisocial personality
(D) Histrionic personality
(E) Schizotypal personality

7.   The term "hysterical" has been dropped as a diagnostic label because

(A) it has become too pejorative
(B) it refers only to women
(C) it has been replaced by the term "conversion"
(D) it refers to a neurosis not a personality
(E) it has become too nonspecific

8.   Which of the following disorders is thought by many to be strongly influenced by cultural roles?

(A) Avoidant personality
(B) Passive–aggressive personality
(C) Antisocial personality
(D) Dependent personality
(E) Borderline personality

Directions: Each question below contains four suggested answers of which **one or more** is correct. Choose the answer

    A   if **1, 2, and 3** are correct
    B   if **1 and 3** are correct
    C   if **2 and 4** are correct
    D   if **4** is correct
    E   if **1, 2, 3, and 4** are correct

9. Personality traits may become a personality disorder when they

(1) are inflexible
(2) are unstable
(3) cause impairment in social functioning
(4) do not involve a genetic predisposition

10. Patients with personality disorders may

(1) lose touch with reality transiently
(2) often be irritating and infuriating
(3) tolerate stress poorly
(4) elicit strong negative reactions in physicians

11. Individuals with one of the cluster A personality disorders tend to use defense mechanisms of projection and fantasy. These disorders include

(1) antisocial personality
(2) paranoid personality
(3) histrionic personality
(4) schizoid personality

12. The disorders often associated with the dramatic, emotional, and erratic group of personality disorders include

(1) schizophrenia
(2) mania
(3) alcoholism
(4) somatoform

13. When someone with borderline personality disorder is hospitalized with a medical illness the most common coping reactions (defense mechanisms) likely to be demonstrated include

(1) regression
(2) denial
(3) splitting
(4) isolation of affect

14. Individuals who have a tendency towards high levels of cortical arousal and motor inhibition when stressed are more likely to exhibit

(1) anxiety
(2) acting out
(3) hypochondriasis
(4) dissociation

15. The symptoms associated with cluster B personality disorders may

(1) cause stronger reactions in others than in the individual with the disorder
(2) be severe enough to be briefly psychotic
(3) interfere with all relationships
(4) actually improve work performance

16. Individuals with a paranoid personality disorder are likely to have which of the following traits?

(1) No sense of humor
(2) Acute awareness of power and rank
(3) Pride about being objective
(4) Excessive vanity and concern with appearance

17. When someone with a paranoid personality disorder requires medical treatment, the physician should

(1) avoid setting limits
(2) apologize quickly for mistakes
(3) have a sense of humor
(4) explain everything in detail

18. A 25-year-old man is admitted to the hospital wearing a long white robe and claiming to be a "prophet." He has been wandering the streets preaching about the end of the world. His speech is circumstantial, and he is very anxious. Likely diagnoses include

(1) antisocial personality disorder
(2) schizophrenia
(3) paranoid personality disorder
(4) schizotypal personality disorder

19. To make the diagnosis of antisocial personality disorder in adults, one should see evidence of a conduct disorder in childhood, the features of which include

(1) truancy
(2) initiating physical fights
(3) setting fires
(4) drug abuse

20. Behaviors seen in individuals with an antisocial personality disorder include

(1) significant unemployment
(2) taking pleasure in the suffering of others
(3) failure to arrange for a caretaker for the children when away
(4) fascination with weapons or torture

21. Medications found to be clinically useful in the management of borderline patients include

(1) Benzodiazepines
(2) Carbamazepine
(3) Lithium
(4) Tranylcypromine

22. When a person with an obsessive–compulsive personality disorder is hospitalized with a medical disorder, which of the following interventions may be helpful?

(1) Consistent reassurance of the patient that the staff cares
(2) Setting limits with the help of the nurses
(3) Use of low-dose neuroleptics
(4) Allowing the patient active participation in decisions

23. A patient with a self-defeating (masochistic) personality disorder who becomes ill and needs medical care is likely to

(1) be uncomfortable with others caring for him or her
(2) demand special treatment
(3) be noncompliant with treatment
(4) be suspicious and quarrelsome

Directions: The group of questions below consists of lettered choices followed by several numbered items. For each numbered item select the **one** lettered choice with which it is **most** closely associated. Each lettered choice may be used once, more than once, or not at all.

Questions 24–28

For each characteristic listed, select the personality disorder most apt to be associated with it.

(A) Paranoid personality disorder
(B) Borderline personality disorder
(C) Narcissistic personality disorder
(D) Antisocial personality disorder
(E) Schizoid personality disorder

24. Takes offense quickly and questions the loyalty of others

25. Has a defective capacity to form social relationships

26. Fails to plan ahead and is impulsive (e.g., may move without a job)

27. Forms relationships that lack empathy; idealizes or devalues others

28. Exudes a sense of entitlement with the expectation of special favors but without assuming reciprocal responsibilities

ANSWERS AND EXPLANATIONS

1. The answer is B. (*I B*) Patients with personality disorders perceive their problem and express their symptoms differently from patients with other psychiatric illnesses. Patients with personality disorders often feel that the disturbances in their lives are caused externally by the outside world (rather than internally), the symptoms of which are called ego-syntonic. Self-induced symptoms that are experienced as internally distressing are called ego-dystonic. Symptoms of a personality disorder are caused by the characterologic style of the patient. Symptoms include feelings of anxiety, depression, and anger, but these symptoms do not meet the criteria for a specific axis I psychiatric illness.

2. The answer is D. (*II A 1 a*) Projection is the defense mechanism whereby an individual attributes to another individual thoughts and feelings that are unacceptable. Fantasy is the creation of an imaginary life. Regression is a retreat to earlier defenses. Splitting is attributing only all good or all bad qualities to an individual, and identification is the unconscious assumption of aspects of another individual's personality.

3. The answer is B. (*II B 3*) Patients with histrionic personality disorder often have a concurrent somatization disorder. Patients with the other personality disorders in cluster B, the dramatic, emotional, and erratic group, may have a number of concurrent problems, but not necessarily somatization disorder. All of the patients with cluster B disorders can be difficult when they become ill, however. Patients with dependent or passive–aggressive personalities may have hypochondriasis, which is a different phenomenon than somatization disorder.

4. The answer is E. (*II C 1 b*) Passive–aggressive behavior is indirect resistance to demands made for social or occupational effectiveness. Examples include failing examinations, clownish conduct, missing appointments, and chronic lateness. This behavior can be distinguished from acting out, the actual motor expression of a thought or feeling, which tends to be actively aggressive. Splitting occurs when patients divide individuals into all good or all bad. Projection is the attribution of one's thoughts and feelings (that are unacceptable) to others, and regression is a retreat to an earlier developmental stage.

5. The answer is C. (*IV A 4*) While the etiology of antisocial disorder is not clear, it is thought that one powerful predictor is a sociopathic or alcoholic father. Antisocial behavior has been associated with closed head injury and encephalitis; however, the proper diagnosis for these behaviors is an organic personality syndrome. Loss of a parent has not been associated with the development of antisocial personality, but inconsistent and compulsive parenting has. While antisocial personality is associated with low socioeconomic status, this is not thought to be a causative but rather the result of this kind of behavior.

6. The answer is A. (*IV B 3*) It is common for individuals with borderline personality disorder to meet the criteria for other *DSM-III-R* diagnoses. In fact, 90% of cases have one other *DSM-III-R* diagnosis, and 40% of cases have at least two other *DSM-III-R* diagnoses. This may be due to the instability of mood and identity that characterizes these patients. The other personality disorders listed in the question—paranoid, antisocial, histrionic, and schizotypal personalities—are not associated to such a striking degree with the presence of other diagnoses.

7. The answer is E. (*IV D 1*) Hysterical is a term that has many meanings in psychiatry and, thus, has lost its usefulness because of this nonspecificity. It has also been used pejoratively when applied to women. Conversion reactions were once called hysterical conversion reactions, referring to both neurosis and a personality disorder. However, it too was dropped because of the lack of specificity.

8. The answer is D. (*V B 1*) Some researchers in psychiatry feel that dependent personality disorder depends to a large extent on cultural roles (i.e., certain individuals or groups are expected to assume dependent roles in the culture based on the gender or ethnic background). To some extent, this may be changing, but it can still be observed.

9. The answer is B (1, 3). (*I A*) When a stable pattern of response leads to problems in functioning, a personality disorder may be present. Alternatively, when personality traits become inflexible and maladaptive, causing either significant impairment in social or occupational functioning or subjective distress, then a personality disorder may be present. Some personality disorders appear to involve genetic factors.

10. The answer is E (all). (*I C 1–4*) Symptoms of personality disorders almost always effect other individuals. Occasionally, the symptoms can be so severe that the patient appears to lose touch with reality transiently and is unable to function for a brief period of time. Individuals with personality disorders are usually irritating and infuriating to others and can elicit strong negative reactions in the physicians who care for them. Because these patients tolerate stress poorly when ill, they tend to regress and become more symptomatic.

11. The answer is C (2, 4). (*II A*) The cluster A personality disorders include paranoid, schizoid, and schizotypal personality disorders. Individuals with these disorders use defense mechanisms of projection and fantasy and tend toward psychotic thinking. Individuals with antisocial and histrionic personality disorders tend to use the defense mechanisms of dissociation, denial, splitting, and acting out.

12. The answer is D (4). (*II B*) Somatoform disorder, which is characterized by a preoccupation with pain in the absence of any clinical findings, is often associated with the histrionic personality disorder, one of the disorders in the dramatic, emotional, and erratic group (cluster B). Additionally, mood disorders, particularly depression, are common in this cluster and, indeed, may be the chief complaint. Mania and schizophrenia are not common in this group of patients. Alcoholism is seen in all personality disorders but is not particularly associated with this group.

13. The answer is A (1, 2, 3). [*II B 1; IV B 5, 6 a (1)*] When individuals with a borderline personality disorder become ill, stress is increased, and they are likely to demonstrate exacerbations of their defense mechanisms. The most prominent defenses are regression and splitting. Denial is also seen in this kind of personality disorder. Intensification, not isolation, of affect, is likely to be seen.

14. The answer is B (1, 3). (*II B 1 d, C 1 c*) Individuals who have high levels of cortical arousal and increased motor inhibition when stressed are likely to exhibit anxiety and hypochondriasis as a result. Patients with low cortical arousal and decreased motor inhibition are likely to act out and also exhibit dissociation.

15. The answer is A (1, 2, 3). (*II B 1–3; IV A–D*) Cluster B personality disorders interfere with both work and social relationships. They often cause strong reactions in those around them. Occasionally, they are severe enough to cause a transient psychosis when the person is under great stress. They clearly interfere with all relationships.

16. The answer is A (1, 2, 3). (*III B 2*) Individuals with a paranoid disorder tend to have a pervasive and unwarranted suspicion and mistrust of others. This is associated with a lack of a sense of humor, being very aware of power and rank, particularly in others, and a sense of pride in themselves for being rational and objective. Vanity and concern with appearance are seen in narcissistic and histrionic personality disorders.

17. The answer is C (2, 4). (*III B 4*) Illness tends to exacerbate the personality traits of paranoid personalities. They become even more guarded and suspicious. If the patient becomes agitated or threatening, limits must be set. It is not usually helpful to use humor with these patients since they lack an ability to appreciate humor. Physicians should always apologize immediately for any untoward events. It is important to explain everything in a straightforward and detailed way.

18. The answer is C (2, 4). (*III C 1, 2*) Patients who are strange or odd in appearance, behavior, and thinking, but who are not schizophrenic, often have schizotypal personalities. However, schizophrenia has not been ruled out in the patient described in the question. Patients with an antisocial personality disorder or a paranoid personality disorder rarely exhibit strange or odd behavior.

19. The answer is A (1, 2, 3). (*IV A 2*) Features of a conduct disorder in childhood are associated with an antisocial personality disorder diagnosis in adulthood; these do not necessarily include drug abuse. Substance abuse may be a primary diagnosis that leads to problems in behavior, but it should be considered a separate diagnosis. Truancy, initiating physical fights, and setting fires are all symptoms of a conduct disorder.

20. The answer is B (1, 3). (*IV A 2 b*) Individuals with an antisocial personality disorder do not particularly care about the feelings of others. They have a long history of frequent job changes, serious absenteeism, or walking off the job, leading to significant unemployment. They also make poor parents, which is manifested in their children by a lack of adequate nutrition, poor hygiene, lack of medical care as well as failure to arrange for caretakers when they are away from their children. People with sadistic personality disorder take pleasure in the suffering of others. They are also fascinated by weapons and torture. These features are not features of antisocial personality disorder.

Tegretol , Parnate

21. The answer is C (2, 4). (*IV B 6 b*) Medications that are useful in the treatment of borderline personality disorder include carbamazepine and tranylcypromine, one of the monoamine oxidase inhibitors. Tranylcypromine appears to improve the patient's mood without effecting changes in behavior. Carbamazepine appears to improve some of the symptoms of behavioral dyscontrol. Lithium has not been effective in the treatment of borderline patients, and benzodiazepines can often make symptoms worse.

22. The answer is D (4). (*V C 5*) Patients with obsessive–compulsive personality disorders, when ill, generally tend to intensify their symptoms of obstinacy and a need for control. This sometimes can lead to a struggle with the physician about who is in charge. It is useful to allow the patient as much active participation in the decisions and details of his or her medical care as possible. Reassuring the patient that the staff cares is generally not helpful; it is more useful with dependent patients. Setting limits is a generally useful technique but is rarely needed with obsessive–compulsive patients. Neuroleptics are also not indicated for this kind of personality disorder.

23. The answer is B (1, 3). (*VI A 5*) Patients with self-defeating personality disorder tend to be martyrs and self-sacrificing. They find it difficult to allow others to care for them. They also tend to covertly sabotage treatment, often by being noncompliant. They rarely demand special treatment and are not likely to become suspicious or quarrelsome, which is more typical of a paranoid patient.

24–28. The answers are: 24-A, 25-E, 26-D, 27-C, 28-C. (*III A 1, B 1, 2; IV A 2, B 1, C 2*) Individuals with paranoid personality disorder exhibit a pervasive and unwarranted suspicion and mistrust of others. They are usually hypersensitive and unable to deal with feelings. They may take offense quickly and question the loyalty of others.

Schizoid individuals have defects in their ability to form social relationships. They have few close friends, maybe only one or two, including family members. Individuals are characterized by emotional coldness and aloofness, lacking warm, tender feelings. They are indifferent to praise, criticism, and the feelings of others.

Individuals with antisocial personality disorder have a history of continuous and chronic antisocial behavior that has violated the rights of others. Individuals appear to be unable to control their impulses and postpone immediate gratification. Problem behavior begins in adolescence. A failure to plan ahead, such as moving without a clear goal or prearranged job, or honor financial obligations, are characteristic.

Individuals with narcissistic personality disorder have a grandiose sense of their own importance. They have little ability to empathize with others and appear to be more concerned with appearance than substance. Individuals are likely to overidealize as well as devalue others. Narcissistic individuals tend to exude a sense of entitlement and expect to be acknowledged as special.

12

Psychiatric Emergencies

James H. Scully

I. OVERVIEW. A **psychiatric emergency** or crisis **is a stress-induced pathologic response** that physically endangers the affected individual or others or that significantly disrupts the functional equilibrium of the individual or his or her environment. The pathologic response may manifest as an acute alteration in the individual's thought, mood, or behavior. Either the individual, the environment, or both may experience or react to the situation as emergent.

A. Evolution of a crisis

1. **Stressors** from any source present an individual with a situation or problem to resolve; however, in a crisis the usual **coping mechanisms** of the individual are insufficient and are overwhelmed.

2. **Increased anxiety and disorganization** may follow, which can further impair the individual's functional integrity and problem-solving capacity.

3. **Failure of adaptation** may result in an increasing sense of helplessness, accompanied by panic, depression, or both and then in further disorganization.

4. **Impulsive, maladaptive, and even desperate attempts by the individual to regain any equilibrium** are likely in this spiraling situation. The new equilibrium may reorganize the individual and reduce dysphoria but still be maladaptive in the limitations in function of the individual or disruption of the environment required to maintain it. For example, an individual may diminish the anxiety and reduce the nightmares following a traumatic event by using alcohol but eventually may develop medical, social, and occupational complications from excessive use.

5. **A request for help** may occur at any time during this cycle, depending on the individual's response to the crisis and the current social context. An individual with any psychiatric diagnosis or an individual without any preexisting psychopathology can present with a psychiatric emergency. A diagnosis of a major mental disorder may be the result of an individual's maladaptive responses.

B. Components of stress-induced responses. There is a dynamic interplay among the stressor, the affected individual, and the social matrix that influences the response of the individual. It is the severity of the psychopathologic response that creates a psychiatric emergency out of a particular crisis.

1. **Stressors** always depend on the interplay of individual and social factors, but they may be considered predominantly either internal or external.
   a. **Internal stress** results when a person faces a normal developmental task for which he or she is ill-equipped or ill-prepared. A seemingly minor environmental event may have massive personal psychological meaning for the individual, causing that individual to experience a disruptive increase in needs, a loss, or a conflict. Examples include an anxious adolescent who becomes disorganized upon leaving his or her family for college or an aging, lonely woman who becomes suicidal following the death of her cat.
   b. **External stress** results from a life event that is readily recognized as a source of stress, such as the death of a family member, a divorce, or a major illness. (A major illness may be an endogenous psychiatric illness, such as mania; this can be an external stressor.)

2. **Affected individuals** are crucial determinants of whether the stress is major or minor and whether the response is adaptive or maladaptive.
   a. Healthy individuals may resolve the crisis in an adaptive, growth-promoting fashion.

b. Healthy individuals may become so overwhelmed by massive trauma as to manage only a pathologic adaptation, which leaves them more vulnerable to future stress.

c. Individuals with significant psychopathology may decompensate with even minor environmental stress.

3. Social matrix. Each individual varies in his or her need for external support and structure and in his or her capacity to accept them. Both the type of stress and kind of response influence the amount of environmental support that can be recruited.

a. Individuals may have multiple supportive resources that facilitate an adaptive resolution to the crisis.

b. Individuals may have several reliable sources of support that are insufficient in the face of severe stress.

c. Individuals may have a few supports that are easily overwhelmed and withdrawn or are even actively intolerant of their attempts at reconstitution. Rather than being a source of support, the external environment becomes another source of stress.

II. PRINCIPLES OF EVALUATION

A. Immediate assessment of the condition and the dangerousness of the patient's behavior is essential. Such an assessment can be made on the basis of the following:

1. Patient's behavior. Loud, agitated, angry, and threatening behavior requires limit-setting and control before further evaluation.

2. Arrival in the emergency department. A patient who is brought in handcuffed or otherwise restrained requires cautious assessment despite calm or withdrawn behavior. The patient may be calm as a result of external control, and withdrawing this control prematurely may result in an escalation of the agitated behavior.

3. Reports on behavior. Reports of dangerousness from family members and others must be investigated even though there may be inconsistencies in the patient's history or behavior.

B. Thorough evaluation. Secure surroundings that provide safety and comfort for both the evaluator and patient should be available for a more extensive evaluation. The first three steps listed below should be routine. The remaining three may not be immediately necessary with a cooperative patient. However, if indicated by the history or by an escalation of the patient's behavior, the remaining steps should be initiated before the evaluation can proceed safely.

1. The physical setting should be quiet, open, and sparsely furnished. There should be a minimum of objects that could be used as weapons. The interviewer and the patient should have an unobstructed exit from the room. A call button to summon immediate help must be easily accessible to the interviewer.

2. Trained help who provide a show of force and can subdue an agitated patient should be readily available. It may be necessary to have help in or just outside of the interview room.

3. Mental status examination. The physician should observe the patient's appearance, manner, and behavior during the evaluation (see Chapter 1).

4. A search for weapons may be indicated by the history or the patient's behavior before further evaluation takes place.

5. Verbal and nonverbal expressions of expectation of the patient to control him- or herself and to be responsible for his or her behavior may help the patient cooperate with the task at hand. The patient may need to be reminded that external control is also available.

6. Physical restraint in the form of 2- or 4-point leather restraints is indicated if the patient cannot respond to verbal limit-setting and reassurance. The need for safety for all concerned must supersede the patient's requests, but the clinician must recognize the restrained patient's vulnerability and helplessness and treat him or her with respect and compassion.

a. If the patient arrives in restraints or handcuffs, adequate evaluation must take place before any change in status is permitted.

b. If an unrestrained patient cannot be controlled, he or she should be placed in leather restraints until the evaluation is completed. A patient should not be restrained supine but on the side or with the head elevated to prevent aspiration if vomiting occurs. In addition, a patient in restraints requires constant monitoring.

C. Identification of a crisis situation

    1. Overt. Evidence of a crisis may be immediately apparent from the patient's behavior or the circumstances surrounding his or her arrival in the emergency department.

    2. Covert. The patient may be quite calm and superficially cooperative; he or she may present with relatively minor somatic complaints and deny any serious emotional disturbances. Nevertheless, the patient may be potentially lethal to him- or herself or others. Empathic, detailed history-taking with a high level of suspicion often reveals the true nature of the emergency. The following factors should raise the index of suspicion:

        a. Risk factors. Certain historic data and mental status findings increase the probability of particular emergencies occurring and should serve as red flags to guide assessment.

        b. Vague, evasive, and qualified answers to questions in crucial areas, such as suicide, homicide, and impulse control, must be vigorously pursued. A patient's attempt to minimize or ignore the consequences of observed or reported behavior should not be accepted without investigation. Discrepancies between the patient's history and the reports of others must be explored, which may involve meeting alone with the other parties to ascertain their true concerns.

        c. Feelings of unease or discomfort on the part of the physician should be examined. An intuitive, experienced physician may read between the lines of a patient's communication, detect subtle discrepancies between affect and content, and accurately uncover a latent but emergent situation.

D. Chief complaint and present illness

    1. Patient. Rapport is facilitated by allowing the patient to tell his or her own story as much as possible. The examiner should elicit relevant information by using the following questions:

        a. What are the symptoms or problems that led the patient to seek help?

        b. Why is the patient requesting help now?

        c. Why are these symptoms a problem at this particular time?

        d. What are the individual's normal coping mechanisms in times of stress?

        e. What is his or her level of functioning in general?

        f. How did he or she cope previously with similar stresses?

        g. What attempts is he or she presently making to resolve the problem?

    2. Others. Family members, friends, employers, and co-workers may be able to answer many of these questions if the patient will not or cannot answer them accurately. Different individuals may accurately describe a particular aspect of the patient's situation or level of function; the physician must then compose an integrated picture.

E. Patient history. The more detailed the history available, the more complete is the picture of the patient. In a crisis situation, detailed history-taking may not be feasible; however, the following areas must be explored in all patients.

    1. Previous psychiatric illnesses. The symptoms, circumstances, treatment, and response to treatment of previous illnesses should be outlined.

    2. Dangerous behavior. Previous episodes of self-destructive or assaultive behavior must be carefully explored as they have significant predictive value.

    3. Medical history

        a. Significant medical illnesses may have direct bearing on the current crisis, may color the presentation, or may produce chronic vulnerability to stress.

        b. Drugs. Prescribed medication, alcohol, and illicit drugs can profoundly affect thinking, feeling, and behavior. They may cause the crisis or significantly impair the patient's adaptive capacity.

F. Physical examination should be thorough with particular attention paid to evidence of drug intoxication, withdrawal symptoms, and acute and chronic neurologic disease.

G. Laboratory tests should be guided by other findings and by the differential diagnosis. Blood and urine tests for toxic agents may be particularly helpful in the emergency setting.

III. SUICIDE

A. Epidemiology (Table 12-1)

Table 12-1. Risk Factors for Suicide

Male
Caucasian
Divorced, widowed, or separated
Older age
Poor health in past 6 months
Loss of job
Presence of depression, schizophrenia, or organic brain
    disease
History of a suicide attempt

1. **Rate.** The annual suicide rate for the general population in the United States has remained relatively constant over the years at 11–13/100,000 population.
   a. In 1985, approximately 285,000 deaths by suicide were reported in the United States. There were 8–10 times as many suicide attempts.
   b. Suicide is the eighth overall cause of death in the United States.
   c. Suicide is underreported in part because of the stigma attached to it and because deaths from self-destructive behavior, such as accidents (particularly drunk driving), alcoholism, and medical noncompliance, are not counted as suicide deaths.

2. **Age.** In general, suicide rates increase with age; however, recent trends show a slight decline in suicide rates in the elderly and a rise in suicide rates in the young.
   a. Suicide rates for men peak around age 45 then continue to rise slowly. Suicide rates for men over 75 are twice that for men aged 45–54. Although elderly people make up 10% of the population, they account for 25% of all suicides. In women, suicide rates peak after age 55.
   b. While the overall rates for suicide have been stable, there have been dramatic changes in the suicide rates for young people.
      (1) In 1960, the suicide rate for 15–24-year-olds was 5.2/100,000 population, but by 1984, the suicide rate was 12.5/100,000.
      (2) The rates are highest in young white males followed by young nonwhite males and then young white females.
      (3) Suicide among children 5–14 years of age, although still uncommon (0.7/100,000), has also doubled in recent decades.
      (4) Death by violent means (e.g., suicide, homicide, or accidents) accounts for over 75% of all deaths for individuals 15–24 years of age.

3. **Sex**
   a. Men *commit* suicide three times more often than women, and suicide is the seventh leading cause of death in men of all ages. Men are also more likely to use firearms than women.
   b. Women *attempt* suicide four times more often than men, and suicide is the eleventh leading cause of death in women overall. Women are also more likely to ingest drugs than men.

4. **Marital status**
   a. Married individuals with children have the lowest suicide rates.
   b. Individuals who have never married have almost double the suicide rates of married individuals (22/100,000).
   c. The highest suicide rates occur in previously married (especially divorced) men at 69/100,000 as compared to divorced women at 18/100,000.

5. **Physical health**
   a. As many as 70% of individuals who commit suicide have some active, usually chronic, illness.
   b. Approximately 50% of patients who die by suicide have sought medical help within 1 month or less of their deaths, and 80% have seen their physicians within 6 months of their deaths.
   c. Illnesses that cause loss of mobility, disfigurement, or chronic pain are associated with an increased suicide risk. Renal dialysis patients, for example, are at particular risk.

6. **Mental health.** Almost no one commits suicide who does not have a psychiatric disorder. Depression, alcoholism, and schizophrenia are the most common diagnoses.
   a. **Depression** is present in over 50% of suicide victims. Patients with delusional depressions are at the highest risk. For example, men who have suffered a severe impairment due

to depression are 500 times more likely to kill themselves than men who have no psychiatric illnesses.
   b. **Alcoholism** is present in 25% of suicide victims.
   c. **Schizophrenia** is present in 10% of suicide victims. It is not clear whether these patients are also depressed; they may not be.
   d. **Delirium and dementia** account for about 5% of suicide victims.

7. **Occupation.** In general, suicide rates are higher among professionals in high-stress jobs, such as physicians, lawyers, dentists, and policemen. Among physicians, specialities particularly at risk change with each study, but, in general, the risks are about the same. Female physicians have suicide rates as high as or higher than male physicians.

B. Common presentations

1. **Overt**
   a. **Suicidal behavior.** The patient may have ingested drugs or attempted suicide by wrist-slashing, shooting, jumping, or other means that result in injury. Thus, the patient often requires medical or surgical intervention (e.g., gastric lavage or suturing) before a psychiatric assessment can be completed. The patient should be considered acutely suicidal until proven otherwise. Close observation is required to prevent another attempt or to prevent the patient from leaving the emergency department.
   b. **Suicidal ideation.** The patient may be obviously depressed, revealing concerns with little prompting, and in considerable pain and distress. He or she may ask for help in controlling the suicidal impulses and for relief from depression.

2. **Covert**
   a. **Suicidal behavior.** Although the patient may minimize or deny the implications of his or her behavior, he or she may have "accidents," which range from suspiciously to obviously suicidal. The patient who is unconscious of his or her self-destructive impulses is no less dangerous because the suicidal intent may be missed or ignored. A similar kind of patient is one who appears homicidal or assaultive but whose behavior is primarily an attempt to provoke others, such as the police, to kill him or her.
   b. **Suicidal ideation.** The patient may present for medical evaluation of minor or severe somatic complaints. He or she may appear depressed or may disguise the distress. Empathic questioning may reveal the patient's feelings. The patient may show distress out of proportion to objective findings or may make a series of visits to the emergency department over a short period of time. Although hoping to find help, he or she may take the medication given for somatic complaints in a suicide attempt.

3. **Chronic suicidal ideation and behavior.** The patient repeatedly calls or presents to the emergency room with suicidal ideation and attempts. Self-destructive behavior may be a means by which to manipulate the environment or to relieve internal discomfort rather than a means by which to die. These patients evoke tremendous frustration and hostility in caregivers and are at great risk to be ignored or actively rejected. Because they are also at great risk to kill themselves ultimately by design, miscalculation, or impulsiveness, careful evaluation is required.

C. Biologic factors. While most research on suicide has focused on epidemiology and social or psychological correlates in recent years, biologic studies, particularly of the biogenic amines, has been undertaken.

1. **Biogenic amines**
   a. Studies of brains of suicide victims have revealed low levels of 5-hydroxyindoleacetic acid (5-HIAA) and serotonin.
      (1) Low levels of 5-HIAA have also been found in the cerebrospinal fluid of a group of depressed patients who attempted suicide but survived.
      (2) One study reported that patients with low levels of 5-HIAA who attempted suicide were 10 times more likely to commit suicide than individuals with high 5-HIAA levels.
      (3) Lower levels of 5-HIAA and serotonin were found in suicide victims who used violent methods (e.g., guns) than those who did not use violent methods.
   b. Monoamine oxidase activity in both the brain and platelets also appears to be diminished in suicidal patients.

2. **Genetics.** Most studies of families have involved mood disorders where suicide is a factor rather than studies of suicide alone.
   a. In one study of twins, the only suicides that occurred were in monozygotic pairs. There were no suicides among dizygotic twins.

    b. Family studies of an Amish community also found increased suicide rates in families with heavy genetic loading for unipolar, bipolar, and other mood disorders.

D. Assessment of lethality (suicide risk)

    1. Episodic suicidal ideation and behavior. Suicidal behavior may remit and relapse both in response to the patient's changing internal emotional and cognitive states and his or her environment. Either the patient, the environment, or both may require intervention to protect the patient.

    2. Ambivalence of the suicidal patient. The balance between the patient's wish to live and wish to die must be evaluated, including the factors that tip the balance one way or the other. Prior warning is given in 8 of 10 eventual suicides.

    3. Risk factors (predictors). The patient's ambivalence and the episodic nature of suicidal behavior allow for identification and prevention in many cases. The following predictors may aid the physician in determining both who is at risk and to what extent.

        a. Demographic indicators. Unemployed, divorced, Caucasian men over the age of 45 years are at particularly high risk. Any of these factors, occurring singly or in combination, should alert the physician to investigate. [Younger men are also at high risk (see section III A 2).]

        b. Historic indicators. A recent loss, real or symbolic, or a change in the status of the affected individual may precipitate a crisis with feelings of anxiety and depression.

           (1) Present illness. Reports of hopelessness, helplessness, loneliness, and exhaustion are worrisome. An unexpected change in behavior, such as giving away possessions, or an unexpected change in attitude, such as calm or resignation in the midst of a distressing situation, must be investigated. Overt or indirect talk of death must be followed up with specific questions about fantasies, wishes, plans, and means. In the case of an unsuccessful suicide attempt, the following additional issues are important:

                (a) The patient's perception of the lethality of the attempt, his or her expectations of rescue, and his or her relief or disappointment at being alive are often more important than the objective dangerousness of the attempt, particularly in cases of apparent minimal danger.

                (b) The extent to which the precipitating crisis is resolved or is being resolved may influence the patient's wish to remain alive and his or her attitude towards the future.

           (2) History of suicide attempts increases the risk of suicide, particularly if the attempts have been multiple. The circumstances and lethality of the previous attempts should be determined.

           (3) Medical history. A history of chronic illness or an acute change in physical health increases the risk of suicide.

           (4) Family history. A family history of suicide is important both in terms of the patient's identification with the individual who died and the possibility of inheritance of an affective disorder. The anniversary date of the death or the patient reaching the same age of the person who died may be particularly stressful times.

        c. Diagnostic indicators include conditions of depression, thought disorder, and impairment of impulse control, especially secondary to alcohol or drug abuse.

        d. Present mental status. The physician should assess the severity of depression, the presence of psychosis (especially command hallucinations), and any problems of impulse control. In addition, the physician should be aware of the patient's response to the interview. Does the patient feel understood, experience some relief, and express more hopefulness, or does the patient remain angry, pessimistic, and desperate?

        e. Resources. The availability and support of family and friends are crucial; it is essential to get their perceptions of the patient's lethality. They may need to be interviewed away from the patient to feel comfortable revealing their concerns. Additionally, in planning for disposition and treatment, the physician must be sure of their support and willingness to assume some responsibility for the patient. In particular, the physician must ascertain that there is no collusion with or covert encouragement of the patient's suicidal behavior.

E. Countertransference reactions to suicidal patients. Countertransference refers to the emotional reactions that the physician has to the patient; these reactions may be unconscious or only dimly conscious. They may have a powerful influence on the physician's attitude towards the patient, his or her approach to the patient, and even his or her clinical judgment.

    1. The physician has his or her own particular attitudes towards suicide and death, his or her own set of personal and clinical experiences in these matters, and conflicts about his or her own aggressive or self-destructive impulses. Unless the physician is aware of these reactions, he or she may minimize or distort clinical data from the patient to fit personal feelings or beliefs. The physician may fear being overwhelmed or at loss if the patient admits to suicidal ideation. He or she may even fear (wrongly) that he or she will influence the patient to commit suicide by talking about it.

2. **The patient**, depending on his or her behavior, evokes varying degrees of frustration, anger, and helplessness in most caregivers. At times the patient evokes so much hostility that the physician wishes that the patient were dead. Such a reaction is extremely serious because it is likely that others in the patient's environment feel similarly.

F. Principles of emergency treatment

1. The patient must be protected.

2. A psychiatric consultation is necessary if there is any question about the patient's lethality.

3. Treatment options include the following:
   a. **Hospitalization.** A patient should be hospitalized if the lethality of his or her ideation or behavior is high. Lethality might be high because of the persistence of the patient's wish to die, the severity of his or her concurrent psychopathology, or the absence of reliable supports in the patient's social environment.
      (1) A patient can be hospitalized voluntarily if he or she concurs with the need for inpatient treatment.
      (2) A suicidal patient can also be hospitalized involuntarily on a mental health hold if voluntary hospitalization is refused. (The length of time that a patient can be held initially for treatment varies from state to state but is often in the range of 72 hours.) A severely suicidal patient who resists treatment may require one-to-one observation to prevent escape or self-injury.
   b. **Outpatient treatment** is less restrictive than hospitalization and is indicated when there is some crisis resolution, mild concurrent psychopathology, mobilization of environmental resources, and a therapeutic response to the interview. It usually involves a follow-up appointment within 48 hours and intensive crisis treatment thereafter. Somatic treatment can be started on an outpatient basis, but only limited quantities of medication should be dispensed because of the potential for overdose.

IV. THE VIOLENT PATIENT

A. Etiology of violence. Violent behavior is a result of the interplay between innate psychobiologic factors and the external environment.

1. **Biologic factors**
   a. **Neurotransmitters.** Serotonin metabolism appears to be involved in violent behavior in the same way it is involved in suicidal behavior, that is, lower levels of 5-HIAA have been found in the cerebrospinal fluid of offenders who killed with unusual cruelty than in the cerebrospinal fluid of nonviolent offenders.
   b. **Limbic-system.** The role of partial complex seizures and violence remains controversial; however, there appears to be no overall difference in the levels of violent behavior between patients with epilepsy and those without.
   c. **Chromosomal abnormalities.** Sex chromosome abnormalities, particularly XYY, were thought to influence criminal behavior because there was an increased number of men with that abnormality in prison. However, recent studies do not support this hypothesis. Low intelligence is more likely to be linked to arrests for violence than a chromosomal abnormality.
   d. **Endocrine abnormalities**
      (1) Since such a high percentage of violence is committed by men, there has long been speculation that androgens may be involved; however, no studies have been able to demonstrate this connection. With the exception of pedophilic behavior, anti-androgen treatment has not been effective in decreasing violence.
      (2) Premenstrual syndrome has also been implicated in aggressive behavior in women and has even been used as a legal defense for violence, but scientific evidence of a causal link is lacking.
   e. **Alcohol and drugs.** Alcohol decreases impulse control and inhibition and impairs judgment. There is a clear association between alcohol intoxication and violent behavior. Other drugs that have a simliar effect on the brain and behavior include amphetamines, cocaine, phencyclidine, and sedative-hypnotics. The aggressive and

criminal behavior associated with obtaining these and other illegal drugs also is an indirect cause of violent behavior.

2. **Psychosocial factors**
   a. **Developmental.** A history of being a victim of child abuse is now well known to be associated with becoming an abusive adult. Witnessing abuse is also associated with increased violent behavior. Spouse abuse and family violence, even if not directed at the child, can influence later behavior.
   b. **Guns.** Perhaps 80 million handguns are owned by Americans. The number of deaths due to firearms continues to rise, especially over the past 25 years. It is crucial for the physician to be aware of the presence of firearms in the home of any patient being evaluated for violent behavior.
   c. **Environment**
      (1) Crowding appears to be a factor in the increased potential for violence.
      (2) Weather also has an effect on violence. Increased ambient temperature to the point of discomfort may produce increased aggression; however, if it becomes very hot, aggressive behavior diminishes.
   d. **Socioeconomic factors.** Studies of race and violence have led to contradictory and controversial findings.
      (1) Nonwhite populations experience higher rates of violence, both as victims and aggressors, than white populations.
      (2) The best studies show that race and economic inequality are not related to homicide but that **absolute poverty and marital disruption** are related to violence in these groups. It appears that the socioeconomic factors that disrupt the family structure increase the risk of aggression and violence in the children of these families.

B. **Differential diagnosis.** While any patient is potentially dangerous, there are certain diagnoses that are more likely to be associated with violence. Furthermore, an accurate diagnosis enables the institution of specific treatment measures.

1. **Psychotic disorders**
   a. **Bipolar disorder–manic type.** Manic patients are often irritable and angry rather than amusing. They are pressured and hyperactive and may become aggressive if their grandiose, unrealistic plans are blocked. Their behavior may also be disorganized and unintentionally violent.
   b. **Schizophrenic disorders.** These psychotic disorders may be accompanied by considerable panic and agitation as well as deficient reality testing and impulse control. Although infrequently seen now, a state of catatonic excitement may occur during which the patient may be extremely dangerous. More commonly seen are patients with paranoid schizophrenia, who are extremely hostile and fearful of attack and who may act aggressively to defend themselves. Schizophrenic patients may experience command hallucinations, ordering them to hurt others.
   c. **Paranoid disorders.** Patients with these disorders generally present with stable, well-developed delusions but with better reality testing and impulse control than do those with schizophrenia. However, the overly controlled and often denied hostility may break through as murderous rage if the individual feels particularly threatened or experiences diminished impulse control.

2. **Nonpsychotic disorders**
   a. **Intermittent explosive disorder.** People with this disorder, usually men, episodically lose control and commit serious assaults or destruction of property. Their behavior is grossly out of proportion to any precipitating psychological stressors. While they may have genuine remorse about their actions afterwards, many of these people end up in jails or mental hospitals. A family history of violence is common.
   b. **Post-traumatic stress disorder.** In trauma victims who have committed acts of violence, such as combat veterans, there is often a fear of loss of control. Explosions of aggressive behavior may be unpredictable. They may be associated with the experience of flashbacks, which are triggered by something in the environment. Drugs and alcohol can complicate the situation, especially when there are chronic feelings of rage and frustration.
   c. **Personality disorders**
      (1) **Borderline patients** have difficulty in regulating mood and behavior. Impulsive behavior, including violence as well as sexual promiscuity, suicide gestures, and difficult and intense interpersonal relationships are seen.
      (2) **Antisocial personalities** exhibit not only outbursts of violence but also pervasive

antisocial behavior, such as lying, stealing, and reckless behavior that may endanger others.

(3) **Paranoid personalities** are easy to insult and are quick to react to any imagined or real insult. When two people with paranoid personality disorders are placed together, violence can easily result. Substance abuse makes people with any sort of personality disorder more likely to act out.

3. Organic mental disorders

   a. Substance abuse. Alcohol intoxication is probably the most common precipitating cause of violent behavior in our culture. Other drugs that are associated with violence include sedative-hypnotics, such as barbiturates and benzodiazepines, and stimulants, such as cocaine, amphetamines, and phencyclidine (PCP), glue sniffing, and even steroids. The physician should check for dysarthria, nystagmus, unsteady gait, and tremors. Patients with PCP intoxication are particularly likely to present with confusion, disorientation, rage, and violent behavior.

   b. Central nervous system disorders. Traumatic injuries to the brain, including birth injury, have been associated with violent behavior. Postconcussion syndrome, which can be caused by apparently minor head injury, involves increased irritability and impulsive behavior. Any other organic mental disorder, including infections, degenerative processes, or poisons, can affect behavior.

   c. Partial complex seizures. Temporal lobe epilepsy has long been thought a cause of violence, although violence during a seizure is rare. Increased violent behavior between seizures is a controversial issue. If there are poorly directed episodes of violence with a repetitive pattern, whether or not they are associated with other seizure activity, then the patient should receive an electroencephalogram with nasopharyngeal leads.

   d. Adult attention-deficit disorder. Some adults continue to have symptoms of attention-deficit disorder after childhood. These symptoms include hyperactivity, poor concentration, easy frustration, and poor impulse control. Methylphenidate may be an effective treatment for these individuals.

C. Assessment of dangerousness. Although making a clinical diagnosis is important, it is only one factor that goes into an overall assessment of imminent and ongoing dangerousness. Future violent behavior is extremely difficult to predict, but consideration of the following issues is helpful.

1. Episodic violent behavior. For most people, violent behavior is an infrequent event; this increases the difficulty in predicting future occurrences. However, there is always a balance between the individual's internal state, including the degree of tension and the controls over expression of aggression, and the environment. Certain combinations of internal and external factors may produce an assaultive crisis. An astute clinician can often identify when a patient is escalating beyond an acceptable expression of anger and frustration towards loss of control and assaultiveness. Appropriate interventions at various points of this cycle may prevent the crisis or minimize the chances of serious injury.

2. Internal control of violent impulses. Factors that impair impulse control either transiently or chronically may be crucial in determining whether or not an individual only fears a loss of control or actually acts on his or her impulses. In addition, there are certain contexts in which violence is more likely to occur; the extent to which the current situation recreates a previous one that resulted in a loss of control should be examined. The patient's perception of external danger, whether real or imagined, and the need to protect him- or herself are important factors.

3. Risk factors

   a. Demographic indicators. Young men in the range of 16–25 years of age are particularly at high risk for violent behavior. Since domestic violence is so prevalent, parents and spouses are at risk.

   b. Historic indicators

      (1) **A recent major life change** may place an individual under increased stress, leading to increased internal tension and frustration. The patient's feelings of internal pressure, frustration, anger, and potential explosiveness should be carefully explored.

         (a) Situations and individuals that increase or decrease the feelings of tension should be identified. The attempts that the patient has made to cope with these feelings and the results achieved should be discussed.

         (b) Attention should be given to the patient's level of optimism or pessimism about prevention of a violent action.

(c) The patient's thoughts and fantasies about violence are also extremely important; in particular, there may be certain sadistic fantasies or violent ruminations directed towards a specific individual or individuals. Specific threats require investigation of the patient's relationship with and accessibility to the threatened individual.

(d) Specific plans and the availability of and familiarity with weapons increase the danger.

(e) The patient's perception of what keeps him or her from carrying out the action is also important.

(f) Current use of drugs and alcohol should be explored.

(2) **History of violence**

(a) A history of violent behavior is the most reliable predictor of future violence. This includes fighting, assaults, arrests, and sanctioned violence (e.g., violence sanctioned for soldiers and police).

(b) A history of impulsive or self-destructive behavior, including accidents, arrests for speeding or reckless driving, and self-mutilation, puts the individual at increased risk.

(3) **Childhood history**

(a) A history of witnessing or experiencing neglect or abuse in childhood increases the likelihood of abuse and brutality directed towards the patient's own children.

(b) A childhood history of cruelty to animals may be associated with continuing aggressiveness.

c. **Diagnostic indicators.** The common diagnostic denominator is the degree to which impulse control and judgment are impaired in the contexts of hostility, irritability, and distorted perceptions of reality.

d. **Present mental status.** Fluctuation in the patient's levels of tension and agitation throughout the interview should be noted. The patient's impulse control and judgment during the examination may contradict the content of his or her speech. Command hallucinations to hurt others are particularly worrisome as are escalating delusional perceptions of external danger because these may be accompanied by frantic attempts at self-preservation. Sometimes delusional thinking may place others in danger in the guise of protecting them. For example, a psychotic mother may believe that she must bathe her child in scalding water to purify and cleanse him or her. Any evidence of confusion and organic mental disorders is also crucial as it suggest impairment of impulse control and judgment.

e. **Social matrix.** The thoughts of family and friends concerning the patient's violence potential should be sought in separate interviews, especially if they are potential victims. The family may provide a reliable history about the patient's access to weapons. The clinician should assess if the potential victim behaves in a challenging or provocative way towards the patient. If the patient appears to be calm, an interview with both the patient and the intended victim may be necessary to observe their behavior towards each other and to determine if there has been any resolution of the crisis. Possible use of available community resources beyond those offered by family and friends, such as safe houses, should be assessed.

f. **Physician's feelings.** Persistent feelings of fear or unease on the part of the physician may be important clues that further investigation and evaluation are necessary.

D. **Countertransference reactions to violent patients**

1. **Physician's reaction.** An angry, agitated, and threatening patient is likely to frighten and disorganize the physician. The physician's lack of awareness of this fear, previous personal experiences with violence, and conflicts over his or her own aggressive impulses may adversely influence his or her response to the patient.

a. **No reaction.** The physician may ignore or minimize the patient's concern with loss of control.

b. **Anger.** The physician may become angry and argue with the patient in response to the fear that he or she experiences. He or she may challenge and humiliate the patient, further escalating a dangerous situation.

c. **Counterphobic reaction.** The physician may act as though he or she is in control in response to unconscious fear and feelings of lack of control.

d. **Overly frightened reaction.** The physician may overestimate the patient's violent potential with the result that the physician is unnecessarily anxious and self-protective.

2. **Consequences.** Intense, unacknowledged countertransference reactions can interfere with

clinical judgment and treatment. The extremes range from being overly concerned with control and even punitive to releasing the patient prematurely or "permitting" him or her to escape in order to avoid dealing with the patient. Either way, the patient may receive an inadequate evaluation and inappropriate treatment. Potential victims may remain in considerable danger.

E. Principles of managing the violent patient

1. Safety is paramount.
   a. There must be an adequate number of trained staff to restrain the patient physically if necessary.
   b. Staff should approach the patient as both caring and able to set limits.

2. Behavioral techniques can be effective.
   a. Act calmly.
   b. Speak softly in a nonauthoritarian way.
   c. Have both the patient and examiner sit.
   d. Check for the presence of and confiscate all weapons.
   e. Be sure there is immediate access to an exit from the examining room.
   f. Use seclusion and restraint to prevent imminent harm to others.

3. Psychopharmacologic approach
   a. Neuroleptics are the most commonly used medications in an emergency situation. Haloperidol is given 5–10 mg intramuscularly every 30 minutes until agitation is controlled to a maximum of 100 mg/day. Neuroleptics should be avoided in alcohol or drug toxicity or withdrawal.   *Haloperidol*
   b. Benzodiazepines are used for the treatment of alcohol withdrawal. Diazepam (5–10 mg) and sodium amobarbital (200 mg) can be diluted and given intravenously. Oral administration of phenobarbital can be used when there is time to determine the daily dose of the sedative-hypnotic to which the patient is addicted.
   c. Phenobarbital in dosages of up to 640 mg/orally has been effective in managing aggressive behavior in patients with brain seizures. Side effects include decreased pulse and blood pressure.
   d. Other medications that are useful in managing violent patients include lithium, carbamazepine, phenytoin, and β-blockers, such as propranolol.
      (1) Lithium is useful in mania but has not been shown to be effective for other conditions.
      (2) Carbamazepine (600 mg/day) has shown some effectiveness in decreasing aggressive behavior in schizophrenics and in patients with partial complex seizures.
      (3) Phenytoin has been effective in patients with episodic dyscontrol syndrome, although carbamazepine may be even more effective.
      (4) Propranolol has been effective in patients with brain damage.

4. Duty to warn and protect others
   a. In our society, an individual is held responsible for his own actions, and what is said to a physician is considered confidential. However, as a result of the *Tarasoff* decision (*Tarasoff v. Regents of University of California,* 1976) and other legal cases involving attacks on third parties, clinicians are now expected to weigh the need for confidentiality against the need to protect others. In *Tarasoff,* the clinician was found liable for not breaking confidentiality and warning Miss Tarasoff that the patient had specifically threatened her.
   b. If the patient has made a credible threat to do physical harm to a specific person, the clinician has a duty to warn that person. Good medical practice may also require involuntary treatment of the patient.

V. THE VICTIMS. Many victims present to the emergency department. Some are obviously victims, while others, particularly victims of family violence, may be less obvious; their predicament may be missed, denied, or rationalized, and they may return home to face further abuse and trauma.

A. Child abuse. Although child abuse continues to be underreported in the United States, at least 500,000 children are significantly injured each year. Physical injuries can range from welts or contusions to multiple fractures to death. Concomitant emotional trauma is more difficult to measure but is no less disabling. Physicians may be tempted to rationalize abuse as severe discipline but in the range of normal or to feel that they do not have the right to interfere in family business. This attitude may be particularly prevalent in cases involving middle- and upper-class families; however, abuse is just as prevalent in middle- and upper-class families as in lower-class families.

1. **Clues.** There are a number of clues that can guide the physician's exploration of potential abuse despite denials by parents or reluctance on the part of the child to admit to the abuse.
   a. **Unexplained trauma** should raise the question of abuse, especially if there is evidence of multiple injuries at different stages of healing.
   b. **Delay** in seeking treatment, especially if poorly explained, may reflect parental fears of detection. Despite being the source of the injury, the parent may be overly concerned, and the child may be clingingly dependent on the parent.
   c. **Evidence of role reversal** between parents and child may be apparent, reflecting unrealistic expectations on the part of the child to meet parental needs and a lack of empathic understanding of the child's needs on the part of the parents.
   d. **Pseudomature behavior** on the part of the child may be an adaptation to the parents' unrealistic expectations.
   e. **Vague somatic complaints or behavioral symptoms**, such as nightmares, phobias, and enuresis, which reflect stress stemming from an abusive home situation, may be the presenting complaints.
   f. **Parental stress** should be evaluated with regard to child abuse, particularly if there is a history of abuse in the parent's childhood.

2. **Evaluation.** In addition to observing the child and parents together, the clinician should interview the child and parents separately, depending on the age of the child.
   a. **Evaluation of the child.** The type of examination varies depending on the age of the child and his or her ability to talk about him- or herself and the family. After a careful physical examination, x-rays of the long bones and skull to detect old fractures may be indicated for a young child. If the child is able to talk, a description of the family situation may be helpful, particularly of how discipline is carried out on both the affected child and on his or her siblings. A child may be reluctant to talk about this directly, which must be respected; a child may communicate indirectly through expression of wishes, fears, fantasies, and play. Sometimes it is helpful to talk with siblings, especially older ones.
   b. **Evaluation of the parents.** The parents should be interviewed separately as well as together. Even if only one parent is abusive, there is always collusion (if only out of fear) by the nonabusing partner. Questioning may begin concerning the general stress at home and that caused by the children. How the parents respond to the child's crying and conduct discipline is informative. Description of the pregnancy, labor, and delivery defines the extent to which the child was wanted or unwanted. The current perception of the child and his or her role reveals whether or not the parents have an accurate empathic understanding of the child's needs. An investigation of the quality of the marital relationship and some history of the parents' childhoods, especially their own experiences with discipline and abuse, is helpful. Specific questions about fear of loss of control or actual loss of control, anger, and aggression towards the child are necessary.
   c. **Assessment** of the extent of abuse and potential dangerousness should be made. The specifics should guide the treatment intervention. The clinician should be aware that both parents and children may resist any intervention, no matter how dangerous the situation is.

3. **Emergency treatment.** The goal is to protect the child and to initiate treatment that will prevent future abuse.
   a. The child should be given immediate necessary medical treatment.
   b. The child welfare agency and a psychiatric consultant should be consulted about how to protect this child and other children in the home. Protection may involve:
      (1) Hospitalizing the child
      (2) Placing the child and the siblings out of the home temporarily
      (3) Hospitalizing the abusive parent
   c. The parents should be informed that the abuse has been reported and what this entails. Although initially angry, the parents may also be relieved at the prospect of help.
   d. Under no circumstances should the child be released to the parents, regardless of the intensity of their protests, unless the physician is confident that the child will be safe and unless a treatment alliance has been developed.

B. **Sexual abuse (including incest).** Sexual molestation of children and adolescents ranges from petting to intercourse. It may involve a single event by a stranger or episodes repeated over a period of years by a family member or friend of the family. There may be little pain, evidence of trauma, or significant injury. Father- (or stepfather-) daughter incest is the most common;

it is the example used in the following discussion. Mother–son incest is rare and suggests serious psychopathology, often psychosis, in the mother. Overall, at least 200,000 cases of incest are reported each year, and up to 90% of incidents are not reported.

1. Clues
   a. If a young daughter appears to have the central role in the family, she may also have replaced the mother as the sexual partner for her father. Overly close and stimulating physical contact between a father and daughter should be discussed, particularly if the mother is absent either physically or emotionally.
   b. Perineal or vaginal trauma at any age requires investigation of sexual abuse. The suspicion of any physical abuse should raise the question of sexual abuse.
   c. Vague somatic complaints or frequent visits to physicians may reflect the child's distress and her search for help.
   d. Antisocial behavior, including sexual promiscuity, truancy, and running away, may be responses to sexual abuse at home. Over 50% of female runaways give sexual molestation as a reason for leaving home.
   e. Any psychiatric symptoms, including suicidal behavior, may stem from sexual abuse. The specific symptom reflects the developmental age of the child or adolescent.
   f. Pregnancy and venereal disease, especially in girls under the age of 12 years, should be evaluated for evidence of sexual abuse.

2. Evaluation. The age of the child determines the extent to which the child, the parent, or both are the focus of interviews. The child will be more hesitant to talk if she has been molested by a family member rather than a stranger.
   a. Evaluation of the child
      (1) Interview. The physician should talk with the child and examine her carefully. Questions must be phrased to match her developmental age. If possible, details of the event, including the identity of the molester, threats made, fear of harm, extent of injury, and feelings, should be obtained. In addition, it is helpful to elicit the child's perception of the reaction of others; children may experience significant shame and guilt and assume responsibility for the situation. In a case of incest, talking about issues of privacy, sleeping arrangements, physical intimacy, and the parental relationship may provide a lead into talking about sexual contact. Also, appreciating the child's fantasies and fears about the consequences of disclosure is important. The child should be reminded that she is not at fault.
      (2) Physical examination should be done carefully and nonintrusively. However, the physician must be aware that he or she is also gathering evidence for what may be a criminal proceeding. As with other cases of abuse and rape, specimens and pictures may be necessary.
   b. Evaluation of the parents
      (1) If a child has been molested by a stranger, the parents may need to ventilate their outrage away from the child so that they can be available to support the child and not confuse, frighten, and overwhelm her with their own feelings.
      (2) In a case of incest, questioning should go from general to specific. Inquiring about sleeping arrangements, privacy, physical contact, and the marital relationship may lead to specific questions about sexual activity. The extent of the sexual activity should be determined, including whether other daughters are involved. The father may deny, minimize, or rationalize his behavior, and it is important to be nonjudgmental. The mother may have colluded with the incest and may have even promoted it; she will not necessarily be an ally early in the treatment process. If both parents deny such activity, they should be confronted with the child's report.
   c. Consequences. There are serious consequences for all family members following disclosure of incest. Disclosure significantly disrupts the existing family equilibrium, however pathologic it may have been. All participants may develop psychiatric symptoms, especially anxiety and depression, and may be at risk for suicide.

3. Treatment
   a. The indicated medical treatment and follow-up for the victim, including that for venereal disease and pregnancy, must be provided.
   b. The child protection team and a psychiatric consultant must be contacted to plan further intervention. All cases of suspected or actual incest must be reported to the local child welfare agency, which can determine if legal charges and court involvement are indicated.
   c. The child should be protected from further abuse, which may involve hospitalization or placement out of the home. If there are other children at risk, the least disruptive option may be to have the father leave home until treatment is under way.

d. It may be necessary to hospitalize one or both of the parents, depending on their re-action to the disclosure.

e. Outpatient treatment is begun by breaking through the denial and conveying the expectation that the problem is treatable if all participate.

C. Spouse abuse. Violence in the home is pervasive, involving all socioeconomic classes. The most frequent pattern is husbands battering wives. At least one-fourth of all homicides occur among family members, and one-half of these involve spouse killing spouse. Husbands and wives kill each other with about equal frequency.

1. Clues. The physician may be inclined to rationalize the situation as private family business and avoid involvement. As it may be a chronic situation with a certain equilibrium, both partners may resist intervention. Also, the distinction between victim and perpetrator may not always be clear. The following are red flags for further investigation.

   a. Unusual or unexplained trauma may point to abuse; this is especially true during pregnancy, which is often a time of particular stress.

   b. Vague somatic complaints may reflect underlying psychological distress in either part-ner.

   c. Threats of violence from either spouse must be completely investigated.

   d. Evaluation of any psychiatric symptoms, especially those of chronic stress and depression, may result in disclosure of abuse at home.

   e. Overconcern of a spouse or boyfriend, to the extent that the patient is not allowed to be alone or is rushed out of the emergency department, may disguise ongoing abuse and a fear of exposure.

   f. Behavioral problems or psychiatric symptoms in the children may reflect chaos and violence in the home.

2. Evaluation

   a. Evaluation of the victim. After establishing a supportive relationship, the physician should ask increasingly specific questions about violence, both past and present. The physician should not be put off by evasive answers or initial denial but should appreciate the vulnerable position of the victim (i.e., she may fear abandonment or retaliation if she is candid and may see no alternatives for herself). Some discussion of resources and alternatives, such as safe houses, may be helpful early in the interview if the victim is fearful of cooperating.

   b. Evaluation of the abusive partner. If present, the abusing spouse should be evaluated with respect to dangerousness (see section IV). If he is not present, some assessment of the level of lethality of the situation should still be made. This should include an evaluation of impulse control, the availability of weapons, the provocativeness of the victim, and the homicidal potential of both partners.

3. Treatment. The goal is to prevent further injury to either partner.

   a. If there is any question about the lethality of the situation or the psychopathology of the partners, **psychiatric consultation** should be requested.

   b. If lethality or risk of future injury is high, the **wife should not return home**. Options include staying with friends or family, referral to a safe house, or hospitalization. If the victim refuses treatment, the physician should make her aware of resources and options but should not exert further stress by pressuring her to accept help that she does not want unless she is returning to a life-threatening situation.

   c. The physician should support the wife's decision not to return home, although he or she should not make the decision for her, except in the most serious of circumstances. Further treatment is often helpful to the wife during the process of separating from her spouse and establishing herself independently. There may be a tendency on her part to repeat the situation by finding another abusive partner.

   d. If the lethality of the present situation is low (i.e., the abusive partner wants help to prevent a recurrence), both husband and wife can be referred for treatment as a couple or individually as indicated. In any case, treatment should be offered to the abusing spouse.

   e. The child welfare agency should be notified as there may be concurrent abuse, emo-tional if not physical, of the children.

D. Rape. Rape is a crime of violence not of sexuality. It is the most common violent crime in the United States and one of the most underreported. As many as 70%–90% of rapes go un-reported for a variety of reasons, not the least of which is continued victimization of affected women by police, courts, hospital staff, and even family and friends.

1. **Characteristics of the crime**
   a. **Location.** Rape can take place anywhere from a deserted city street at night to a supermarket parking lot at midday to a woman's own home.
   b. **Violence.** In all rapes, the woman's life is implicitly threatened. Explicit force is used 85% of the time, and victims are struck or choked 50% of the time. Five percent of women are severely beaten.
   c. **Victims.** Although rape of men is increasing, women are victims in the majority of cases. In addition, this is the only violent crime, except perhaps spouse abuse, in which the victim's story is suspect unless she fought back. There is frequently the implication and even accusations that the victim invited or encouraged the assault.
   d. **Assailants.** The rapist is male, usually under 24 years of age, with a prior record. He has often been sexually impotent prior to the rape.

2. **Clinical presentation.** The response of an individual to a rape has much in common with stress response syndromes in general and response to other assaults in particular. However, there are many issues specific to rape, which intensify the conflicts and impair resolution. The following stages can usually be observed, and an accurate diagnosis of where the victim is in the process guides appropriate treatment.
   a. **Denial.** The first stage is one of shock and disbelief. The woman may describe a feeling of numbness and disbelief, which can last from minutes to hours to days. Though appearing shaken and drained, she may not show much overt emotion. This should not be mistaken for a lack of concern or lack of distress about the assault.
   b. **Emotional disorganization.** In this stage, the denial alternates with periods of intense feelings of fear, anger, humiliation, and depression. These feelings may be associated with intrusive memories of the event, nightmares, phobias, hypervigilance, and anxiety. This stage may have varying degrees of intensity and continue for months or years.
   c. **Resolution.** The victim naturally attempts some resolution to her disorganized state, which is distressing in itself and disruptive to normal functioning.
      (1) **Maladaptive resolution.** The victim's attempts at resolution may be maladaptive, resulting in the establishment of chronic symptoms or creating new problems as bad as or worse than the initial event. Victims may make drastic changes in life-style, which serve to diffuse anxiety about future attacks but which are professionally and socially crippling. There may be loss of relatedness to others and especially a loss of sexual interest. There may be abuse of drugs and alcohol to decrease anxiety and suppress intrusive memories and nightmares. The result may be suicide unless there is active intervention.
      (2) **Adaptive resolution.** In this case, the victim, with or without treatment, gradually integrates the event with a decrease in intrusive recollections and feelings and returns to normal functioning in work and relationships. Future similar situations or particular reminders of the attack may trigger transient reemergence of symptoms but usually with less intensity and distress as time passes.

3. **Evaluation and treatment.** It is particularly difficult to separate evaluation and treatment in cases of rape. Above all, the physician, especially if male, must guard against repeating the humiliation by an intrusive interview and examination. If is helpful if the vicitm is treated and counseled by a female practitioner.
   a. **The rape crisis team** or a psychiatric consultant should be called immediately to help assess the patient's current needs and support her through the examination.
   b. **The patient's wishes and requests** must be respected. If the patient is alone and wants family or friends contacted, she should be helped in doing this. If she prefers not to contact anyone, this must be honored.
   c. If the patient **presents in a stage of denial**, her distress should not be underestimated. With reassurance about her present security, the patient may begin to express the feelings and disorganization of the next stage. If she continues to maintain denial, it should be explained that it is natural to have feelings and thoughts that may cause considerable distress and that talking about these will help her master them.
   d. If the patient is **disorganized and upset**, she may feel considerable pressure to review the details of the event and to ventilate feelings, which may include associated feelings of guilt, shame, responsibility, vulnerability, and helplessness.
   e. If the patient arrives in the emergency department following a recent rape, an **empathic medical examination** should be done once the patient is prepared. Details of the event are necessary to guide the physical examination. Specimens must be collected should the patient want to press charges immediately or at a later date. There must be discussion, treatment, and follow-up due to the possibility of venereal disease and pregnancy.
   f. **The patient's resources** should be assessed. Meeting with family and friends separately

(especially husbands and boyfriends) may help them vent their outrage and conflicting feelings away from the patient and, as a result, be more supportive of her.

g. **The patient's own decision** about returning home and subsequent treatment should be supported unless it is grossly unreasonable or dangerous. If the patient appears to be placing herself in jeopardy, physically or emotionally, it may be necessary to insist on further crisis intervention immediately.

h. **Psychiatric follow-up** should be arranged as indicated. If the patient is particularly resistant to treatment, some outreach at a later date by a rape crisis center may be helpful.

VI. TELEPHONE CALLS

A. **General issues.** People may call the emergency department for a variety of reasons, some of which may be covert or overt requests for help for any of the crises previously described. The physician is quite limited as to what he or she can do over the telephone, but there are general principles of management.

1. The patient's name, telephone number, and address should be obtained as soon as possible in the conversation.

2. The physician should try to develop an alliance with the patient without becoming too involved over the telephone.

3. Acknowledging the limits of the telephone, the physician should encourage the patient to come to the emergency department as the next step in treatment.

4. If the patient refuses to come in, the physician's assessment of potential dangerousness dictates how active he or she must be in getting the patient to the hospital.

B. **Covert presentation.** Whatever the request by telephone, it may be a subtle clue to a more serious problem. Use of the telephone may reflect the patient's conflict, discomfort, or embarrassment in seeking help. If the underlying reasons for the call are revealed, the patient may feel understood, less alone and isolated, and receptive towards coming to the emergency department or to being referred to the appropriate resources. The physician should follow up his or her referral, both with the patient and the agency or clinic involved, to make sure that they have made contact with each other.

C. **Overt presentation**

1. **The cooperative patient** may describe a crisis overtly and simply be requesting help to get into treatment. In other cases, the patient's ambivalence may make it necessary for the physician to make arrangements with family, friends, or the police to get the patient to the hospital.

2. **The uncooperative patient.** If the physician is concerned about imminent danger and the patient refuses to provide information, the physician may be forced to trace the call and follow up any leads that the patient gives. Although it can be extremely frustrating, the physician should try to build an alliance with that part of the patient desiring help, and he or she should remind the patient of the limitations of telephone contact.

D. **Chronic callers.** Every emergency department has a contingent of chronic callers. Some of these people are lonely and need reassurance; some are consciously or unconsciously expressing their anger and rage by repeatedly frustrating the staff.

1. **Approach.** Whatever the motivation for the calls, an attempt should be made to get the caller into the appropriate treatment setting.

2. **Plan.** Whether or not they go into treatment, a plan for handling them, which identifies these individuals by name, aliases, and content of call, should be written down. This prevents new staff from becoming tangled in a frustrating situation and minimizes the maladaptive gratification that these individuals receive from making their calls.

STUDY QUESTIONS

Directions: Each question below contains five suggested answers. Choose the **one best** response to each question.

1. All of the following statements regarding a psychiatric emergency are true EXCEPT

(A) it is stress-induced
(B) the usual coping mechanisms reestablish equilibrium
(C) there is a pathologic response
(D) there is physical danger
(E) problem-solving ability is decreased

2. Internal stress is illustrated by which of the following examples?

(A) An episode of mania in a person with bipolar illness
(B) A myocardial infarction suffered by a 60-year-old man
(C) A divorce after 15 years of marriage of a 40-year-old woman
(D) Disorganization in an 18-year-old college freshman away from home for the first time
(E) Irritability and loss of impulse control in a 20-year-old man following minor head injury

3. An individual who unsuccessfully attempts suicide by overdose is most likely

(A) not really serious about dying
(B) a girl younger than 20 years of age
(C) just trying to get attention
(D) a manipulative individual with few friends
(E) without a family history of suicide

4. What percentage of patients who die by suicide have sought medical help within 6 months of their deaths?

(A) 40%
(B) 50%
(C) 60%
(D) 70%
(E) 80%

5. An example of a *covert* presentation of suicidal behavior is

(A) an overdose with sleeping pills
(B) superficial cuts in the wrist
(C) a single-car accident
(D) alcoholism
(E) mountain climbing

6. Which of the following clinical presentations are associated with violent behavior?

(A) The XYY chromosomal abnormality
(B) Low intelligence
(C) The XO chromosomal abnormality
(D) Epilepsy
(E) None of the above

7. Which of the following disorders is most likely to present as violent behavior?

(A) Bipolar disorder–manic type
(B) Anxiety disorder
(C) Major depressive episode
(D) Somatoform disorder
(E) Obsessive–compulsive personality disorder

8. The most common drug associated with violent behavior is

(A) phencylidine
(B) cocaine
(C) amphetamines
(D) steroids
(E) alcohol

9. In evaluating potentially violent patients, all of the following are important EXCEPT

(A) obtaining a complete history of drug and alcohol abuse
(B) assessing the patient's capacity for impulse control
(C) determining those situations that result in violent behavior
(D) feeling relaxed and comfortable with the patient
(E) contacting family and friends for further information

10. All of the following statements about child abuse are true EXCEPT

(A) children are often reluctant to admit to abuse
(B) physicians may be hesitant to intervene in family matters
(C) abuse is more prevalent in families of lower socioeconomic status
(D) any unexplained trauma should raise the question of abuse
(E) abusive parents may appear overly concerned about the child's welfare

11. Specific clues to potential child abuse include all of the following EXCEPT

(A) strict religious beliefs in the family
(B) a parent under stress
(C) a child with frequent nightmares
(D) a child with pseudomature behavior
(E) a parent who experienced abuse as a child

12. In the emergency treatment of child abuse, it is most important to

(A) keep the family together
(B) avoid offending the parents
(C) educate the parents as to acceptable discipline
(D) encourage the child not to disobey his or her parents
(E) notify the local child protection team

Directions: Each question below contains four suggested answers of which **one or more** is correct. Choose the answer

    A   if **1, 2, and 3** are correct
    B   if **1 and 3** are correct
    C   if **2 and 4** are correct
    D   if **4** is correct
    E   if **1, 2, 3, and 4** are correct

13. An agitated 24-year-old man is brought to the emergency room in handcuffs by the police after he was found wandering along the highway in a confused state. The patient becomes mute and appears to be calm. The first steps in managing this patient include

(1) taking a history from the police
(2) removing the handcuffs to make the patient comfortable
(3) talking with the patient about his impulse control
(4) administering a 5-mg dose of haloperidol intramuscularly

Questions 14–17

A 27-year-old man comes to the emergency department in a slightly intoxicated state to have a laceration on his forearm sutured. He becomes increasingly belligerent as he is questioned about the cause of his injury and grabs a pair of scissors from the suture tray.

14. Appropriate responses by the physician include

(1) continuing to suture the laceration and calmly redirecting the patient's attention
(2) insisting that the patient regain self-control and put down the scissors
(3) confronting the patient with his alcohol problem and instructing the nurse to determine the alcohol level in the blood
(4) calling for other staff and security guards

15. Inappropriate responses to this situation reflect various countertransferences to the violent patient. These include

(1) a counterphobic reaction
(2) no reaction
(3) an angry reaction
(4) a limit-setting reaction

16. Further management of this patient requires

(1) inquiring about the details of the injury
(2) searching the patient for weapons
(3) obtaining a history of violent behavior
(4) performing a mental status examination

17. If the patient escapes from the emergency department, the physician should

(1) pursue the patient
(2) assume that the patient will return when he is ready for treatment
(3) assume that the patient will be all right once he sobers up
(4) notify family and friends about the patient's potential dangerousness

(end of group question)

18. Factors that increase the risk of dangerous behavior in an emergency situation include

(1) a history of mania
(2) a history of a suicide attempt
(3) alcohol abuse
(4) the presence of head trauma

19. Factors that increase the statistical risk of suicide include being

(1) married
(2) female
(3) a schoolteacher
(4) on renal dialysis

20. Depression has long been thought to be a cause of suicide. Correct statements about the relationship of depression and suicide include which of the following?

(1) About half of the people who commit suicide are suffering from depressive illness
(2) Schizophrenic patients who kill themselves are also suffering from depressive illness
(3) Men who have suffered a severe depressive illness are 500 times more likely to kill themselves than men who have no psychiatric illness.
(4) Female physicians attempt suicide three times more frequently than male physicians, but male physicians complete suicide three times more frequently than female physicians.

21. Disorders of the brain that have been associated with increased violent behavior include

(1) encephalitis
(2) birth injury
(3) minor head trauma
(4) grand mal seizures

22. Behavioral techniques that can be effective in managing a potentially violent patient include

(1) speaking authoritatively
(2) allowing the patient to move freely
(3) letting the patient know that he is upsetting you
(4) checking for weapons

23. Important aspects of the treatment of sexual abuse of a child may include

(1) maintaining confidentiality so that the abusive parent will open up
(2) hospitalizing either the child or one or both parents
(3) avoiding involvement of the legal system so that therapy can be effective
(4) evaluating and treating any venereal disease

24. A maladaptive resolution of a victim's attempt to deal with a rape include which of the following symptoms?

(1) Shock and disbelief
(2) Nightmares
(3) Anxiety
(4) Alcohol abuse

25. Occasionally, a patient becomes a chronic caller to emergency rooms. Important aspects in managing these patients include

(1) having the patient come in for a planned appointment
(2) conducting a thorough mental status examination
(3) limiting the time during which the staff talks with the patient
(4) telling the patient that his or her calls are a way of expressing rage

Directions: The group of questions below consists of lettered choices followed by several numbered items. For each numbered item select the **one** lettered choice with which it is **most** closely associated. Each lettered choice may be used once, more than once, or not at all.

Questions 26–29

Match each patient history with the diagnosis that is most appropriate.

(A) Post-traumatic stress disorder
(B) Schizophrenic disorder
(C) Pathologic intoxication
(D) Intermittent explosive disorder
(E) Bipolar disorder–manic type

26. A 42-year-old man is brought to the emergency department by his family after becoming threatening when they confronted him about his excessive spending. He bought $5000 worth of clothing in the preceding week and then gave it away. He explains that this is part of his presidential campaign, which he has been working on night and day for several weeks.

27. A 23-year-old woman is brought to the emergency department by the police after assaulting her younger sister. She accused the sister of being "a witch" and said that she was ordered by "the voices" to destroy her. She has no friends and has gradually become preoccupied with witchcraft over a period of several years.

28. A 36-year-old Vietnam War veteran is brought into the emergency department in an anxious, tremulous, and diaphoretic state. While coming out of a bar, he attempted to grab a police officer's revolver after hearing a car backfire. He was shouting incoherently about "the enemy."

29. A 20-year-old man is brought to the emergency department after tearing up a restaurant and assaulting his companions. He is confused and agitated. His friends deny any history of violence or prior psychiatric history. They state that he had become violent quite suddenly and that they have been unable to calm him.

ANSWERS AND EXPLANATIONS

1. The answer is B. (*I A*) When a psychiatric emergency exists, there is a crisis. The usual coping mechanisms that the individual uses to solve a crisis are insufficient or are overwhelmed, thus, causing a pathologic response, such as changes in mood, thought, or behavior. Psychiatric emergencies place an individual or those around him or her in physical danger due to a loss of control. Problem-solving ability is decreased because of the lack of equilibrium and failure of adaptation. Stress from any source can cause a problem that the individual cannot solve by the usual coping mechanisms.

2. The answer is D. (*I B 1 a, b*) Internal stress may result in an individual who is faced with a normal developmental task, such as leaving home for the first year of college. When the individual is unable to accomplish this developmental task, there may be massive psychological disruption, and a psychiatric emergency may result. While it is appropriate to have some anxiety upon leaving home for college, disorganization in thinking is a result of an extreme internal stress. Mania and myocardial infarction are major illnesses and, thus, external stressors. Divorce is an obvious external stress as is irritability and loss of impulse control following minor closed head trauma.

3. The answer is B. (*III A 2, 3, D*) Women **attempt** suicide four times more often than men; men successfully **commit** suicide three times more often than women. The suicide rate among women gradually increases from the teenage years and peaks between 40 and 60 years of age. All suicidal patients are ambivalent; a lack of success does not necessarily suggest a nonlethal intention. An unsuccessful suicide attempt may indeed mobilize support from family and friends, but the self-destructiveness and dangerousness of the behavior must be taken very seriously. Unsuccessful suicide attempts may be a chronic manipulative pattern for some patients with severe character pathology, but for the majority, an attempt reflects a significant crisis of desperate proportions from which the individual can fully recover. A family history of suicide puts an individual at a greater risk both to attempt and actually commit suicide.

4. The answer is E. (*III A 5*) Approximately 50% of suicide victims have sought medical help within 1 month of their deaths, and 80% have seen physicians within 6 months of their deaths. "Medical help" does not mean psychiatric help; rather, most patients go to their family physicians looking for help but in a covert fashion. As many as 70% of patients who commit suicide have some active medical illness that keeps them in contact with their physicians. They may not reveal feelings of depression or suicidal ideation unless directly asked. Furthermore, many depressed patients initially present to nonpsychiatric physicians with various somatic complaints, fatigue, and insomnia; again they may not describe depression or suicidal ideation unless asked. If the diagnosis is missed, these patients may attempt suicide with the prescriptions that they are given for anxiety or sleeplessness.

5. The answer is C. (*III B 1, 2*) Covert suicidal behavior is unconscious, self-destructive behavior. Accidents, particularly single-car accidents, are examples of covert suicidal behavior. Overdosing with sleeping pills and superficial cuts on the wrist are overt suicidal acts. While alcoholism is associated with suicidal behavior, it is not considered a covert suicidal act. Mountain climbing can be a healthy behavior and is not suicidal unless the person doing it takes unreasonable risks.

6. The answer is B. (*IV A 1 c*) Despite the increased percentage of persons with chromosomal abnormalities, particularly XYY, in prison populations, recent studies do not support the hypothesis that chromosomal abnormalities, either XYY or XO, are associated with criminal behavior. Epilepsy has not been demonstrated to increase the risk of violent behavior. However, low intelligence from whatever cause is likely to be associated with violence in the general population.

7. The answer is A. (*IV B 1 a*) Bipolar patients in the midst of a manic episode are frequently extremely irritable and have a low frustration tolerance in conjunction with great pressure in their thinking and activity. They may quickly become aggressive if they are slighted or frustrated in their plans. Patients with the other diagnoses mentioned may present with considerable psychomotor agitation (e.g., those with anxiety disorder or major depressive episodes) or dramatic demands (e.g., those with somatoform disorder), but they are far less likely to strike out at others. An individual with an obsessive–compulsive personality disorder tends to be overly controlled and avoids direct expression or acknowledgment of anger.

8. The answer is E. (*IV B 3 a*) Alcohol is the most common precipitating cause of violent behavior in our culture and is the drug most widely used. Cocaine, especially its new variety of crack, is associated with a very high incidence of violence among users, but together with amphetamines and phencylidine, the number of people who use it is much smaller than the number who use alcohol. Steroids can be associated with violent behavior when used medically or when abused by individuals seeking to build their muscle mass but not with the same frequency as alcohol.

9. The answer is D. *(IV C, D)* While it is essential to insure one's safety when evaluating a potentially violent patient, it is unlikely that the physician will feel relaxed and comfortable. Some degree of anxiety and tension is expected, and its absence suggests a countertransference denial of the patient's dangerousness. The patient's capacity to control his or her aggressive impulses is central to the evaluation; both drug and alcohol intoxication may significantly impair this capacity. The patient may be unable or unwilling to provide the necessary information; family and friends may be able to describe more accurately the patient's behavior and the precipitants for violence. Not only is the patient's impulse control important, determination of the likelihood of his or her returning to a situation that previously produced violent behavior is also crucial.

10. The answer is C. *(V A)* Child abuse is as prevalent in upper- and middle-class families as it is in lower-class families, but the physician may find that he or she has a more difficult time addressing the issue in the former groups, particularly if they are similar to his or her own socioeconomic group. In addition, the physician may feel reluctant to raise questions about the severity of family discipline and make a judgment as to what is too severe. He or she may mistakenly interpret the parents' overly concerned attitude or the child's reluctance to talk as evidence of a close, happy family. Vague or evasive answers from either children or parents about the cause of the trauma should never be accepted at face value but always should be investigated further.

11. The answer is A. *(V A 1)* Although many religious groups may emphasize obedience and discipline, this does not in itself suggest an abusive home situation. Parents under stress may take out their hostilities on the children; they may attempt to exercise the absolute control that they do not have elsewhere at the expense of the children. A parent who was abused as a child may see such abuse as acceptable or may be unable to control his or her rage, much as his or her own parent could not. Children may show pseudomature behavior in response to the chaos in the home and to the needs of their parents. Any symptomatic behavior in the child, including but not limited to frequent nightmares, may originate from an abusive situation.

12. The answer is E. *(V A 3)* The physician is required by law to notify the local child protection agency of any **suspected** abuse; the agency decides how complete an investigation is indicated. While it is hoped that, with treatment, the abuse can be stopped and the family can stay together, the immediate goal is to protect the child. Although the questioning should be done in an empathic, nonjudgmental way to build a treatment alliance with the parents, an accurate assessment of the dangerousness of the home situation must take precedence over the parents' feelings. Education about alternative ways of discipline may be an important long-range goal, but it is not helpful in the emergency situation. Lastly, although the child's behavior may be problematic and require treatment, the central issue in the emergency situation is the parents' capacity to control aggressive behavior towards the child.

13. The answer is B (1, 3). *(II A, B; IV C)* Although the patient appears to be calm, his muteness prevents taking the initial history, but it should still be attempted. The observations of the police are crucial to the diagnostic process; the patient's confusion and muteness suggest serious psychopathology. The patient's calmness may be the result of the external control exerted by the police and the handcuffs. Removal of the handcuffs without adequate precautions may lead to a re-escalation of agitated behavior. Although external control may be necessary, administration of haloperidol at this point without a diagnosis might confuse the picture and even make the patient worse [e.g., neuroleptics are contraindicated in cases of phencyclidine (PCP) intoxication]. This patient might be best managed with 2- or 4-point leather restraints until he cooperates with the history-taking, physical examination, and mental status examination.

14. The answer is C (2, 4). *(II A–C; IV)* Despite the patient's initial cooperation, he has escalated to overt threatening behavior with minimal provocation. The patient's behavior must be dealt with before anything else. Firm verbal limits that encourage self-control but that do not challenge the patient should be given. If the patient does not respond, the security guards should be called. If the patient still does not calm down, preparations to disarm him safely must take place. Any discussion with the patient about his alcohol problem must wait until he is sober and in control.

15. The answer is A (1, 2, 3). *(IV D)* A firm limit-setting response on the part of the physician would be appropriate in this situation. A counterphobic reaction, an angry reaction, and no reaction represent countertransference, which can impair clinical judgment and even further increase the danger in dealing with a violent patient. Ignoring the patient's behavior may frighten him because he fears that no one will help him maintain control. An angry response may challenge and humiliate the patient, leading to further escalation. A counterphobic reaction may place the physician in considerable danger since he or she will not take appropriate self-protective measures.

16. The answer is E (all). (*II A, B, E; IV D*) Once the patient has been controlled (i.e., the scissors have been taken away and restraints applied if necessary), he or she should be searched for other weapons, and the medical treatment should be completed. At this point, the patient must be evaluated in terms of ongoing dangerousness. The details of the injury and history of violent behavior are crucial. These data together with a mental status examination will help to determine if the patient requires psychiatric treatment, treatment for alcoholism, or if legal charges for attempted assault should be filed.

17. The answer is D (4). (*IV E*) This patient may be all right once he sobers up, but at present, he is volatile and assaultive. To ignore this is a serious countertransference as is pursuing an angry, injured, intoxicated man with a weapon without adequate help. The patient may return, but given his impairment in impulse control and judgment, this seems unlikely. The police and any family or friends who can be reached should be fully apprised of the situation as they too may be in danger if the patient returns home.

18. The answer is E (all). (*II E 1–3*) A history of a psychiatric illness should alert the clinician to potential recurrences of that illness. Furthermore, a history of any kind of dangerous behavior, whether self-destructive or assaultive, increases the risk of violent behavior. Drugs and alcohol, which decrease impulse control, and neurologic conditions, which can affect central nervous system function, can also increase the risk of dangerous behavior.

19. The answer is D (4). (*III A 3–5, 7*) Individuals with a chronic illness, such as kidney failure, appear to be at an increased risk statistically for suicidal behavior. Being divorced or single rather than married is also a risk factor as is being male rather than female. Teaching school, while more stressful than it used to be, is still not considered a high-stress job.

20. The answer is B (1, 3). (*III A 6, 7*) About 50% of the people who commit suicide have a depressive illness, although almost everybody who kills him- or herself has some psychiatric disorder. Alcoholism is seen in about 25% of suicide victims, and schizophrenia in about 10%. Schizophrenics who kill themselves may or may not be depressed. Men with a severe depression are 500 times more likely to kill themselves than men who have no psychiatric illness. While women generally attempt suicide four times more frequently than men, men are three times more likely to complete the act. This is not true for physicians where the suicide rates for women are at least as high as the suicide rates for men.

21. The answer is A (1, 2, 3). (*IV B 3 b, c*) Injury to the brain has been associated with violent behavior. Postconcussion syndromes, which can be caused by minor head injury or even injury at birth, and infections of the brain, such as encephalitis, have also been associated with changes in behavior. Seizures, particularly the grand mal type, are not associated with violent changes, although there is some question about partial complex seizures having an effect on behavior.

22. The answer is D (4). (*IV E 2*) Behavioral techniques can be effective in managing potentially dangerous patients. The physician should act calmly so as not to escalate the situation and speak softly in a nonauthoritarian way. It is important to have the patient sit and not move about. Checking for weapons is mandatory, especially in the emergency room.

23. The answer is C (2, 4). (*V B 3*) With sexual abuse of a child, it is important to protect the child from any further abuse. This may be accomplished by separating the child from the family and the abusive parent by placing him or her outside of the home or in the hospital. It may also be necessary to hospitalize one or both of the parents, depending upon their reactions to the disclosure of the sexual abuse. Medical treatment for the victim of sexual abuse includes the assessment and treatment of any venereal disease that may be present. Rather than maintaining confidentiality, it is mandatory that sexual abuse be reported to legal authorities; the legal system may be the only way in which the abusive parent can be made to seek treatment.

24. The answer is D (4). [*V D 2 c (1)*] Rape is an intense stress and leads to a stress response in all victims. The first stage is one of shock and disbelief. Normal reactions include nightmares, anxiety, and hypervigilance for months after the event and as the victim works through the event. Alcohol abuse to decrease anxiety and suppress intrusive memories is a maladaptive resolution to the trauma.

25. The answer is B (1, 3).(*VI D 1, 2*) Chronic callers to emergency services or physicians may have a number of reasons for this behavior. It is important to have the patient come in for a planned appointment to initiate appropriate treatment. These patients often resist an appointment, but it is important to limit the reinforcement chronic callers receive from talking with staff. It is inappropriate to conduct a mental status examination over the telephone. While some patients are expressing rage by calling emergency rooms, others are lonely and need reassurance.

26–29. The answers are: 26-E, 27-B, 28-A, 29-C. (*IV B*) The most likely diagnosis of the 42-year-old man described in the question is bipolar disorder–manic type. The affected individual's poor judgment and unrealistic behavior motivated by grandiose ideas were sustained over some time, ruling out post-traumatic stress disorder, pathologic intoxication, and intermittent explosive disorder. The specific symptoms of insomnia, hyperactivity, grandiosity, and irritability are consistent with a diagnosis of bipolar disorder rather than schizophrenia.

The most likely diagnosis of the 23-year-old woman is schizophrenic disorder. The violent behavior was the culmination of chronically developing delusional beliefs and ultimately the result of command hallucinations. While hallucinations and delusions can occur in bipolar disorder–manic type, there is no evidence of other manic symptoms. In fact, the patient's chronic deteriorating course with poor social relationships suggests schizophrenia.

The most likely diagnosis of the Vietnam War veteran is post-traumatic stress disorder. This patient had a flashback to a combat situation triggered by the sound of a car backfiring. The patient is essentially in a dissociative state and experiences his current situation as though he were back in combat. Despite his appearing anxious and incoherent at the moment, there is nothing else to suggest mania. Although he had been drinking, his violent behavior was not triggered directly by alcohol as occurs with pathologic intoxication.

The most likely diagnosis of the 20-year-old man is pathologic intoxication, which is a dramatic violent behavioral response triggered by a small amount of alcohol and often accompanied by confusion and disorientation. There are no symptoms or previous history in this case to suggest schizophrenia or bipolar disorder–manic type. The diagnosis of intermittent explosive disorder, while more common in men, requires a history of violent behavior and clearly directed violence. There is no history of a traumatic event, post-traumatic symptoms, or a triggering stimulus.

Challenge Exam

Introduction

One of the least attractive aspects of pursuing an education is the necessity of being examined on what has been learned. Instructors do not like to prepare tests, and students do not like to take them.

However, students are required to take many examinations during their learning careers, and little if any time is spent acquainting them with the positive aspects of tests and with systematic and successful methods for approaching them. Students perceive tests as punitive and sometimes feel that they are merely opportunities for the instructor to discover what the student has forgotten or has never learned. Students need to view tests as opportunities to display their knowledge and to use them as tools for developing prescriptions for further study and learning.

A brief history and discussion of the National Board of Medical Examiners (NBME) examinations (i.e., Parts I, II, and III and FLEX) are presented in this preface, along with ideas concerning psychological preparation for the examinations. Also presented are general considerations and test-taking tips as well as how practice exams can be used as educational tools. (The literature provided by the various examination boards contains detailed information concerning the construction and scoring of specific exams.)

National Board of Medical Examiners Examinations

Before the various NBME exams were developed, each state attempted to license physicians through its own procedures. Differences between the quality and testing procedures of the various state examinations resulted in the refusal of some states to recognize the licensure of physicians licensed in other states. This made it difficult for physicians to move freely from one state to another and produced an uneven quality of medical care in the United States.

To remedy this situation, the various state medical boards decided they would be better served if an outside agency prepared standard exams to be given in all states, allowing each state to meet its own needs and have a common standard by which to judge the educational preparation of individuals applying for licensure.

One misconception concerning these outside agencies is that they are licensing authorities. This is not the case; they are examination boards only. The individual states retain the power to grant and revoke licenses. The examination boards are charged with designing and scoring valid and reliable tests. They are primarily concerned with providing the states with feedback on how examinees have performed and with making suggestions about the interpretation and usefulness of scores. The states use this information as partial fulfillment of qualifications upon which they grant licenses.

Students should remember that these exams are administered nationwide and, although the general medical information is similar, educational methodologies and faculty areas of expertise differ from institution to institution. It is unrealistic to expect that students will know all the material presented in the exams; they may face questions on the exams in areas that were only superficially covered in their classes. The testing authorities recognize this situation, and their scoring procedures take it into account.

Scoring the Exams

The diversity of curriculum necessitates that these tests be scored using a criteria-based normal curve. An individual score is based not only on how many questions were answered correctly by a specific student but also on how this one performance relates to the distribution of all scores of the criteria group. In the case of NBME, Part I, the criteria group consists of those students who have completed 2 years of medical training in the United States and are taking the test for the first time and those students who took the test during the previous four June sittings.

Since this test has been constructed to measure a wide range of educational situations, the mean, or average, score generally can be achieved by answering 64% to 68% of the questions correctly. Passing the exam requires answering correctly 55% to 60% of the questions. The competition for acceptance into medical school and the performance levels necessary to stay in school are so high that many students who have always achieved these high levels naturally assume they must perform in a similar fashion and attain equivalent scores on the NBME exams. This is not the case. In fact, among students who are accustomed to performing at levels exceeding 80% to 90%, fewer than 4% taking these tests perform at that high level. Unrealistically high personal expectations leave students psychologically unprepared for these tests, and the anxiety of the moment renders them incapable of doing their best work.

Actually, **most students have learned quite well**, but they fail to display this learning when they are tested because they do not understand the construction, purpose, or scoring procedures of board exams. It is imperative that they understand that they are **not** expected to score as well as they have in the past and that the measurement criteria is group performance, not only individual performance.

While preparing for an exam, it is important that students learn as much as they can about the subject they will be tested on as well as prepare to discover just how much they may not know. Students should study to acquire knowledge, not just to prepare for tests. **For the well-prepared candidate, the chances of passing far exceed the chances of failing**.

Materials Needed for Test Preparation

In preparation for a test, many students collect far too much study material only to find that they simply do not have the time to go through all of it. They are defeated before they begin because either they cannot get through all the material leaving areas unstudied, or they race through the material so quickly that they cannot benefit from the activity.

It is generally more efficient for the student to use materials already at hand; that is, class notes, one good outline to cover or strengthen areas not locally stressed and for quick review of the whole topic, and one good text as a reference for looking up complex material needing further explanation.

Also, many students attempt to memorize far too much information, rather than learning and understanding less material and then relying on that learned information to determine the answers to questions at the time of the examination. Relying too heavily on memorized material causes anxiety, and the more anxious students become during a test, the less learned knowledge they are likely to use.

Positive Attitude

A positive attitude and a realistic approach are essential to successful test taking. If concentration is placed on the negative aspects of tests or on the potential for failure, anxiety increases and performance decreases. A negative attitude generally develops if the student concentrates on "I must pass" rather than on "I can pass." "What if I fail?" becomes the major factor motivating the student to **run from failure rather than toward success**. This results from placing too much emphasis on scores rather than understanding that scores have only slight relevance to future professional performance.

The score received is only one aspect of test performance. Test performance also indicates the student's ability to use information during evaluation procedures and reveals how this ability might be used in the future. For example, when a patient enters the physician's office with a problem, the physician begins by asking questions, searching for clues, and seeking diagnostic information. Hypotheses are then developed, which will include several potential causes for the problem. Weighing the probabilities, the physician will begin to discard those hypotheses with the least likelihood of being correct. Good differential diagnosis involves the ability to deal with uncertainty, to reduce potential causes to the smallest number, and to use all learned information in arriving at a conclusion.

This same thought process can and should be used in testing situations. It might be termed **paper-and-pencil differential diagnosis**. In each question with five alternatives, of which one is correct, there are four alternatives that are incorrect. If deductive reasoning is used, as in solving a clinical problem, the choices can be viewed as having possibilities of being correct. The elimination of wrong choices increases the odds that a student will be able to recognize the correct choice. Even if the correct choice does not become evident, the probability of guessing correctly increases. Just as differential diagnosis in a clinical setting can result in a correct diagnosis, eliminating incorrect choices on a test can result in choosing the correct answer.

Answering questions based on what is incorrect is difficult for many students since they have had nearly 20 years experience taking tests with the implied assertion that knowledge can be displayed only by knowing what is correct. It must be remembered, however, that students can display knowledge by knowing something is wrong, just as they can display it by knowing something is right. **Students should begin to think in the present as they expect themselves to think in the future**.

Paper-and-Pencil Differential Diagnosis

The technique used to arrive at the answer to the following question is an example of the paper-and-pencil differential diagnosis approach.

> A recently diagnosed case of hypothyroidism in a 45-year-old man may result in which of the following conditions?
>
> **(A)** Thyrotoxicosis
> **(B)** Cretinism
> **(C)** Myxedema
> **(D)** Graves' disease
> **(E)** Hashimoto's thyroiditis

It is presumed that all of the choices presented in the question are plausible and partially correct. If the student begins by breaking the question into parts and trying to discover what the question is attempting to measure, it will be possible to answer the question correctly by using more than memorized charts concerning thyroid problems.

- The question may be testing if the student knows the difference between "hypo" and "hyper" conditions.
- The answer choices may include thyroid problems that are not "hypothyroid" problems.
- It is possible that one or more of the choices are "hypo" but are not "thyroid" problems, that they are some other endocrine problems.
- "Recently diagnosed in a 45-year-old man" indicates that the correct answer is not a congenital childhood problem.
- "May result in" as opposed to "resulting from" suggests that the choices might include a problem that **causes** hypothyroidism rather than **results from** hypothyroidism, as stated.

By applying this kind of reasoning, the student can see that choice **A**, thyroid toxicosis, which is a disorder resulting from an overactive thyroid gland ("hyper") must be eliminated. Another piece of knowledge, that is, Graves' disease is thyroid toxicosis, eliminates choice **D**. Choice **B**, cretinism, is indeed hypothyroidism, but it is a childhood disorder. Therefore, **B** is eliminated. Choice **E** is an inflammation of the thyroid gland—here the clue is the suffix "itis." The reasoning is that thyroiditis, being an inflammation, may **cause** a thyroid problem, perhaps even a hypothyroid problem, but there is no reason for the reverse to be true. Myxedema, choice **C**, is the only choice left and the obvious correct answer.

Preparing for Board Examinations

1. **Study for yourself**. Although some of the material may seem irrelevant, the more you learn now, the less you will have to learn later. Also, do not let the fear of the test rob you of an important part of your education. If you study to learn, the task is less distasteful than studying solely to pass a test.

2. **Review all areas.** You should not be selective by studying perceived weak areas and ignoring perceived strong areas. This is probably the last time you will have the time and the motivation to review **all** of the basic sciences.

3. **Attempt to understand**, **not just to memorize**, **the material.** Ask yourself: To whom does the material apply? When does it apply? Where does it apply? How does it apply? Understanding the connections among these points allows for longer retention and aids in those situations when guessing strategies may be needed.

4. Try to **anticipate questions that might appear on the test.** Ask yourself how you might construct a question on a specific topic.

5. **Give yourself a couple days of rest before the test.** Studying up to the last moment will increase your anxiety and cause potential confusion.

Taking Board Examinations

1. In the case of NBME exams, be sure to **pace yourself** to use the time optimally. As soon as you get your test booklet, go through and circle the questions numbered 40, 80, 120, and 160. The test is constructed so that you will have approximately 45 seconds for each question. If you are at a circled number every 30 minutes, you will be right on schedule. A 2-hour test will have 150–170 questions and a 2½-hour test will have approximately 200 questions. You should use all of your allotted time; if you finish too early, you probably did so by moving too quickly through the test.

2. **Read each question and all the alternatives carefully** before you begin to make decisions. Remember the questions contain clues, as do the answer choices. As a physician, you would not make a clinical decision without a complete examination of all the data; the same holds true for answering test questions.

3. **Read the directions for each question set carefully.** You would be amazed at how many students make mistakes in tests simply because they have not paid close attention to the directions.

4. It is not advisable to leave blanks with the intention of coming back to answer the questions later. Because of the way board examinations are constructed, you probably will not pick up any new information that will help you when you come back, and the chances of getting numerically off on your answer sheet are greater than your chances of benefiting by skipping around. If you feel that you must come back to a question, mark the best choice and place a note in the margin. Generally speaking, it is best not to change answers once you have made a decision, unless you have learned new information. Your intuitive reaction and first response are correct more often than changes made out of frustration or anxiety. **Never turn in an answer sheet with blanks**. Scores are based on the number that you get correct; you are not penalized for incorrect choices.

5. **Do not try to answer the questions on a stimulus–response basis.** It generally will not work. Use all of your learned knowledge.

6. **Do not let anxiety destroy your confidence.** If you have prepared conscientiously, you know enough to pass. Use all that you have learned.

7. **Do not try to determine how well you are doing as you proceed.** You will not be able to make an objective assessment, and your anxiety will increase.

8. **Do not expect a feeling of mastery** or anything close to what you are accustomed. Remember, this is a nationally administered exam, not a mastery test.

9. **Do not become frustrated or angry** about what appear to be bad or difficult questions. You simply do not know the answers; you cannot know everything.

Specific Test-Taking Strategies

Read the entire question carefully, regardless of format. Test questions have multiple parts. Concentrate on picking out the pertinent key words that might help you begin to problem solve. Words such as "always," "all," "never," "mostly," "primarily," and so forth play significant roles. In all types of questions, distractors with terms such as "always" or "never" most often are incorrect. Adjectives and adverbs can completely change the meaning of questions—pay close attention to them. Also, medical prefixes and suffixes (e.g., "hypo-," "hyper-," "-ectomy," "-itis") are sometimes at the root of the question. The knowledge and application of everyday English grammar often is the key to dissecting questions.

Multiple-Choice Questions

Read the question and the choices carefully to become familiar with the data as given. Remember, in multiple-choice questions there is one correct answer and there are four distractors, or incorrect answers. (Distractors are plausible and possibly correct or they would not be called distractors.) They are generally correct for part of the question but not for the entire question. Dissecting the question into parts aids in discerning these distractors.

If the correct answer is not immediately evident, begin eliminating the distractors. (Many students feel that they must always start at option A and make a decision before they move to B, thus forcing decisions they are not ready to make.) Your first decisions should be made on those choices you feel the most confident about.

Compare the choices to each part of the question. **To be wrong**, a choice needs to be incorrect for only part of the question. **To be correct**, it must be **totally** correct. If you believe a choice is partially incorrect, tentatively eliminate that choice. Make notes next to the choices regarding tentative decisions. One method is to place a minus sign next to the choices you are certain are incorrect and a plus sign next to those that potentially are correct. Finally, place a zero next to any choice you do not understand or need to come back to for further inspection. Do not feel that you must make final decisions until you have examined all choices carefully.

When you have eliminated as many choices as you can, decide which of those that are left has the highest probability of being correct. Remember to use paper-and-pencil differential diagnosis. Above all, be honest with yourself. If you do not know the answer, eliminate as many choices as possible and choose reasonably.

Multiple True–False Questions

Multiple true–false questions are not as difficult as some students make them. These are the questions in which you must mark:

> **A** if **1, 2, and 3** are correct,
> **B** if **1 and 3** are correct,
> **C** if **2 and 4** are correct,
> **D** if only **4** is correct, or
> **E** if **all** are correct.

Remember that the name for this type of question is multiple true–false and then use this concept. Become familiar with each choice and make notes. Then concentrate on the one choice you feel is definitely incorrect. If you can find one incorrect alternative, you can eliminate three choices immediately and be down to a fifty–fifty probability of guessing the correct answer. In this format, if choice 1 is incorrect, so is choice 3; they go together. Alternatively, if 1 is correct, so is 3. The combinations of alternatives are constant; they will not be mixed. You will not find a situation where choice 1 is correct, but 3 is incorrect.

After eliminating the choices you are sure are incorrect, concentrate on the choice that will make your final decision. For instance, if you discard choice 1, you have eliminated alternatives A, B, and E. This leaves C (2 and 4) and D (4 only). Concentrate on choice 2, and decide if it is true or false. Rereading and concentrating on choice 4 only wastes time; choice 2 will be the decision maker. (Take the path of least resistance and concentrate on the smallest possible number of items while making a decision.) Obviously, if none of the choices is found to be incorrect, the answer is E (all).

Comparison-Matching Questions

Comparison-matching questions are also easier to address if you concentrate on one alternative at a time. Choose option:

    A if the question is associated with **(A) only**,
    B if the question is associated with **(B) only**,
    C if the question is associated with **both (A) and (B)**, or
    D if the question is associated with **neither (A) nor (B)**.

Here again, the elimination of obvious wrong alternatives helps clear away needless information and can help you make a clearer decision.

Single Best Answer–Matching Sets

Single best answer–matching sets consist of a list of words or statements followed by several numbered items or statements. Be sure to pay attention to whether the choices can be used more than once, only once, or not at all. Consider each choice individually and carefully. Begin with those with which you are the most familiar. It is important always to break the statements and words into parts, as with all other question formats. **If a choice is only partially correct, then it is incorrect**.

Guessing

Nothing takes the place of a firm knowledge base, but with little information to work with, even after playing paper-and-pencil differential diagnosis, you may find it necessary to guess at the correct answer. A few simple rules can help increase your guessing accuracy. Always guess consistently if you have no idea what is correct; that is, after eliminating all that you can, make the choice that agrees with your intuition or choose the option closest to the top of the list that has not been eliminated as a potential answer.

When guessing at questions that present with choices in numerical form, you will often find the choices listed in an ascending or descending order. It is generally not wise to guess the first or last alternative, since these are usually extreme values and are most likely incorrect.

Using the Challenge Exam to Learn

All too often, students do not take full advantage of practice exams. There is a tendency to complete the exam, score it, look up the correct answers to those questions missed, and then forget the entire thing.

In fact, great educational benefits can be derived if students would spend more time using practice tests as learning tools. As mentioned earlier, incorrect choices in test questions are plausible and partially correct or they would not fulfill their purpose as distractors. This means that it is just as beneficial to look up the incorrect choices as the correct choices to discover specifically why they are incorrect. In this way, it is possible to learn better test-taking skills as the subtlety of question construction is uncovered.

Additionally, it is advisable to go back and attempt to restructure each question to see if all the choices can be made correct by modifying the question. By doing this, four times as much will be learned. By all means, look up the right answer and explanation. Then, focus on each of the other choices and ask yourself under what conditions they might be correct? For example, the entire thrust of the sample question concerning hypothyroidism could be altered by changing the first few words to read:

> "Hyperthyroidism recently discovered in. . . ."
> "Hypothyroidism prenatally occurring in. . . ."
> "Hypothyroidism resulting from. . . ."

This question can be used to learn and understand thyroid problems in general, not only to memorize answers to specific questions.

The Challenge Exam that follows contains 180 questions and explanations. Every effort has been made to simulate the types of questions and the degree of question difficulty in the various licensure and qualifying exams (i.e., NBME Parts I, II, and III and FLEX). While taking this exam, the student should attempt to create the testing conditions that might be experienced during actual testing situations. Approximately 1 minute should be allowed for each question, and the entire test should be finished before it is scored.

Summary

Ideally, examinations are designed to determine how much information students have learned and how that information is used in the successful completion of the examination. Students will be successful if these suggestions are followed:

- Develop a positive attitude and maintain that attitude.
- Be realistic in determining the amount of material you attempt to master and in the score you hope to attain.
- Read the directions for each type of question and the questions themselves closely and follow the directions carefully.
- Guess intelligently and consistently when guessing strategies must be used.
- Bring the paper-and-pencil differential diagnosis approach to each question in the examination.

- Use the test as an opportunity to display your knowledge and as a tool for developing prescriptions for further study and learning.

National Board examinations are not easy. They may be almost impossible for those who have unrealistic expectations or for those who allow misinformation concerning the exams to produce anxiety out of proportion to the task at hand. They are manageable if they are approached with a positive attitude and with consistent use of all the information the student has learned.

Michael P. O'Donnell

QUESTIONS

Directions: Each question below contains five suggested answers. Choose the **one best** response to each question.

1. When evaluating patients in a psychiatric emergency, it is always necessary to

(A) search patients for weapons
(B) restrain patients
(C) tell patients to control themselves
(D) ask patients to change into hospital clothes
(E) have trained help available

2. A 35-year-old man with an obsessive–compulsive personality disorder is likely to exhibit all of the following symptoms EXCEPT

(A) perfectionism that interferes with performance
(B) compulsive checking behavior
(C) preoccupation and concern for rules
(D) indecisiveness
(E) stinginess with compliments

3. Premature ejaculation is defined most accurately by which of the following statements?

(A) The cause is usually psychological, and the disorder has been "learned" by the patient
(B) The disorder has become relatively uncommon
(C) It is the inability of the partner to achieve orgasm more than 50% of the time
(D) It can be diagnosed if the man cannot sustain intercourse for more than 30 minutes
(E) It is generally associated with arousal of the parasympathetic nervous system

4. A 41-year-old man has suffered from dissatisfaction and unhappiness over the past 9 years and complains that he is not getting all he wants out of life. He was depressed briefly 12 years ago after he stopped seeing a girlfriend. The most likely diagnosis is

(A) major depression
(B) secondary dysthymia
(C) bipolar disorder, depressed
(D) primary dysthymia
(E) cyclothymia

5. A psychiatrist is asked to speak to a pair of identical twins. One of the twins has developed schizophrenia, and the psychiatrist is aware that the chances of the other twin developing schizophrenia are

(A) 95%
(B) no greater than the risk for the general population
(C) the same as they would be for a nontwin sibling
(D) between 35% and 70%
(E) almost certain

6. Early in the psychiatric interview, it is most important for the physician to

(A) inform patients of the fee
(B) obtain details of past psychiatric illnesses
(C) let patients talk about what is bothering them
(D) ask patients about legal issues associated with their problems
(E) inquire about the patients' feelings as well as historic facts

7. Someone who exhibits pathologic jealousy, is overly concerned about hidden meanings, and expects to be tricked is demonstrating signs of

(A) a schizotypal personality
(B) a paranoid personality
(C) a schizoid personality
(D) an antisocial personality
(E) none of the above

8. While a detailed history cannot always be obtained in crisis evaluations, the physician should always ask about

(A) previous violence
(B) previous hospitalizations
(C) truancy in school
(D) abuse in childhood
(E) none of the above

9. A 60-year-old man is brought to the emergency room by relatives who had just come to visit him from out of town. For a number of weeks, or perhaps longer, the relatives believe that he has been hearing and seeing things that were not there, particularly visions of people. His level of self-care has deteriorated markedly. He has no history of treatment for psychiatric disorders, although the relatives noted that after his wife died a decade ago he became somewhat withdrawn and isolated and less social than previously. All of the following diagnoses are possible EXCEPT

(A) delirium
(B) schizophrenia
(C) dementia
(D) major depressive episode
(E) organic mental syndrome with mixed features

10. All of the following statements about gender identity are true EXCEPT

(A) gender identity is set by 1 year of age
(B) the early embryo is undifferentiated sexually (i.e., it is bisexual)
(C) gender identity refers to one's sense of being masculine or feminine
(D) an infant is assigned a gender identity on the basis of genitalia
(E) the Y chromosome is necessary for the development of male genitalia

11. Anaclitic depression is most apt to result

(A) when an attachment relationship is disrupted during the first 6 months of life
(B) from the absence of attachment in the first year of life
(C) when an attachment relationship is disrupted between the ages of 7 and 30 months
(D) when an attachment relationship is disrupted anytime during childhood
(E) None of the above

12. A 23-year-old woman reports that she has been troubled by episodes during which she feels apprehensive and which usually occur in the morning. Her heart rate increases. She sweats excessively. Agitation and restlessness are prominent. Which of the following laboratory tests should be ordered?

(A) Thyroid function tests
(B) A toxicologic screen
(C) Measurement of serum sodium level
(D) Measurement of serum glucose level
(E) Measurement of serum ammonia level

13. Which of the following abnormalities is a manifestation of barbiturate intoxication but not of barbiturate withdrawal?

(A) Confusion
(B) Nystagmus
(C) Postural hypotension
(D) Disorientation
(E) Agitation

14. In a family therapy session for a patient with anorexia nervosa, the father reveals that he has sexually molested the 13-year-old patient. You should

(A) let the family know that this is inappropriate behavior that must be stopped and follow up on the family's compliance within 1 week
(B) immediately leave the session to report the abuse to the child protective service agency
(C) recommend individual psychiatric treatment for the father
(D) tell the family that you and they should continue discussing the problem, reporting it only if it persists
(E) none of the above

15. Recent studies indicate that the highest suicide rates are among

(A) young white women
(B) young white men
(C) young black men
(D) elderly white women
(E) elderly white men

16. Which of the following statements concerning the course and prognosis of schizophrenia is true?

(A) The slower the onset of symptoms of schizophrenia, the better the long-term prognosis
(B) Patients with hebephrenic symptoms tend to do better than those with paranoid symptoms
(C) The outcome on schizophrenia tends to be better in Third World countries than in developed countries.
(D) Male patients with schizophrenia tend to do better than female patients
(E) None of the above

17. Personality disorders are almost always

(A) Manifested during adolescence
(B) worse in old age
(C) free of genetic–biologic influences
(D) associated with good occupational functioning
(E) seen intermittently in adult life

18. All of the following conditions are considered disorders of bonding and attachment EXCEPT

(A) autistic disorder
(B) hospitalism
(C) anaclitic depression
(D) vulnerable child syndrome
(E) child abuse

19. A 40-year-old businessman from another city arrives in the emergency room complaining of severe, chronic migraine headaches, which are relieved only by meperidine. His primary physician is unavailable by telephone. The emergency room physician should ask about all of the following conditions EXCEPT

(A) hallucinations and delusions
(B) legal problems
(C) losing prescriptions
(D) loss of consciousness
(E) use of alcohol

20. Slow wave activity on the electroencephalogram is commonly present in

(A) dementia
(B) delirium
(C) schizophrenia
(D) alcohol withdrawal
(E) human immunodeficiency virus

21. A 34-year-old woman visits her physician in December and describes another recurrence of depression in late autumn. The most likely mechanism for her depression is

(A) excess of noradrenergic activity
(B) diminished serotonergic activity
(C) disruption of circadian rhythms
(D) aberrant patterns of family relationships
(E) none of the above

22. A 15-year-old boy with a history of recurrent tonsillitis is brought to his physician with complaints of irritability, difficulty in school, and emotional outbursts. He is observed to grimace often. The indicated medical treatment is

(A) salicylates
(B) lithium carbonate
(C) penicillin
(D) L-dopa
(E) haloperidol

23. A young woman with anorexia nervosa steadfastly refuses to eat. She is not yet in imminent medical danger from starvation, and she remains an outpatient. A logical approach at this point would be to

(A) break off treatment with the patient, refusing to treat her unless she agrees to eat
(B) set a critical weight for the patient below which she will be hospitalized if necessary and forced to gain weight
(C) insist that the patient must increase her caloric intake or she will be hospitalized
(D) try to curtail her physical activities (e.g., running and dancing)
(E) none of the above

24. What percentage of patients who commit suicide have a concurrent medical illness?

(A) 20%
(B) 45%
(C) 50%
(D) 70%
(E) 85%

25. Symptoms of mania include all of the following EXCEPT

(A) pressured speech
(B) creativity
(C) expansiveness
(D) homicidal ideation
(E) paranoid delusions

26. A 6-year-old boy presents with acute onset of hyperactivity of 1-month duration. It is noted in the history that the behavioral change followed a few days after the child's first grand mal seizure. The next step in the physician's evaluation should be to

(A) perform a sleep-deprived electroencephalogram with N-P leads
(B) take a medication history
(C) prescribe a CT scan of the head
(D) consult a pediatric neurologist
(E) add carbamazepine to the drug regimen

27. A 28-year-old woman presents with complaints of irritability and moodiness. She gives a history of brief episodes during which she hears voices and is excessively suspicious of others. Her speech is slightly slurred. Which of the following conditions is the most likely diagnosis?

(A) Hyperparathyroidism
(B) Lead intoxication
(C) Wilson's disease
(D) Folate deficiency
(E) Sydenham's chorea

28. A 25-year-old woman who has been hospitalized for 5 years in the state hospital complains that men are constantly telling her to perform sexual acts. She hears these men in the room with the examiner. At other times, she stands in front of a mirror for hours at a time, smearing lipstick over much of her face and grinning in an unusual way. She believes that the ward staff can read her thoughts and puts inappropriate thoughts into her mind. At other times, she feels her thoughts leave her head and go out to objects in the room. Her speech is almost incomprehensible and is filled with made-up words. When she is confronted with subjects that may be difficult or painful for her, she tends to giggle and often runs away. Presuming that no other significant patterns of symptoms have been observed other than those noted above, the most likely diagnosis is schizophrenia

(A) paranoid type
(B) residual type
(C) undifferentiated type
(D) catatonic type
(E) disorganized type

29. Paraphilias are best characterized by which of the following statements?

(A) Patients feel little shame or guilt
(B) These disorders occur with equal frequency in men and women
(C) The etiology is thought to be genetic
(D) Depression is a common finding
(E) Patients see themselves as "sick"

30. Recent biologic studies of patients who attempt suicide by violent means have demonstrated

(A) low levels of epinephrine in the cerebrospinal fluid
(B) low levels of 5-hydroxyindoleacetic acid in the cerebrospinal fluid
(C) high levels of norepinephrine in the cerebrospinal fluid
(D) low levels of dopamine in the brain
(E) high levels of most biogenic amines in the brain

31. The hospital management of anorectic patients commonly includes all of the following EXCEPT

(A) restriction of privileges
(B) nasogastric alimentation
(C) locked seclusion
(D) weight monitoring
(E) ketone monitoring

32. A routine psychiatric evaluation of a patient consists of all of the following steps EXCEPT

(A) a careful physical examination is conducted
(B) data are gathered from the interview
(C) a history of the problem is obtained
(D) a differential diagnosis is developed
(E) a treatment plan is constructed

33. A middle-aged woman has been treated for a number of years by various physicians for insomnia. On the night of admission to the hospital for elective surgery, she becomes anxious and agitated. There is no evidence of bleeding, infection, or neurologic disease, but the patient develops postural hypotension and fever. Administration of which of the following substances might be appropriate at this point?

(A) Diazepam
(B) Haloperidol
(C) Disulfiram
(D) Phenobarbital
(E) Thiamine

34. A 58-year-old man is brought to the hospital for evaluation of an acute confusional state. He is noted to be tachycardic and has dry skin and mucous membranes. He is restless and agitated. The most likely cause for this syndrome is

(A) reserpine toxicity
(B) scopolamine toxicity
(C) L-dopa toxicity
(D) disulfiram toxicity
(E) benzodiazepine toxicity

35. Diagnostic findings consistent with anorexia nervosa include all of the following EXCEPT

(A) normal serum protein and albumin levels
(B) hyperkalemia
(C) normal serum cortisol
(D) bradycardia, hypotension, hypothermia
(E) hypercarotenemia

36. All of the following statements concerning autistic disorder are true EXCEPT

(A) incidence appears to be highest in upper socioeconomic strata
(B) it occurs more commonly in boys than in girls
(C) it appears to be a neurologically based syndrome
(D) Mental retardation may or may not occur
(E) Grand mal seizures frequently occur

37. A 26-year-old woman presents to the emergency room with shortness of breath, dizziness, and tingling in her fingers for which no organic cause can be found. The psychiatric diagnosis that would most immediately explain her symptoms is

(A) situational reaction
(B) endogenous anxiety
(C) caffeinism
(D) hyperventilation syndrome
(E) post-traumatic stress disorder

38. During an interview with a patient, the physician makes the following statement: "During the past month, you have increased your drinking to a pint of alcohol per day, and in the past 3 days, you have been contemplating suicide." This is an example of

(A) facilitation
(B) clarification
(C) summarization
(D) interpretation
(E) open-ended question

39. A 27-year-old schizophrenic woman suffers from an increased frequency of psychotic episodes and rehospitalization when attempts are made to return her to her family. A therapist believes the family to be typical of a high expressed emotionality family. Reasonable treatment approaches to reduce this risk factor for rehospitalization include all of the following EXCEPT

(A) encouraging the family to join the Alliance for the Mentally Ill
(B) initiating a psychoeducational program for the family around managing the illness of schizophrenia
(C) decreasing the frequency of contact between the patient and family by arranging a placement outside the home
(D) encouraging the patient's mother to enter psychotherapy
(E) encouraging the family to go into therapy to reduce deviant communications

40. Which of the following prognoses is most accurate for anorexia nervosa?

(A) Most patients recover
(B) Most girls recover, but very few boys recover
(C) The earlier the onset in life, the better the outcome of the disease
(D) By the age of 30 years, 30%–40% of patients die
(E) None of the above

41. Amphetamine psychosis is characterized by all of the following EXCEPT

(A) mania
(B) loose associations
(C) clear sensorium
(D) tactile hallucinations
(E) paranoia

42. All of the following drugs are contraindicated in patients who are intoxicated with alcohol EXCEPT

(A) diazepam
(B) phenobarbital
(C) disulfiram
(D) glutethimide
(E) haloperidol

43. The classic psychosomatic illnesses include all of the following EXCEPT

(A) essential hypertension
(B) rheumatoid arthritis
(C) hyperventilation
(D) thyrotoxicosis
(E) neurodermatitis

44. Individuals who episodically lose control and assault another person with little or no provocation but who are then genuinely remorseful most likely have

(A) a bipolar disorder–manic type
(B) an antisocial personality
(C) a paranoid disorder
(D) an intermittent explosive disorder
(E) an organic mental disorder

45. Common medical complications of bulimia nervosa include all of the following EXCEPT

(A) metabolic acidosis
(B) parotitis
(C) caries
(D) esophagitis
(E) oligomenorrhea

46. Echolalia is an example of

(A) psychomotor retardation
(B) an uncooperative attitude
(C) a speech impairment
(D) monotone speech
(E) a rapid rate of speech

47. An individual with a schizoid personality disorder may do well in which of the following circumstances?

(A) When hospitalized for a medical illness
(B) In social situations, such as dating
(C) If others reach out to them affectionately
(D) If treated with antidepressants
(E) In jobs that require social isolation

Questions 48 and 49

An attractive 32-year-old single woman has come to the emergency department accompanied by a friend. With prompting, she reports having been raped at knife point several hours earlier. Although her friend is quite upset, the patient is telling her story with considerable composure and detachment. She is acting as though she is not particularly concerned about the whole matter.

48. The patient's behavior indicates that she

(A) wants to forget about the attack
(B) has put the episode behind her and wants to get on with her life
(C) was not really raped but probably encouraged the man
(D) is in a protective state of numbing and denial
(E) needs to be pushed to reveal her true feelings

49. Two months later, the same patient returns to the emergency department complaining of difficulty sleeping. She requests medication to help her sleep and fears that she might be going crazy because of repetitive nightmares. The most appropriate treatment at this time would be to

(A) give the patient 1 month's supply of sleeping pills and have her return at the end of the month if she is still having trouble sleeping
(B) encourage the patient to talk about the traumatic experience before she leaves the emergency room
(C) refer the patient for psychological testing to determine if she has evidence of a psychotic depression
(D) reassure the patient that her symptoms are expected and recommend psychotherapy to work through the event
(E) confront the patient about the addictive potential of sleeping medication and encourage her to try to sleep without it

(end of group question)

50. A 14-year-old girl with anorexia nervosa is at risk for serious medical complications from starvation. She refuses to be hospitalized. The physician's next step should be to

(A) continue the efforts at outpatient treatment
(B) place a hold on the patient and force her to come into the hospital against her will
(C) refer the patient to a colleague with the hope that he or she will have more success
(D) have the parents sign a release absolving you of responsibility for the case
(E) trick the patient into being admitted by telling her that you will not say anything about food or weight while she is an inpatient

51. The treatment of bulimia nervosa is most accurately described by which of the following statements?

(A) Hospitalization is regularly indicated
(B) Adjunctive medications are regularly prescribed
(C) Individual psychodynamic psychotherapy is seldom adequate
(D) Group psychotherapy is usually the treatment of choice
(E) Mixed modality treatment appears to offer promising results

52. Tactile hallucinations of insects crawling under the skin are called

(A) hypnagogic
(B) hypnopompic
(C) formication
(D) kinesthetic
(E) gustatory

53. The first measure that should be taken in the treatment of encopresis is to

(A) determine if the child has an impaction
(B) help the child understand his or her anger
(C) perform a rectal examination to rule out Hirschsprung's disease
(D) assure the parents that the child is not soiling deliberately
(E) recommend negative reinforcement for soiling behavior

54. The diagnosis of self-defeating personality disorder should not be made if the individual

(A) is in a setting of physical abuse
(B) provokes rejection from others
(C) is not interested in a caring relationship
(D) avoids pleasure
(E) rejects attempts by others to help

55. All of the following statements regarding electroconvulsive therapy (ECT) are true EXCEPT

(A) ECT is an effective treatment in more than 90% of appropriately treated patients
(B) the mechanism of action of ECT is unknown
(C) ECT is an accepted treatment for patients with mania who are not responsive to other treatment
(D) previous successful treatment with ECT is an indication for subsequent ECT
(E) depressed patients with psychotic features do not respond to ECT

56. Failure to thrive is most often caused by

(A) psychological factors
(B) hypothyroidism
(C) fetal alcohol syndrome
(D) constitutional factors
(E) Addison's disease

57. The dexamethasone suppression test can be used to

(A) diagnose schizophrenia
(B) follow the treatment course in bipolar illness
(C) treat refractory depression
(D) follow the treatment course in depression
(E) diagnose the presence of depression

58. A 20-year-old man is admitted to an inpatient unit with a first episode of hallucinations, delusions of a persecutory nature, agitation, combativeness, and a history of these symptoms building over a 3-week period. Depending on what other information is available from relatives, history from friends, and laboratory testing, possible diagnoses include all of the following EXCEPT

(A) brief reactive psychosis
(B) organic mental syndrome
(C) borderline personality disorder
(D) schizophrenia
(E) schizophreniform disorder

59. Treatment modalities that are usually helpful for post-traumatic stress disorder include all of the following EXCEPT

(A) patient discussion of the precipitating event
(B) relaxation techniques
(C) biofeedback techniques
(D) use of propanediols
(E) use of monoamine oxidase inhibitors

60. The concurrent presence of a mood disorder is more likely in which of the following personality disorders?

(A) Schizoid personality
(B) Paranoid personality
(C) Borderline personality
(D) Avoidant personality
(E) Antisocial personality

61. The most important reason to monitor lithium levels is

(A) to check on patient compliance
(B) because the toxic dose is similar to the therapeutic level
(C) because lithium is rapidly excreted from the body
(D) because lithium is a salt rather than a drug
(E) none of the above

Questions 62 and 63

62. A patient hospitalized for gastritis is found during his last outpatient appointment to have a slightly enlarged liver. Appropriate initial blood tests would include all of the following EXCEPT

(A) hemoglobin
(B) blood alcohol level
(C) blood cultures
(D) drug screen
(E) liver function tests

63. Although the blood alcohol level of the patient is 10 mg/100 ml, there is no evidence of intoxication. It is a reasonable assumption that the patient

(A) has a tolerance to narcotics
(B) is dependent on alcohol
(C) has pancreatitis
(D) is impotent
(E) has cerebral atrophy

(end of group question)

64. Which of the following statements concerning neuroleptic medications is true?

(A) Neuroleptics are equally effective in treating positive and negative symptoms of schizophrenia
(B) All neuroleptics run the risk of causing tardive dyskinesia
(C) If a patient fails to respond to a particular neuroleptic, it is accepted practice to add one or more different neuroleptics to the treatment regimen
(D) "Drug holidays," consisting of an number of days on a neuroleptic with several days off, have been shown to be an effective way to reduce the risk of tardive dyskinesia
(E) For acute psychotic episodes, there is substantial evidence that rapid neuroleptization to high dosage levels is likely to produce much more rapid and effective control of symptoms than moderate sustained neuroleptic dosages

65. A 35-year-old man is found to have injected himself with foreign matter for no apparent reason, but he denies this. The most likely diagnosis is

(A) hypochondriasis
(B) malingering
(C) somatization disorder
(D) conversion disorder
(E) factitious disorder

66. Homosexuality is characterized by all of the following statements EXCEPT

(A) approximately 4% of men in the United States are exclusively homosexual
(B) over one-third of males have had an orgasm with a partner of the same sex at least once
(C) there is a higher incidence of some mental illnesses, such as mood disorders, in homosexuals than in heterosexuals
(D) there is a higher incidence of some physical illnesses, such as hepatitis, in homosexuals than in heterosexuals
(E) treatment aimed at changing homosexual to heterosexual preference is generally unsuccessful

67. All of the following statements concerning family interactional research in schizophrenia are correct EXCEPT

(A) families with high expressed emotionality appear to present a risk for relapse for schizophrenic family members, approximately four times that of low expressed emotionality families
(B) communications deviance and affective style appear to be better predictors for the development of schizophrenia spectrum disorders in family members than expressed emotionality
(C) double-bind communications from mothers has been found to produce schizophrenia in children with prolonged exposure to it
(D) the Finnish Adoption Study has produced preliminary data, which support the contention that children of schizophrenic mothers bear a genetic vulnerability to disordered interactions in the rearing environment
(E) psychoeducational approaches appear to be able to reverse the effects of high expressed emotionality on the relapse rates for schizophrenic family members

68. Cluster A, the odd or eccentric group of personality disorders, includes schizoid, schizotypal, and

(A) histrionic personalities
(B) borderline personalities
(C) paranoid personalities
(D) passive–aggressive personalities
(E) antisocial personalities

69. When a sexual history must be taken from a patient, it is most important that the physician

(A) find out about family attitudes towards sex
(B) evaluate the status of the patient's relationship with his or her spouse
(C) diagnose any medical condition that might interfere with sex
(D) overcome nervousness and embarrassment
(E) take an open, nonjudgmental stance in listening to the patient

70. Precipitating events for psychotic episodes that are later diagnosed as part of a schizophrenic illness include all of the following EXCEPT

(A) alcohol abuse
(B) major psychosocial stressors
(C) a major depressive episode
(D) traumatic life events
(E) use of psychomotor stimulants

71. Psychotherapy of the schizophrenic should include all of the following elements EXCEPT

(A) a warm, open relationship aimed at promoting the patient's self-esteem and educating the patient about his or her illness
(B) a supportive psychotherapeutic technique that focuses on resolving problems in the daily life of the schizophrenic patient
(C) setting concrete limits on the behavior of the patient, including the consequences of violent or threatening actions
(D) encouraging increased socialization with people in the community to build more extensive social networks
(E) encouraging the patient to express anger and hostility as much as possible in the therapeutic relationship in order to reduce affective pressure for relationships outside of the therapeutic setting

Directions: Each question below contains four suggested answers of which **one or more** is correct. Choose the answer

A	if **1, 2, and 3** are correct
B	if **1 and 3** are correct
C	if **2 and 4** are correct
D	if **4** is correct
E	if **1, 2, 3, and 4** are correct

72. Established psychotherapeutic treatments for depression focus on

(1) addiction to drugs and alcohol
(2) maladaptive interpersonal relationships
(3) difficulty with social standards
(4) incorrect perceptions and thinking

73. The mental status examination differs from the psychiatric history in that the mental status examination evaluates

(1) the patient at one point in time
(2) interpersonal relationships
(3) observable signs of mental illness
(4) developmental milestones and their effect on current functioning

74. The withdrawal–conservation behavioral response is characterized by

(1) decreased activity
(2) increased susceptibility to illness
(3) decreased metabolism
(4) depression

75. Causes of secondary enuresis include

(1) juvenile-onset diabetes mellitus
(2) a urinary tract infection
(3) psychological factors
(4) spina bifida occulta

SUMMARY OF DIRECTIONS

A	B	C	D	E
1, 2, 3 only	1, 3 only	2, 4 only	4 only	All are correct

76. A 25-year-old man has had longstanding fears of humiliating himself in social interactions. As a result, he has become increasingly isolated and shy. Recently, he has found himself wishing he were dead and has been waking up early in the morning. Appropriate drug treatments might include

(1) benzodiazepines
(2) atenolol
(3) antihistamines
(4) monoamine oxidase inhibitors

77. A 43-year-old man is hospitalized for foot surgery. When he is interviewed by the nursing staff he states that he is married, has three children, and lives with his family. He had previously told his physician that he has been living with his father since separating from his girlfriend and her two children. When asked about this discrepancy, he becomes flustered and confused. Then he tells the questioner that he will be returning to his home in another state after surgery. Conditions that are likely to account for this patient's confabulation include

(1) Korsakoff's psychosis
(2) diabetes mellitus
(3) presenile dementia
(4) Addison's disease

78. Anticholinergic poisoning is characterized by

(1) warm, dry skin
(2) mydriasis
(3) psychosis
(4) tachycardia

79. Current research demonstrates a likely role in schizophrenia for which of the following neurotransmitter systems?

(1) Dopamine
(2) Neuropeptides
(3) γ-Aminobutyric acid (GABA)
(4) Dopamine optical isomers

80. The ethical and legal principles of medical care involved in the *Tarasoff* decision include which of the following?

(1) Whatever is said in therapy is confidential
(2) Patients who threaten violence must be hospitalized
(3) Potential victims of violence must be warned
(4) Sexual relations between therapists and patients are prohibited

81. Perceptual abnormalities include

(1) hallucinations
(2) depersonalizations
(3) illusions
(4) perseverations

82. Correct statements about the management of somatoform pain disorder include which of the following?

(1) It benefits from a multidisciplinary approach
(2) Sedatives are used to decrease anxiety
(3) Success is related to the duration of symptoms
(4) Behavior therapy decreases the patient's perception of pain

83. A 62-year-old man visits his physician with complaints of fatigue, inactivity, weight loss, and abdominal discomfort. He appears to be depressed. Possible causes for this presentation include

(1) dementia
(2) aspirin abuse
(3) pancreatic cancer
(4) hyperthyroidism

84. Treatment approaches to substance abuse and dependence include

(1) detoxification
(2) controlled use of the substance
(3) family therapy
(4) visits at the patient's discretion

Questions 85–87

A 17-year-old boy was brought to the emergency room by his father after admitting that he had taken three of his father's sleeping pills [30 mg of flurazepam (Dalmane)] in a suicide attempt. He was medically cleared with the physicians and nurses making jokes about "a three Dalmane overdose." The patient appeared depressed, but he minimized the episode, saying that he was just upset about school. The father was angry about "running up a bill for nothing" and was impatient to take his son back home. Both were resistant to a psychiatric evaluation.

85. Since neither the patient nor his father wanted to stay and since the overdose was not life-threatening, the most apppropriate treatment at this time would include

(1) calling other family members to come to the hospital
(2) referring the boy to the school counselor to discuss his academic problems
(3) insisting that the father and son stay to be interviewed individually
(4) encouraging the father to watch out for his son

86. Additional treatment approaches at this point would include

(1) beginning antidepressant therapy since the medication takes 10–14 days to be effective
(2) encouraging the father to hide his sleeping pills and other medications
(3) giving the son an excuse from school for a couple of days so that he may rest
(4) suggesting family counseling to help to relieve tensions

87. The boy remained silent, and the father continued to insist on going home. The decision was made to send the boy home with his father. He was brought in the following morning dead from a self-inflicted gunshot wound to the head. The father had left his loaded revolver in his dresser before going to work. This case represents errors in suicide evaluation, including

(1) not adequately evaluating the son's feelings about being alive
(2) not appreciating the meaning of the suicide attempt for both the son and the father
(3) not assessing adequately the father's capacity to be a resource and support
(4) not immediately hospitalizing the patient against his will

(end of group question)

88. Risk factors for somatization disorder include

(1) female gender
(2) alcoholism in first-degree male relatives
(3) unstable early environment
(4) Caucasian race

89. Paraphilias are thought to be etiologically related to

(1) excessive sexual drive
(2) learned behavior
(3) family history of antisocial personality
(4) early developmental problems

90. Conditions that increase the risk for subdural hematomas include

(1) hypertension
(2) senility
(3) atherosclerosis
(4) alcoholism

91. The relationship between anxiety and depression is characterized by which of the following statements?

(1) Many depressed people are also anxious
(2) Many patients with panic disorder become depressed
(3) The same treatments may be effective for panic anxiety and depression
(4) There is familial transmission of panic and depression

92. The sleep lab (polysomnography) has been useful in studying which of the following conditions?

(1) Seizure disorders
(2) Impotence
(3) Depression
(4) Schizophrenia

93. Disorders characterized by the voluntary control of symptoms include

(1) malingering
(2) conversion disorder
(3) factitious illness
(4) somatization disorder

SUMMARY OF DIRECTIONS

A	B	C	D	E
1, 2, 3 only	1, 3 only	2, 4 only	4 only	All are correct

---

94. A 35-year-old man comes into the emergency room complaining that he has heard a voice at night telling him that he is a bad and guilty person. With no further information, the clinician should seriously consider which of the following possibilities in the differential diagnosis?

(1) Brief reactive psychosis or schizophreniform disorder
(2) A mood disorder
(3) A personality disorder
(4) A normal cultural variant of a certain culture

95. A 27-year-old woman who recently moved to a new city becomes depressed with symptoms of weight loss and suicidal ideation. In planning the initial phase of treatment, it is crucial to consider which of the following factors?

(1) The possibility of weight gain on tricyclic antidepressants
(2) A history of spending sprees and hypersexuality
(3) A family history of alcoholism
(4) Social supports available to the patient in her new home

96. Biofeedback treatment of essential hypertension is characterized by which of the following statements?

(1) It involves learning awareness of blood pressure changes
(2) It results in significant changes in blood pressure
(3) It uses relaxation techniques
(4) It is a practical treatment for hypertension

97. Antidepressant medications thought to have a therapeutic window, that is, a therapeutic response that increases to a certain blood level then decreases, include

(1) nortriptyline
(2) imipramine
(3) amitriptyline
(4) desipramine

98. Methods of treating autistic disorder include

(1) electroconvulsive therapy
(2) behavior modification
(3) imipramine administration
(4) psychotherapy

99. Correct statements about transsexualism include which of the following?

(1) It is an expression of homosexuality
(2) Crossdressing is necessary for sexual arousal
(3) Biologic factors are significant in its etiology
(4) It is associated with early developmental disturbance

100. The clinical laboratory is important in the diagnosis and treatment of mental disorders. Important functions include

(1) identifying biologic markers of psychiatric illness
(2) monitoring blood levels of psychotropic medications
(3) screening for other medical illnesses
(4) assessing the severity of psychiatric illness

101. Interventions that are effective in protecting a child when physical abuse is suspected include

(1) hospitalizing the child
(2) placing the child outside the home
(3) hospitalizing the abusive patient
(4) initiating family therapy

102. Common complications of alcoholism include

(1) brain damage
(2) gastritis
(3) hypertension
(4) suicide

103. Conditions that may cause an organic anxiety syndrome include

(1) sedative–hypnotic withdrawal
(2) pheochromocytoma
(3) caffeine use
(4) hypoparathyroidism

104. A few days after a mastectomy, an attractive 45-year-old woman is heavily made-up, wearing a flimsy negligee, and making seductive comments to her 25-year-old intern. She was remarried 1 year previously after divorcing her first husband for seeing a younger woman. She has no previous psychiatric history. Factors attributable to her behavior that should be considered first include

(1) anxiety that her new husband may no longer find her attractive
(2) acute schizophrenic psychosis
(3) acute organic mental syndrome
(4) stranger anxiety

histrionic person. disorder

105. Complications of somatization disorder include

(1) excessive use of medication
(2) iatrogenic illness secondary to invasive diagnostic procedures
(3) overuse of health resources
(4) frequent physician disengagement

106. Correct statements concerning the epidemiology of schizophrenia include which of the following?

(1) The outcome for schizophrenia tends to be better in the industrialized nations than in Third World countries
(2) In the Third World, women appear to suffer from schizophrenia at a rate higher then men
(3) Mortality rates for schizophrenia tend to be roughly that of the general population
(4) The sex ratio for the incidence of schizophrenia is roughly 1:1 in the industrialized countries

107. Projective tests used in psychological evaluations include the

(1) Rorschach Test
(2) Thematic Apperception Test
(3) Sentence Completion Test
(4) Draw-a-Person Test

108. Erectile failure is common in men who have

(1) a prostatectomy
(2) coronary artery disease
(3) an orchiectomy
(4) lupus erythematosus

109. Signs and symptoms found in the syndrome of hospitalism include

(1) severe inanition in infancy
(2) absence of bonding
(3) susceptibility to infection
(4) jaundice

110. Night terrors are characterized by which of the following statements?

(1) Children are characteristically inconsolable during night terrors
(2) They are characterized by vivid recall of the content of the dream
(3) They may be successfully treated with sedative-hypnotic medications
(4) They occur only rarely in children of preschool age

111. The concept of a type A personality is associated with which of the following characteristics?

(1) Impatience
(2) Hostility
(3) Driven quality
(4) Increased incidence of coronary artery disease

112. Individuals with personality disorders in the emotional, dramatic, and erratic group (cluster B) often use which of the following defense mechanisms?

(1) Dissociation
(2) Denial
(3) Splitting
(4) Acting out

113. Results of the Epidemiologic Catchment Area (ECA) study include which of the following?

(1) At least 25% of the general public will suffer from a psychiatric illness sometime during their lifetime
(2) Women have higher rates of psychiatric illness during their lives than men
(3) Men have more difficulty with substance abuse than women
(4) Men and women have the same rates of depressive illness

SUMMARY OF DIRECTIONS

A	B	C	D	E
1, 2, 3 only	1, 3 only	2, 4 only	4 only	All are correct

114. Common causes of inhibited female orgasm include

(1) lack of information
(2) major psychopathology
(3) disturbance in the primary relationship
(4) side effects of medications

115. Medications useful in the treatment of withdrawal from alcohol or other sedative-hypnotic drugs include

(1) diazepam
(2) haloperidol
(3) amobarbital
(4) lithium

116. Psychological theorists postulate that anorexia nervosa represents a symptomatic expression of

(1) psychosexual conflicts
(2) psychological conflicts with the mother
(3) disordered self-regulation
(4) psychological conflicts with the father

117. The widespread use of positron emission tomography is limited by

(1) nonspecific biochemical activity in the brain
(2) lesions less than 0.5 cm, which cannot be seen
(3) a lack of anatomic detail of the brain scans
(4) an expensive cylotron, which is needed to prepare compounds for the study

118. The initial treatment of conversion disorder involves

(1) education about the effect of stress on the symptoms
(2) suggestion that the symptoms will improve
(3) reassurance about the prognosis
(4) confrontation about psychological issues

119. Problems that are the hallmark of the borderline personality disorder include

(1) an instability of self-image
(2) a sense of entitlement
(3) impulsive behavior
(4) interpersonal exploitation

120. In families with a history of schizophrenia, there is also an increase in the number of relatives with which of the following personality disorders?

(1) Schizoid personality
(2) Antisocial personality
(3) Paranoid personality
(4) Schizotypal personality

121. True statements about sexual abuse include

(1) father– (or stepfather–) daughter incest is most common
(2) sexual abuse often precipitates running away from home
(3) sexual abuse may present as vaginal trauma
(4) children are often ashamed of their incestuous activity

Questions 122–124

Match each disorder with its most likely etiology.

(A) Reactive etiology
(B) Genetic/neurologic etiology
(C) Both
(D) Neither

122. Autistic disorder

123. Attention-deficit hyperactivity disorder

124. Symbiotic psychosis

Questions 125–130

For each clinical characteristic listed below, select the eating disorder with which it is most likely to be associated.

(A) Anorexia nervosa
(B) Bulimia nervosa
(C) Both
(D) Neither

125. Cathartic abuse

126. Male predominance

127. Significant mortality

128. Preoccupation with weight

129. Pharmacologically responsive

130. Concomitant substance abuse

Directions: The groups of questions below consist of lettered choices followed by several numbered items. For each numbered item, select the one lettered choice with which it is most closely associated. Each lettered choice may be used once, more than once, or not at all. Choose the answer

Questions 131–135

Match the conditions listed below with the most appropriate medication.

(A) Thioridazine
(B) Imipramine
(C) Methylphenidate
(D) Phenobarbital
(E) No medication

131. Childhood schizophrenia

132. Hyperactivity

133. Enuresis

134. Autistic disorder

135. Idiopathic grand mal epilepsy

Questions 136–140

For each of the neurotransmitters and neurochemical systems listed below, select the evidence used to support their role in the pathophysiology of schizophrenia.

(A) Naloxone is reported to reverse schizophrenic symptoms in some patients
(B) Dopamine-β-hydroxylase levels in cerebrospinal fluid correlates with levels of functioning in schizophrenics
(C) Benzodiazepines may help control acute psychotic symptoms of schizophrenics
(D) The neurotransmitter most commonly implicated in the pathophysiology of schizophrenia; other neurotransmitters may modulate this system
(E) Hallucinogens, which produce schizophrenia-like symptoms, are thought to exert their influence through this neurotransmitter system

136. γ-Aminobutyric acid

137. Serotonin

138. Norepinephrine

139. Dopamine

140. Endorphins

Questions 141-145

Match each clinical situation listed below with the medication most likely to be associated with it.

(A) Benzodiazepines
(B) Tricyclic and tetracyclic antidepressant drugs
(C) Monoamine oxidase inhibitors
(D) Barbiturates
(E) Antihistamines

141. Used as a hypnotic (sleeping pill) in the elderly

142. Tend to produce addiction and tolerance

143. Can be addicting but rarely causes addiction

144. May cause late abstinence syndromes

145. May be effective treatment for phobias and endogenous anxiety

Questions 146-150

For each disorder listed below, select the sign or symptom with which it is most closely associated.

(A) Multiple physical complaints
(B) Preoccupation with fear of illness despite reassurance
(C) May involve alterations in catecholamine neurotransmitters
(D) Psychotic disorders must be ruled out
(E) Modeling is a common characteristic

146. Somatoform pain disorder

147. Hypochondriasis

148. Conversion disorder

149. Body dysmorphic disorder

150. Somatization disorder

Questions 151-155

Match the drug-induced condition with the appropriate treatment.

(A) Haloperidol administration
(B) Forced diuresis
(C) Physostigmine administration
(D) Supportive care
(E) Naloxone administration

151. Narcotic-induced coma

152. Anticholinergic-induced psychosis

153. Amphetamine-induced psychosis

154. Barbiturate intoxication

155. Alcohol intoxication

Questions 156-159

For each causative factor listed below, select the organic mental syndrome with which it is most commonly associated.

(A) Organic amnestic syndrome
(B) Organic mood syndrome
(C) Organic personality syndrome
(D) Delirium
(E) Dementia

156. Progressive arteriosclerosis

157. Phencyclidine use

158. Propranolol therapy

159. Corticosteroid therapy

Questions 160-164

Match each statement below with the type of anxiety that it describes.

(A) Signal anxiety
(B) Situational anxiety
(C) Separation anxiety
(D) Anxiety about dependency
(E) Anxiety about loss of self-esteem

160. It may be associated with fear of loss of control

161. It results in distress when the patient is alone

162. It is manifested in part by a condescending treatment of others

163. It results from rising awareness of an unconscious conflict

164. It may occur immediately or at a later time

Questions 165-169

For each clinical finding or presentation listed below select the disorder with which it is most likely to be associated.

(A) Bipolar disorder
(B) Major depression
(C) Dysthymia
(D) Cyclothymia
(E) None of the above

165. Decreased rapid eye movement latency

166. Sleeplessness

167. Carbamazepine treatment

168. Congestive heart failure

169. Pseudodementia

Questions 170–175

Match each statement below with the sex-related condition it best describes.

(A) Transsexualism
(B) Transvestism
(C) Exhibitionism
(D) Erectile dysfunction
(E) Homosexuality

170. It often occurs for the first time after over-indulgence in alcohol

171. Most men with this disorder have a history of dressing in female clothing before the age of 4 years

172. Psychologically immature young men with hostile feelings towards their "victims" need this behavior to achieve sexual gratification

173. Anxiety about sexual performance is the most common psychological cause

174. The spectrum of psychopathology resembles that of the general population

175. Men with this disorder have excessively close physical and emotional ties to their mothers and have fathers who were absent during their childhoods

Questions 176–180

For each description listed below, select the personality disorder that is most apt to be associated with it.

(A) Passive–aggressive personality
(B) Dependent personality
(C) Sadistic personality
(D) Histrionic personality
(E) Obsessive–compulsive personality

176. Illness is often perceived as a threat to physical attractiveness

177. Pleasure, but not sexual arousal, is derived from the suffering of others

178. Authority is resented, and the efforts of others are obstructed by poor performance

179. Illness is often perceived as a threat to the control of impulses

180. Tasks must be performed in certain ways, but delegation of responsibility is all but impossible because of a fear that others will not perform well

ANSWERS AND EXPLANATIONS

1. The answer is E. (*Chapter 12 II B 1–5*) In a psychiatric emergency, it is always important to have trained help available to provide a show of force or to physically subdue patients, if necessary. It is not necessary to search all patients for weapons but only those who have given some indication from their behavior or prior history that a search is necessary. Physical restraints are needed only when patients cannot respond to reassurance by the clinician. It may be important to tell patients to control themselves, but this may not be necessary and depends on how cooperative patients are. Asking patients to change into hospital clothes is another way of searching for weapons, but this is not necessary in all cases.

2. The answer is B. (*Chapter 11 V C 2*) It is important to remember that the obsessive–compulsive disorder (i.e., the anxiety disorder) is a different illness than the obsessive–compulsive *personality* disorder. Individuals with the obsessive–compulsive personality disorder seem to have perfectionistic and inflexible personalities. These individuals are often indecisive, stingy with compliments and preoccupied by trivial details, but they do not exhibit symptoms of the anxiety disorder, such as compulsive checking and excessive washing.

3. The answer is A. (*Chapter 8 V C 4 c*) Premature ejaculation is the most common sexual dysfunction reported by men. Causes are usually psychological. Often the man has "learned" to ejaculate rapidly from early sexual experiences in which anxiety was high because of fear of getting caught in the act by parents or other authority figures. Defining the disorder is difficult because definitions must take into account the patient's idea about what is the proper duration of sexual intercourse: It is not diagnosed when intercourse lasts less than 30 minutes, although sometimes this is a complaint. It is not defined by the inability of the partner to achieve orgasm more than 50% of the time because this does not take into account the possibility of sexual dysfunction in the partner. Arousal of the sympathetic nervous system, rather than the parasympathetic nervous system, is associated with the dysfunction.

4. The answer is D. (*Chapter 3 IV B 2 b, g*) A clinical picture of chronic depression for several years without severe symptoms as described by the 41-year-old patient in the question is typical of dysthymia. The designation primary dysthymia is made if there is no antecedent, chronic, nonmood psychiatric syndrome or chronic medical illness. The presence of a preexisting chronic condition leads to a secondary designation.

5. The answer is D. (*Chapter 2 III F 1*) Strong evidence for the genetic transmission of the risk for schizophrenia has been obtained from twin studies. While rates of concordance for schizophrenia in dizygotic twins are the same as for any other pair of siblings, rates for schizophrenia in monozygotic or identical twins has been estimated to be between 35% and 70% in most studies.

6. The answer is C. (*Chapter 1 I B 3*) Early in the psychiatric interview, it is important for the physician to let the patients talk about what is bothering them. Only after this point should the interviewer attempt to find out other details, including how these patients feel about what has been happening. Details about previous psychiatric illnesses and about the legal issues associated with these problems, if present, are important as the interview progresses. Informing patients of the fee schedule is generally not done at the beginning of the interview.

7. The answer is B. (*Chapter 11 III B 1, 2*) The central features of a paranoid personality include a pervasive and unwarranted suspicion or mistrust of people, including pathologic jealousy, special concerns about hidden meanings, and expectations of being tricked or harmed. This is not true of the schizotypal personality who is odd and eccentric but does not have a history of expecting to be injured. Schizoid personalities want to stay by themselves and are not routinely concerned about what others are going to do. Individuals with antisocial personality disorder can present with mistrust, but the mistrust is not the core of this disorder.

8. The answer is A. (*Chapter 12 II E 1–3*) The physician should try to obtain as detailed a history as possible, but it is crucial that any previous episodes of self-destructive behavior be elicited because of their predictive value. Previous hospitalizations as well as medications being taken are important but not crucial to an emergency situation. Early childhood experiences, such as truancy from school or abuse, help in the diagnosis of an antisocial personality but are not helpful in an acute situation.

9. The answer is B. (*Chapter 2 III C; VII A, B 2*) Of all the conditions noted, schizophrenia is least likely to appear de novo in a 60-year-old man. Both delirium and dementia are likely diagnoses in this case. It should be remembered that depression with psychotic or melancholic features may present as if it were a "pseudodementia" but may also include hallucinations and delusions suggestive of schizophrenia if the patient's age and course of symptoms are ignored.

10. The answer is A. (*Chapter 8 II A*) Gender identity, which is set by about 2½–3 years of age, is one's sense of being masculine or feminine rather than a biologic state of being. The early embryo is bisexual and requires a Y chromosome for the development of male genitalia. Infants are assigned a sex usually on the basis of their external genitalia and are reared as that sex with the parents' and society's attitudes regarding it.

11. The answer is C. (*Chapter 10 IV A 1*) Anaclitic depression results when an attachment relationship is disrupted during a sensitive phase of development. Between the ages of 7 and 30 months, children are vulnerable to this condition if a lengthy separation from their caregiver with whom they have established an attachment relationship occurs. Prior to the age of 7 months or after the age of 30 months, children appear not to demonstrate this vulnerability. The condition resulting from the absence of attachment relationships in the first year of life is known as hospitalism.

12. The answer is D. (*Chapter 4 VIII B 3 a*) The patient described in the question presents with an episodic disturbance that occurs at a characteristic time of day. Food intake during the day maintains the serum glucose at adequate levels but, without intake overnight, the level drops. Signs and symptoms of hypoglycemia are evident in the morning or after vigorous exercise. This syndrome could easily be mistaken for an anxiety disorder.

13. The answer is B. (*Chapter 5 II B 1 c, 2 e; III B 1*) Both intoxication with and withdrawal from barbiturates may cause confusion, delirium, anxiety, agitation, disorientation, and postural hypotension. If the patient is thought to be withdrawing and a barbiturate is administered, these signs should improve, and nystagmus, which is a sign of intoxication but not withdrawal, may appear.

14. The answer is E. (*Chapter 9 I C 1, 3 b; Chapter 12 V B*) Physicians in all 50 states are required to report to their child protective service agency incidents of actual or suspected child abuse or neglect. These reports should be made within 24 hours of an incident and on an emergent basis if the child is in an ongoing vulnerable situation. A problem of this sort must be reported in every situation. Interrupting the session to make an immediate report is not necessary. Discussing the inappropriateness of the behavior may be helpful, but it is not enough and usually is a long-term treatment objective. In most cases, ongoing intervention with both the family and the perpetrator is indicated.

15. The answer is E. (*Chapter 12 III A 2*) Elderly people make up about 10% of the population, but they account for 25% of all suicides. The highest suicide rates are among elderly white men. Among the young, white men have the highest rates followed by nonwhite men and then white women.

16. The answer is C. (*Chapter 2 III A 2, B, D 1–3; IV C 3*) Schizophrenic patients in Third World countries, for reasons that are not entirely clear, have a better outcome generally than schizophrenics in developed countries. Reasons advanced to account for this include less socioeconomic stress and better family networks in Third World countries and increased social disintegration in industrialized countries. Patients who develop schizophrenic symptoms early in life with a slow onset tend to do worse than those who develop symptoms when they are older or when symptoms develop quickly. Because women tend to develop schizophrenia later in life than men, the outcome of schizophrenia for women tends to be better. Patients with paranoid symptoms have the best prognosis of any type of schizophrenia.

17. The answer is A. (*Chapter 11 I A, C*) Personality disorders are stable, not intermittent, patterns of responses that lead to problems in functioning. They are usually recognized early, that is, by adolescence, and they tend to become less obvious in old age. There is evidence that certain genetic characteristics may make a specific behavioral response more likely to occur. Poor social and occupational functioning are characteristic of personality disorders.

18. The answer is A. (*Chapter 10 II C*) Hospitalism is a disorder in which the child fails to establish any primary attachment relationship. Anaclitic depression is a disorder in which an attachment relationship has developed but is disrupted (usually by parent–child separation) during a sensitive phase of development. Vulnerable child syndrome is characterized by a parent–child bond that is intrusive and overprotective due to an exaggerated concern over the child's vulnerability. Child abuse has its roots in disturbed attachment relationships between parent and child in many cases. Although once postulated to be a result of a disturbed parent–child relationship, autistic disorder has now been shown to be a neurologically based condition.

19. The answer is A. (*Chapter 5 VI C 6 d*) Suspicion of narcotic abuse is increased by demands for a specific opioid; losing prescriptions; requests for prescription refills when the physician who allegedly wrote the prescription is unavailable; legal, occupational, or psychosocial consequences of abuse; and threatening behavior when a requested prescription is not written. A history of loss of consciousness might indicate central nervous system disease, intoxication with any substance, or abstinence from central nervous system depressants. Abuse of multiple drugs is common in narcotic abusers. Psychosis is not a common cause or result of narcotic abuse.

20. The answer is B. (*Chapter 1 II C 1 c (2)*) High voltage slow wave activity is characteristic of delirium when seen on the electroencephalogram (EEG). Delirium associated with alcohol withdrawal or age dementia, however, does not show slow wave activity. As yet, no specific EEG abnormalities have been seen in schizophrenia.

21. The answer is C. (*Chapter 3 V A 2 b*) The 34-year-old woman in the question presents with a recurrent, seasonal depression. This syndrome is hypothesized to be the result of disrupted circadian rhythms in response to diminished hours of daylight. Patients with this so-called seasonal mood disorder have been successfully treated with increased exposure to light (phototherapy).

22. The answer is A. (*Chapter 4 X F*) The history of recurrent tonsillitis is a clue to the presence of Sydenham's chorea, a condition that develops after a recurrent streptococcal infection. Specific features include emotional instability, impaired memory and concentration, irritability, and abnormal movements, including grimacing and jerky movements of the limbs. As with other rheumatic conditions, the indicated treatment is salicylates and bed rest. Sydenham's chorea generally resolves within 3 months of treatment.

23. The answer is B. (*Chapter 9 I E 5 a, b*) The weight of a patient with anorexia nervosa should be followed closely, and limits should be reinforced; that is, weight that is too low should result in hospitalization or curtailment of privileges if the patient is already hospitalized. Although increasing caloric intake would normally result in some weight gain, anorectic patients have learned that they can compensate for ingested calories by vomiting, exercising, or abusing laxatives. Likewise, decreased exercise would be met with vomiting, laxatives, or decreased caloric intake. It is too difficult to eradicate all of the weight-losing maneuvers; therefore, weight should be monitored.

24. The answer is D. (*Chapter 12 III A 5*) As many as 70% of individuals who commit suicide have a concurrent medical illness. Not only are many medical illnesses, especially those with chronic courses, associated with significant pain and disability, but they also represent a loss to be grieved and require that the patient shift his or her self-image and expectations for future professional and social functioning. The patient's future may appear bleak and hopeless in the context of the plans and aspirations of a once healthy and younger person. Chronic medical illness can put a severe strain on families and not only diminish their potential to support the patient but create further pressure on the patient, who may experience increased feelings of personal failure and isolation.

25. The answer is B. (*Chapter 3 IV A 1 a–i*) The essential feature of a manic episode is a distinct period when the predominant mood is elated, irritable, or expansive. Although the expansiveness of mania may lead individuals to feel creative, talented, or gifted, it is not observable in their poorly controlled actions and thought processes. Pressured speech is a readily observable phenomenon in many manics. Delusional thinking and violent ideation may develop during the syndrome.

26. The answer is B. (*Chapter 10 XII B*) Grand mal seizures in children are frequently treated with phenobarbital. Barbiturates, like other sedative-hypnotics, may result in paradoxic excitation in children. In such circumstances, discontinuation of the medication results in resolution of the symptom of hyperactivity. According to the history of the young boy described in the question, the acute onset of hyperactivity would be less likely secondary to a primary neurologic condition than as a side effect to the sedative-hypnotic medication. Selection of an alternative antiepileptic medication would be indicated.

27. The answer is C. (*Chapter 4 VIII A 1*) Wilson's disease (hepatolenticular degeneration) usually presents symptomatically in the second or third decade of life. A personality change in the woman described in the question is evident and is often the first sign of the disease. Transient episodes of psychosis may occur. The disease process involves the putamen and the corpus callosum, resulting in movement or muscular signs, such as the dysarthria manifest here.

28. The answer is E. (*Chapter 2 V A 1–5*) Nothing in the history suggests a catatonic pattern of symptoms for the 25-year-old schizophrenic woman in the question. Likewise, although she may be suspicious and have occasional ideas with a persecutory flavor, there are no systematized or substantial paranoid delusions. She does, however, demonstrate incoherent speech, marked loosening of associations, grossly disorganized behavior, and inappropriate affect, which qualify her for a diagnosis of disorganized type schizophrenia. Undifferentiated type can be ruled out on the basis of the presence of the symptoms of disorganized type. Residual type, characterized by a lack of prominent psychotic symptoms at the time of the evaluation, certainly does not apply in this case.

29. The answer is D. (*Chapter 8 IV A*) Depression is a common finding in the paraphilias, especially when a patient's interpersonal relationships suffer because of the sexual problem. Patients often feel shame and guilt about their impulses to act in deviant ways. Most of these disorders are seen only in men with the exception of masochism. The etiology, which is thought to be psychological rather than biologic in nature, is not known for certain. Despite the distress that the disorders cause, patients do not always see themselves as "sick" and often come to medical attention only after they have been legally apprehended.

30. The answer is B. (*Chapter 12 III C 1*) Recent studies of the central nervous system of suicide victims revealed low levels of hydroxyindoleacetic acid (5-HIAA) in the cerebrospinal fluid. Other studies have reported that low levels of 5-HIAA are found particularly in victims of violent suicides. Norepinephrine and dopamine levels appear to be normal in suicide victims.

31. The answer is C. (*Chapter 9 I E 1 b, 5*) The treatment of anorexia nervosa is aimed at preventing the medical complications secondary to starvation and typically involves behavior modification. With this modality, the medical status of the patient is measured by serially monitoring changes in weight or a catabolic state manifested by ketonuria. As the condition of the patient becomes medically compromised, negative reinforcers, such as restriction of privileges, are invoked. Nasogastric alimentation is provided as needed to reverse the state of starvation either when the condition is life-threatening or when behavior modification approaches have failed. Overtly aggressive or threatening behaviors, requiring locked seclusion, are not common among anorectic patients.

32. The answer is A. (*Chapter 1 I A 1 a–d*) The physical examination may be conducted during a psychiatric examination, but it is not routine. Usually the physical examination is performed if the history leads the physician to suspect a physical illness. A careful history is obtained, and data are gathered from the patient as with any other medical examination. Additionally, the differential diagnosis and treatment plan are constructed on the basis of the data collected.

33. The answer is D. (*Chapter 5 III A, B; VIII*) The history of treatment of insomnia by multiple physicians suggests that the patient probably has been receiving more than one hypnotic (sleeping pill). Since she has been treated for years, she probably has received at least some barbiturates or related compounds, which were in widespread use before benzodiazepines were introduced. It is also possible that she has continued whatever medications have been prescribed over the years in a continued attempt to sleep. If she is dependent on barbiturates, she will experience an abstinence syndrome when they are withdrawn, as would occur upon admission to the hospital and with the prescription of insufficient doses. In view of the rapid onset of symptoms, withdrawal from a short-acting compound is suggested. Phenobarbital would be likely to suppress withdrawal symptoms from any central nervous system depressants if it is administered before the patient becomes delirious. Most neuroleptics, especially haloperidol, lower the seizure threshold and increase the possibility that this manifestation of withdrawal will occur. Diazepam also suppresses a barbiturate abstinence syndrome, but its long duration of action makes it difficult to regulate clinically. Thiamine is appropriate for alcohol withdrawal, which could conceivably be a factor here too. However, the first step is to suppress the abstinence syndrome, which can be accomplished with phenobarbital or pentobarbital administration regardless of whether the cause of the syndrome is alcohol, barbiturates, or benzodiazepines. Disulfiram is not indicated unless alcoholism is diagnosed and discussed.

34. The answer is B. (*Chapter 4 V G 8*) The 58-year-old man described in the question presents with the characteristic findings of anticholinergic toxicity, such as tachycardia, dry skin and mucous membranes, decreased sweating, and acute confusion. Decreased sweating and drying of mucous membranes are not found in the other conditions listed in the question (i.e., reserpine, L-dopa, disulfiram, and benzodiazepine toxicity).

35. The answer is B. (*Chapter 9 I A 2 a–o*) Serum protein and albumin levels in anorectic individuals tend to remain in the normal range until starvation is far advanced. Serum cortisol levels tend to remain normal or slightly high, possibly representing a loss of normal diurnal variation in cortisol secretion. A lowered metabolic rate, which is characteristic of anorexia, is manifested by bradycardia, hypotension, and hypothermia. Increased carotene levels are common among anorectic individuals and tend to distinguish anorexia from other causes of weight loss. Hypokalemia typically becomes a problem during the course of starvation.

36. The answer is A. (*Chapter 10 III A 2, 3, 5, 7*) The fact that autistic disorder is evenly distributed across socioeconomic strata supports its neurologic etiology. Additional support for the neurologic basis of the disorder includes abnormal auditory evoked potentials, abnormal response to vestibular stimulation, and a high incidence of concurrent mental retardation and grand mal epilepsy. The incidence is higher among boys than girls.

37. The answer is D. (*Chapter 6 I E*) Hyperventilation, which may be caused by any type of anxiety, often results in shortness of breath, dizziness, paresthesia, headache, weakness, and occasionally, carpopedal spasm. Situational anxiety, endogenous anxiety, and caffeinism all can cause hyperventilation if the patient becomes sufficiently anxious. Post-traumatic stress disorder more typically causes anxiety and other signs of distress and occurs as a reaction to a traumatic event that has taken place more than 3 months previous to the onset of the psychological disorder. However, hyperventilation could conceivably be caused by anxiety due to post-traumatic stress syndrome.

38. The answer is C. [*Chapter 1 II A 3 b (3)*] The statement in the question, "During the last month, you have increased your drinking to a pint a day, and in the last 3 days, you have been contemplating suicide," is an example of a summarization. Briefly summing up portions of the patient's story shows the patient that the physician is listening and allows the patient to make corrections. An example of facilitation would be, "Tell me more about it," and an example of clarification, which is similar to a summary statement, would be, "During the last month you have increased your drinking. Was this just after your sister died?" Interpretation would be a statement connecting current issues with the past, and an open-ended question would be something like, "Tell me about your home life."

39. The answer is D. (*Chapter 2 VI B; VIII G 1 a; IX G 1–5, H*) Reasonable solutions to the problem of a high expressed emotionality family include encouraging the family to join the Alliance for the Mentally Ill, initiating a psychoeducational program for the family, decreasing the contact between the patient and the family, and encouraging the family to go into therapy to reduce deviant communications. Encouraging the mother to go into psychotherapy is likely to produce substantial disruption in the family's view of itself and of the mother as a scapegoat.

40. The answer is C. (*Chapter 9 I F 1–3*) The earlier the onset in life, the better the prognosis, and the longer the disease course, the worse the prognosis of anorexia nervosa. The prognosis for recovery for boys may be worse than it is for girls, but most girls do not fully recover. The death rate of the disease is listed as 5%–15%; death is usually due to metabolic or electrolyte abnormalities or suicide.

41. The answer is A. (*Chapter 5 II C 3*) Amphetamine psychosis is associated with disturbances, such as paranoia and loose associations, which may make it indistinguishable from schizophrenia; the only means of differentiating the two conditions is to observe the patient in a drug-free state. Tactile hallucinations and delusions of infestation with parasites also may occur. Mania is more likely to be produced by a number of commonly prescribed drugs, including antidepressants, administered to patients with personal histories or family histories of mania.

42. The answer is E. [*Chapter 5 II A 3 a (3), B; V E 4*] Central nervous system depressants, such as diazepam, phenobarbital, and glutethimide, augment the central nervous system depression caused by alcohol. Disulfiram produces severe nausea and vomiting when combined with alcohol, and patients taking this medication must be cautioned against even eating foods cooked in wine. Although restraint is the safest approach to the agitated patient who is intoxicated with alcohol, a nonsedating neuroleptic, such as haloperidol, may be administered if the patient continues to struggle after being restrained.

43. The answer is C. (*Chapter 7 I A 1*) Although essential hypertension, rheumatoid arthritis, hyperventilation, thyrotoxicosis, and neurodermatitis all have psychological components, hyperventilation is generally not considered to be a disease but more of a syndrome that is associated with anxiety. The other distractors (i.e., hypertension, rheumatoid arthritis, thyrotoxicosis, and neurodermatitis) were all originally felt to be the result, at least in part, of psychological conflicts of the patient. These conflicts were believed either to cause or significantly affect the development and course of these illnesses.

44. The answer is D. (*Chapter 12 IV B 2 a*) Intermittent explosive disorder usually occurs in men and is manifested by an episodic loss of control in which these individuals commit serious assaults or destruction of property. This behavior is grossly out of proportion to any psychological stressor. Bipolar patients, on the other hand, can be irritable and angry and may become violent; however, this behavior usually occurs after their plans are blocked. Individuals with an antisocial personality and paranoid individuals show no remorse for their behavior. Patients with organic mental disorders may assault someone without provocation as a result of confusion, but these assaults are not episodic.

45. The answer is A. (*Chapter 9 II D 1–7*) Parotid gland inflammation, dental caries, and esophagitis are all common complications of bulimia nervosa secondary to the effects of vomiting. Menstrual irregularities, including oligomenorrhea, are likewise common. Metabolic disturbances are common, but the *most* common presentations are hypochloremic alkalosis or hypokalemia.

46. The answer is C. (*Chapter 1 II B 7 f*) Echolalia is an example of a speech impairment. The patient repeats like a parrot what the interviewer says. This is not an example of psychomotor retardation in which the patient says little, nor is it considered an uncooperative attitude. The tone and rate of speech are not abnormal.

47. The answer is E. (*Chapter 11 III A 1*) Individuals with a schizoid personality disorder have a defective capacity to form social relationships. When hospitalized, they may become distressed when intruded upon too much by health care professionals. They generally do poorly in social situations, such as dating, and men, in particular, are unlikely to marry. They do not respond to warm, tender feelings of others. There is no evidence that antidepressants improve this disorder. These individuals, however, may do well in jobs that require social isolation.

48. The answer is D. (*Chapter 12 V D 2*) The patient probably does want to forget about the attack, but her apparent composure and detachment reflect the numbing and denial that are often the first stage of a stress-response reaction. The issue for the patient at this moment is survival, not forgetting about the assault or getting on with her life. Her behavior is self-protective and should not be mistaken for a lack of concern about the rape. All victims of life-threatening trauma may wonder if they did something to provoke or cause the assault or accident; this is a reaction to overwhelming helplessness and vulnerability and should not be mistaken for proof that they somehow brought this on themselves. This is particularly true of such a charged issue as rape in which the male physician may tend to blame the victim for her predicament. While it ultimately is helpful for the woman to discuss her feelings with someone, the physician may repeat the trauma and humiliation of the rape by asking unnecessarily probing questions.

49. The answer is D. (*Chapter 12 V D 2, 3*) The patient still may not be able to discuss the details of the assault, of her feelings, or of her symptoms in the emergency department situation, nor is it necessarily therapeutic to pry this open on a one-time visit. Rather, the patient should be reassured that her symptoms, although distressing, are usual following such trauma and are treatable. It probably would be helpful to give the patient a few days' supply of sleeping medication along with a referral for psychotherapy. A 1-month supply of sleeping pills might be used in a suicide attempt, and 1 month is too long to wait for further psychiatric evaluation and treatment. Sleeping medication has some potential for abuse and addiction, but providing this patient with some symptomatic relief at this point is reasonable and humane. Evidence of a psychotic depression would be apparent during the course of treatment, and getting this patient into treatment is the first priority.

50. The answer is B. (*Chapter 9 I E 1 a, 5*) Parents do not have the right to allow their child to starve to death, nor does the child have the right to starve herself to death. In such cases, a hold should be placed on the patient, and she should be hospitalized against her will and her parents' will. This should always be done in compliance with local standards. Trickery or coercion is seldom therapeutic. Consultation with a colleague may be helpful but should not take the place of appropriate medical intervention.

51. The answer is E. (*Chapter 9 II F 1–3*) No one modality of treatment for bulimia nervosa has proven to be universally efficacious. A treatment plan that offers combinations of several treatment modalities (i.e., pharmacotherapy, psychodynamic psychotherapy, and group psychotherapy) appears to be most efficacious. Hospitalization may be indicated for certain medical complications, concomitant suicidal ideation, or severely out of control binging and purging behavior. In most cases, however, bulimics can be managed on an outpatient basis.

52. The answer is C. [*Chapter 1 II B 6 a (3)–(6)*] Tactile hallucinations of insects crawling under the skin are called formication. Hypnagogic and hypnopompic hallucinations occur while either falling or awaking from sleep. Kinesthetic hallucinations are feelings of movement when none occurs, and gustatory hallucinations are hallucinations of taste.

53. The answer is A. (*Chapter 10 VIII C 1*) A significant percentage of children with encopresis have an impaction, and before psychiatric treatment is initiated, the presence of an impaction must be determined. While Hirschsprung's disease should be considered in the differential diagnosis, it would not be the first consideration. Children with encopresis are usually angry, and often these feelings are unconscious. Too early an interpretation of these feelings may cause problems in therapy. Soiling may or may not be a deliberate behavior on the part of the child. Seldom, however, does negative reinforcement eliminate this behavior.

54. The answer is A. (*Chapter 11 VI A 1*) A diagnosis of self-defeating personality should not be made if a person is in a setting of physical or psychological abuse. People in these settings may have little choice about being abused. The other symptoms, such as provoking rejection from others, rejecting attempts by others to help, a lack of interest in a caring relationship, and avoiding pleasure, are hall-marks of the self-defeating personality.

55. The answer is E. (*Chapter 3 VIII A 4*) Electroconvulsive therapy (ECT) has been used for several decades. While it has been viewed as inhumane, it remains an effective treatment for mood dis-orders. Although the precise mechanism of action of ECT is unknown, properly administered, it is associated with a success rate of greater than 90%. Patients selected for ECT fall into four groups: patients with a history of good response to ECT, severely depressed patients with psychotic features, patients who have not responded to medication and cannot take antidepressants, and patients who are manic and who have not responded to other therapy.

56. The answer is A. (*Chapter 9 V B 1*) Although hypothyroidism, fetal alcohol syndrome, con-stitutional factors, and Addison's disease all can cause failure to thrive, psychological causes are most common. A common mistake made by physicians is to defer consideration of psychological causes until all organic causes have been ruled out. Psychological causes should be considered from the beginning of the evaluation: They are not diagnoses of exclusion.

57. The answer is D. [*Chapter 1 II C 1 d (1)*] The dexamethasone suppression test can be used to follow the treatment response in patients who are depressed. It is not particularly useful in diag-nosing the presence or absence of depression or schizophrenia. It is not a treatment for depression, and it is not useful in treating bipolar illness or following the treatment course in bipolar illness.

58. The answer is D. (*Chapter 2 VI D 4; VII A, B 5, 6, 8*) The key to this question is the duration of symptoms of the 20-year-old man described in the question. Under modern diagnostic criteria for schizophrenia, symptoms must be present for a minimum of 6 months. There is no evidence that this durational criterion has been met in the case of the young man.

59. The answer is D. (*Chapter 6 I B 4 b*) Monoamine oxidase inhibitors have been found to ameliorate symptoms in some patients with post-traumatic stress disorder. Antianxiety drugs (e.g., propanediols) are generally useful only if patients are reacting to acute, short-lived stress; post-traumatic stress disorder, on the other hand, may persist for years after the stress has abated. Discussion of the patients' feelings about the stress and its psychological significance is the cornerstone of treatment of all situational anxieties, including both post-traumatic stress disorder and adjustment disorder. Biofeedback, meditation, and related relaxation techniques may be useful; however, behavior therapy, such as systematic desensitization, is more appropriate for the treatment of phobias. It is extremely important to differentiate post-traumatic stress disorder from schizophrenia since the symptoms may become chronic if the patient is approached as a schizophrenic and specific treat-ment for post-traumatic stress disorder is not instituted.

60. The answer is C. (*Chapter 11 II B 2*) The group of dramatic and emotional personality disorders (cluster B) is most often associated with concurrent mood disorders, such as depression. This is particularly true of borderline personality disorder. Schizoid and paranoid patients rarely come to the attention of the physician. Individuals with avoidant and antisocial personality disorders occa-sionally have a concurrent mood disorder but not as commonly as borderline personalities.

61. The answer is B. (*Chapter 1 II C 2 a*) Toxic levels of lithium are very similar to the therapeutic levels, and in some patients, they are the same. For this reason, it is important to monitor lithium levels. While patient compliance and lithium excretion can be checked, these are not the most important reasons for monitoring blood levels of lithium.

62. The answer is C. (*Chapter 5 IV D 1*) The patient has two indicators of possible alcohol abuse—gastritis and an enlarged liver. In addition to investigating these possibilities with hemoglobin and liver function tests, a blood alcohol level test is indicated to provide further evidence of alcohol abuse (i.e., no evidence of impairment with an elevated blood alcohol level). Since many patients abuse multiple drugs, a blood screen is also appropriate. Such investigations are much more com-mon means of uncovering alcoholism in a medical setting than is information volunteered by the patient. Blood cultures would be more appropriate to the workup of an unexplained fever, especially in an abuser of intravenously administered drugs.

63. The answer is B. (*Chapter 5 V C 9*) Absence of intoxication in the presence of a high blood alcohol level indicates that the patient is tolerant to the central nervous system depressant effects of alcohol, thereby meeting a major criterion for alcohol dependency. (It may also be assumed that an abstinence syndrome is likely to occur if alcohol intake is discontinued abruptly). Pancreatitis, impotence, and cerebral atrophy are complications of alcoholism that should be investigated; however, there is as yet no evidence that the patient suffers from them. Since narcotics and alcohol are not cross-tolerant, tolerance to alcohol does not provide any information about tolerance to narcotics.

64. The answer is B. (*Chapter 2 IX J*) Although new neuroleptic agents have not been on the market long enough to cause widespread tardive dyskinesia in comparison with older pharmacologic agents, there is no evidence to support the idea that one neuroleptic or another is less prone to produce tardive dyskinesia than others in spite of claims made by drug companies and others. The use of multiple neuroleptics simultaneously, commonly practiced in some settings, is not supported by studies. In addition to having no demonstrable improvement in therapeutic effect, polypharmacy runs the risk of compounding side effects and creating a clinically confusing symptom picture. Instead, it is common practice with failures of a particular neuroleptic to switch neuroleptics altogether. "Drug holidays," promoted a decade ago, are not effective for a variety of reasons, including the long half-lives of many neuroleptics. Indeed, there is no evidence to support the contention that "drug holidays" prevent tardive dyskinesia. Although neuroleptic medications are effective in controlling various positive symptoms of schizophrenia, they are notoriously ineffective in treating the persistent negative symptomatology.

65. The answer is E. (*Chapter 7 III A*) Factitious disorder is the most likely diagnosis because, although the patient must be aware that he has caused his illness, he probably is not aware of his motivation for doing so. Hypochondriasis is a preoccupation with the sick role but does not usually involve the patient causing harm to him- or herself. Malingering is closer in nature to this case, but the goals of malingering behavior must be apparent. Diagnosis of somatization disorder requires multiple symptoms and that of conversion disorder requires a psychoneurologic loss of function.

66. The answer is C. (*Chapter 8 VIII A*) One of the reasons that homosexuality is no longer considered to be a mental illness is because the incidence and prevalence of mental illness in homosexuals are no higher than in heterosexuals. According to several surveys, conservatively, 4% of the adult male population in the United States is exclusively homosexual; however, a much higher percentage (i.e., approximately 33%) of males have had orgasm with an individual of the same sex at least once, which does not necessarily indicate homosexuality. There is a higher incidence of some illnesses, such as acquired immune deficiency syndrome (AIDS), hepatitis, and venereal disease, in homosexuals who have many sexual partners. Treatment aimed at changing a homosexual preference has been generally unsuccessful.

67. The answer is C. (*Chapter 2 VIII G 1–3, 6, 7 a–c*) Expressed emotionality appears to influence the course of the schizophrenic illness while communications deviance and affective expressivity in families appear to be associated with the development of schizophrenia spectrum disorders. The Finnish Adoption Study does indeed appear to support a model of interaction between biologic vulnerability and communications in families, and, at least in the case of expressed emotionality in the course of schizophrenic illness, a psychoeducational approach has been found to have an ameliorating effect, reducing risks of rehospitalization almost to that of low expressed emotionality families. The concept of the schizophrenigenic mother, which is supported by little clinical evidence, has caused a great deal of damage to the credibility of psychiatry.

68. The answer is C. (*Chapter 11 II A*) Because of the similarities of symptoms and traits, the personality disorders are grouped into three clusters; A, B, and C. Cluster A includes schizoid, schizotypal, and paranoid disorders. These disorders are grouped together because affected individuals use the defense mechanisms of projection and fantasy and may have a tendency toward psychotic thinking. Histrionic, borderline, and antisocial personalities are in cluster B in which affected individuals use the defense mechanisms of dissociation, denial, splitting, and acting out. Passive-aggressive personalities are in cluster C in which affected individuals use the defenses of isolation, passive aggression, and hypochondriasis.

69. The answer is E. (*Chapter 8 V B 2*) The most important aspect in obtaining a complete sexual history is an attitude of openness and impartiality on the part of the physician. Specific questions concerning sexuality are not as important. Family attitudes about sex and the status of the sexual relationship are easier for the patient to talk about if he or she feels that the physician is nonjudgmental. Medical conditions that interfere with sex should be diagnosed but, again, are easier to discuss once the basic relationship with the physician has been established.

70. The answer is C. (*Chapter 2 VI C 1, 2 a–c*) All of the factors listed in the question except a major depressive episode, that is, alcohol abuse, major psychological stressors, traumatic life events, and use of psychomotor stimulants, are commonly associated with the onset of schizophrenic illnesses and brief reactive psychoses. If a patient had a major depression immediately prior to the onset of psychotic symptoms, the most likely diagnosis would be a major depression with psychotic features rather than schizophrenia.

71. The answer is E. (*Chapter 2 IX E 1, 2*) Current thinking about therapeutic relationships with chronic schizophrenic patients suggests that an open, warm relationship that focuses on concrete issues, self-esteem building, and education may be most appropriate for these patients. Although popular a decade ago, encouraging schizophrenic patients to express negative emotions may, if carried to an extreme, interfere with psychosocial functioning outside the therapeutic relationship and may actually produce exacerbations of psychotic symptoms.

72. The answer is C (2, 4). (*Chapter 3 VIII A 6*) Interpersonal and cognitive therapies are effective in the treatment of depression. Some patients require supportive guidance only; others need in-depth exploration of problems, relationships, and conflicts. However, neither addictions nor difficulties with social standards have been shown to be treated effectively with psychotherapy.

73. The answer is B (1, 3). (*Chapter 1 II B*) The psychiatric history reviews the course of a patient's life, while the mental status examination evaluates the patient at one point in time. Additionally, the mental status examination evaluates observable signs of mental illness, such as a patient's appearance and behavior. The mental status examination does not directly evaluate interpersonal relationships or developmental milestones and their effect on current functioning. This is done when the history is taken.

74. The answer is A (1, 2, 3). (*Chapter 7 I A 2 b*) The withdrawal–conservation syndrome describes a physiologic reaction to stress, in which the individual withdraws, thereby conserving energy. However, it has been noted that when the heart rate, body temperature, and metabolism decrease, the immune system is also less reactive, making patients more susceptible to illness, particularly infection. While depression may be a concomitant association with this syndrome, it is not characteristically present.

75. The answer is E (all). [*Chapter 10 VII B 1 a (1), b (2), d, 2*] A variety of organic and psychologic factors cause secondary enuresis. Organic causes include systemic illnesses, such as diabetes, central nervous system disorders, such as spinal cord lesions, and anatomic disorders, such as genitourinary malformations and urinary tract infections. Psychological factors, which include repressed anger, stress, and ambition, account for the majority of cases of secondary enuresis. Treatment is best aimed at the underlying cause. In the case of primary nocturnal enuresis, which may be caused by delayed central nervous system maturation, no treatment is indicated as it is a time-limited condition.

76. The answer is C (2, 4). (*Chapter 6 I B 5; III C 8*) The diagnosis in this case is probably social phobia complicated by the recent development of depression. Benzodiazepines do not improve social phobia and may aggravate depression. Antihistamines are somewhat helpful for older anxious patients and those who may become dependent, but they have no specific action in social phobia. Atenolol may reduce social phobia and is less likely to aggravate depression because it does not cross the blood–brain barrier; it might be combined with an antidepressant. Monoamine oxidase inhibitors have the potential to treat both disorders.

77. The answer is B (1, 3). (*Chapter 4 IV D 2; V F 2 f; VIII B 3 b*) After years of heavy alcohol use, individuals may develop an alcohol amnestic syndrome. In its chronic form, Korsakoff's psychosis, memory loss, and confabulation are prominent. Demented individuals also suffer memory loss. Individuals may be unaware of or need to deny memory loss. Providing inaccurate, but plausible, accounts of life circumstances covers the deficit. Syndromes due to diabetes mellitus tend to be acute in nature, corresponding to a sudden metabolic disturbance. Patients with Addison's disease develop fatigue, lethargy, and depression.

78. The answer is E (all). (*Chapter 5 II F 2*) Because so many psychotropic and over-the-counter drugs have anticholinergic properties, it is extremely important to be able to differentiate anticholinergic toxicity from other types of organic mental syndromes and poisoning. Any psychiatric symptoms, especially delirium and psychosis, that are accompanied by tachycardia, warm, dry skin, and dilated pupils should raise the suspicion of anticholinergic poisoning and prompt a careful history of use of prescription and nonprescription drugs. Intravenous administration of physostigmine temporarily reverses coma and fever but is not a useful treatment for the other manifestations of toxicity.

79. The answer is A (1, 2, 3). (*Chapter 2 VIII B 1 a, b, e*) Current research demonstrates a likely role of dopamine, neuropeptides, and γ-aminobutyric acid in the pathophysiology of schizophrenia. Although there has long been a search for isomers of specific neurotransmitters that may cause schizophrenia, there is currently little evidence to support theories involving isomerism in the pathogenesis of schizophrenia.

80. The answer is B (1, 3). (*Chapter 12 IV E 4 a, b*) The *Tarasoff* decision stated that when a specific threat is made against an individual by a patient, the therapist must break confidentiality and warn that individual. It does not state that the patient must be hospitalized, although that may be a good clinical judgment. While sexual relations between a therapist and patient are prohibited, they are not proscribed by the *Tarasoff* decision.

81. The answer is A (1, 2, 3). (*Chapter 1 II B 6 a–c, 7 e*) Perceptual abnormalities involve the central nervous system and include hallucinations, which are false perceptions of sensory stimuli, depersonalizations, which are altered perceptions of one's own reality, and illusions, which are misinterpretations of true sensory stimuli. Perseverations are abnormalities of the thinking process, which are manifested by repetition of the same word or phrase over and over. They are not considered perceptual abnormalities.

82. The answer is B (1, 3). (*Chapter 7 II C 5, 6*) Patients with somatoform pain disorder complain of pain for which no organic etiology can be found. The longer the duration of the symptoms, the less likely the chance of functional recovery. This condition is notoriously difficult to treat but a multidisciplinary approach offers the best chance for improvement in functioning, including psychotherapy, biofeedback training, and antidepressants. Sedatives can increase the patient's pain perception and decrease activity and, therefore, should be avoided. Behavior therapy may increase the patient's activity level, but it has no effect on the patient's perception of pain.

83. The answer is A (1, 2, 3). (*Chapter 3 VII A 2*) Dementia has many characteristics in common with depression, including apathy, physical complaints, and a depressed mood. In fact, a depressed mood may be one of the early changes in demented individuals. Patients with somatization disorders who are preoccupied with physical complaints (and often abuse aspirin) often experience chronic depression. Patients with pancreatic cancer are most apt to be alcohol abusers, and both pancreatic cancer and alcoholism may present as depression. Hyperthyroidism is associated with elevation in mood and activity.

84. The answer is B (1, 3). (*Chapter 5 IV A, C*) The first step in any effective treatment program is to withdraw the substance completely. Most patients can never use the substance of abuse in moderation; the goal of therapy, therefore, is abstinence. Family members need to be included because they may be drug-dependent themselves, they may covertly encourage substance use in the patient, and they may be important allies. Therapy is more likely to be successful if the patient is required to continue therapy than if he or she is free to drop out at any time.

85. The answer is B (1, 3). (*Chapter 12 III B 1, 2, D–F*) Any suicide attempt must be taken very seriously because the lack of success may reflect ambivalence or a miscalculation, not the lack of a serious intent to die. The suicide rate climbs dramatically for males over 15 years of age. Since this boy has probably not studied pharmacology, one can assume that he did not know that three flurazepam would not be lethal. Rather, his expectations and fantasies about what would happen are more important than the actual pharmacologic toxicity. Both the boy and his father minimized the event based on the outcome, but what of the initial intent? Also, some tension between them and anger on the father's part raises questions about the home situation in general and the father as a support in particular. Given the father's response, it would be important to call other family members and see them in person both to evaluate the family completely and to emphasize the severity of the situation. Both the boy and the father might provide more information individually; the boy, in particular, will be unlikely to talk about his depression and suicidal feelings in the presence of his angry father. Referring the boy to a school counselor is not adequate treatment following an attempted suicide; it does not address the need for evaluation and treatment of depression and assessment of the home situation. Similarly, encouraging the father to watch out for the son is a treatment intervention without adequate evaluation. It assumes that the son must be watched, but without an assessment of ongoing suicidal intent or of the father's interest and ability to be a reliable support.

86. The answer is D (4). (*Chapter 12 III D–F*) Suggesting family counseling assumes that family conflict contributed to the boy's suicide attempt; the counseling must start on the spot with as complete an evaluation of the family as possible if the boy is to go home. Beginning antidepressant therapy immediately in the emergency department suggests first that a complete evaluation for depression in the boy has been done and second that there is a symptomatic depression apparent. There is no evidence that such an evaluation has been done, and if the boy is that depressed, hospitalization should be considered. Encouraging the father to hide the sleeping pills and giving the son an excuse from school suggest that a serious and continuing problem is perceived but is not directly addressed and evaluated. Both interventions reflect an acknowledgment of the boy's depression and suggest an awareness of continuing suicidal ideation. More active intervention is required (i.e., more extensive evaluation of the boy and his support system or hospitalization).

87. The answer is A (1, 2, 3). (*Chapter 12 III D–F*) Outpatient treatment following a suicide attempt is a reasonable option. Not every suicide attempt requires hospitalization, and hospitalization should not be automatic as this may ultimately interfere with an ongoing treatment alliance if it is used prematurely or unnecessarily. However, if the protective environment of the hospital is not used, there should be some crisis resolution, evidence of mild concurrent psychopathology, a mobilization of environmental resources, and a therapeutic response to the interview. There is no evidence from the data that any of these criteria were present. There was neither an adequate evaluation of the son's depression and continuing wish to die nor of the father's understanding of the seriousness of the situation and willingness to be supportive of and responsible for his son. In fact, the father's continuing anger at his son and denial about the suicidal intent was apparent when he left a loaded weapon in the house and in his reluctance to have his son completely evaluated. Eight out of ten eventual suicides give prior warning. The boy had given his, and it was unheeded by the emergency room staff and his father.

88. The answer is A (1, 2, 3). (*Chapter 7 II A 2, 3*) Patients with somatization disorder present with a history of recurrent multiple physical complaints. Approximately 1% of women have somatization disorder, and the ratio of women to men is 10:1. Various etiologies have been proposed, including alcoholism, sociopathy, or somatization disorder in first-degree relatives; a chaotic home life during early development; and an impaired ability to screen out somatic sensation. Race does not seem to play a role.

89. The answer is C (2, 4). (*Chapter 8 IV B 1, 2*) Paraphilias are thought to be related to disturbed early development, leading to an abnormal object choice for sexual stimulation, rather than to genetic or biologic factors. Individuals learn to associate sexual gratification with this behavior and, thus, are reinforced for it. While some cases of paraphiliac behavior may show excessive sex drive or antisocial personality, these features are not general findings.

90. The answer is C (2, 4). (*Chapter 4 IV C 1 e*) Subdural hematomas occur in up to 10% of individuals with head injuries. This condition should be carefully considered in all cases, especially in elderly patients and alcohol abusers. Symptoms include headache, confusion, or focal neurologic signs.

91. The answer is E (all). (*Chapter 6 I B 6 a; III C 2, 3*) About 70% of depressed patients are also anxious, and 20%–30% of apparent cases of anxiety are caused by an underlying depression. There is evidence of familial, probably genetic vulnerability to depression, panic disorder, and mixed depression and anxiety. Approximately 40%–90% of panic patients become depressed at some point, and 20% of depressed patients have panic attacks. Cyclic antidepressants and monoamine oxidase inhibitors are effective in both panic disorder and depression.

92. The answer is A (1, 2, 3). (*Chapter 1 II C 1 e*) Polysomnography, the study of sleep in a laboratory, has been useful in studying medical problems associated with psychiatric symptoms, such as seizure disorders and erectile dysfunctions. Depression has also been studied because of the abnormalities of sleep associated with this illness. Schizophrenia, however, does not demonstrate changes that can be measured by sleep studies.

93. The answer is B (1, 3). (*Chapter 7 III A; IV A; Table 7–2*) Malingering and factitious disorders are classic examples of disorders in which the patient controls the symptoms. Malingering individuals deliberately fake or exaggerate an illness with the conscious intent of deceiving others. Symptoms of the factitious patient range from exaggerated complaints of pain when there is no pain to self-inflicted infection, such as that arising from self-injection with feces or saliva. Lying and exaggerating are common. Conversion disorder involves the unconscious "conversion" of a psychological conflict into a loss of physical functioning.

94. The answer is E (all). (*Chapter 2 VII B 5, 6, 8, C*) All of the diagnostic categories presented in this question should be considered in the differential diagnosis of nocturnal auditory hallucinations. Hypnagogic hallucinations, which have little or no prognostic significance, are not included in the possible answers but should be considered as the most likely item in the differential diagnosis. The clinician should gather information to include or exclude all of these possibilities.

95. The answer is C (2, 4). (*Chapter 3 VIII A 1–3*) The brief history of the 27-year-old woman described in the question strongly suggests major depression. Episodes of elevated mood and hyperactivity reflected in her history of spending sprees and hypersexuality suggest a possible bipolar disorder. This fact raises the possibility of concurrent use of lithium with an antidepressant. Social supports in a new city must be considered when addressing her potential for suicide. Without available supports, hospitalization may be necessary. While a family history of alcoholism is of interest, it adds little to this clinical situation. Possible side effects of tricyclic agents should not deter one from a trial.

96. The answer is A (1, 2, 3). (*Chapter 7 I B 2 b*) The treatment of essential hypertension may involve biofeedback in which the patient is monitored by a machine that provides information about biologic parameters. A tone sounds when the patient's blood pressure goes up, and the patient learns to relax to decrease the tone, and, therefore, the blood pressure. While biofeedback may have short-term benefits for patients whose hypertension is mild and reactive to stress, this treatment is not a practical long-term treatment for the majority of patients with hypertension.

97. The answer is B (1, 3). (*Chapter 1 II C 2 b*) Both nortriptyline and amitriptyline have been shown to have therapeutic windows, that is, the therapeutic effect of these drugs increases as the blood level increases until an upper limit of the blood level is reached at which point the therapeutic effect decreases. Imipramine and desipramine show an increasing or linear response.

98. The answer is C (2, 4). (*Chapter 10 III A 6*) Behavior modification is the most suitable treatment for autistic disorder. It aims to promote social behavior and relatedness, to maximize language skills, and to eliminate idiosyncratic behavior. A structured educational setting with a low student-to-teacher ratio and a constant environment are helpful. Psychotherapy may be helpful when the family is having trouble coping with an autistic child or when environmental factors have complicated the illness. Psychotherapy for the child may be indicated in those children with sufficient language skills and intellect. Neither electroconvulsive therapy nor administration of imipramine is effective in treating autistic disorder.

99. The answer is D (4). (*Chapter 8 III A*) Transsexualism is a disorder of gender identity and should be discriminated for homosexuality in which the sense of gender is consistent with the biologic sex. In transsexualism, there is a persistent belief on the part of affected individuals that despite being normal, they belong to the opposite sex. These individuals wish to be rid of their own genitals and live as members of the other sex. This disorder appears to result from a developmental disturbance in early childhood, not biologic factors. Transvestism is a paraphilia defined by the need for cross-dressing to achieve sexual excitement; however, gender identity is intact.

100. The answer is A (1, 2, 3). (*Chapter 1 II C*) The clinical laboratory is increasingly useful in diagnosing mental disorders. The three main functions include identifying biologic markers of psychiatric illness, monitoring blood levels of psychotropic medications, and screening for any other underlying medical or organic condition that may be causing psychiatric symptoms. Unfortunately, laboratories still cannot assess the severity of psychiatric illness.

101. The answer is A (1, 2, 3). (*Chapter 12 V A 3 b*) The important intervention in the protection of a child when physical abuse is suspected is to separate the abusive parent and the child. This may be accomplished by hospitalizing the child, hospitalizing the abusive parent, or, occasionally, by removing the child from the home temporarily. In all cases, the principle is not to allow the child to go home with the parents. While family therapy may be crucial for the long-term treatment, it is not useful acutely.

102. The answer is E (all). (*Chapter 5 V D 1, 2*) Nervous system complications of alcoholism include cerebral atrophy, Wernicke's encephalopathy, nicotinic acid deficiency, encephalopathy, and peripheral neuropathy. Gastritis, peptic ulcer, and hypertension are frequent presenting complaints of alcoholics. The majority of people who commit suicide are alcoholic, depressed, or both.

103. The answer is A (1, 2, 3). [*Chapter 4 III C 3 d; V B 3 d, C 2 b (2); IX C 2, F*] Organic anxiety syndrome is characterized by severe anxiety caused by a specific organic factor. Typical etiologic factors include caffeine or amphetamines, withdrawal from psychoactive substances, or endocrine disorders, such as hyperthyroidism or pheochromocytoma. Symptoms of anxiety that are frequently present in sedative-hypnotic withdrawal include nervousness, sweating, nausea, and tremor. Patients with pheochromocytoma experience palpitations, lightheadedness, excessive perspiration, and severe anxiety in episodes that often resemble panic attacks. Caffeine produces flushing, tremors, extreme nervousness, and hyperactivity. Hypoparathyroidism leads to hypocalcemia. Typical psychiatric symptoms include confusion, drowsiness, agitation, and depression.

104. The answer is B (1, 3). (*Chapter 6 II C*) A mastectomy may be a threat to a woman who values her beauty and whose first husband found another woman more attractive. However, one must also consider the possibility that a complication of surgery, a drug effect, an action of the illness (e.g., brain metastasis), or a new intercurrent illness is causing an organic mental syndrome. It is unlikely that schizophrenia would appear suddenly for the first time when an individual is in her forties, and signs of psychosis would be expected. Since the patient is exhibiting anxiety in the presence of a familiar caretaker rather than in the presence of someone with whom she is unfamiliar, stranger anxiety is unlikely.

105. The answer is E (all). (*Chapter 7 II A 4*) Complications of the somatization disorder (i.e., a history of multiple complaints) include an excessive number of medical evaluations due to frequent consultations with many different physicians. This, in turn, leads to unnecessary diagnostic procedures and surgery, any iatrogenic illnesses stemming from these procedures, and substance abuse, particularly of prescribed medication.

106. The answer is D (4). (*Chapter 2 III B, D, H*) The sex ratio for schizophrenia in the industrialized world is roughly equal for men and women. In the Third World, however, men appear to suffer from schizophrenia at several times the rate of women. Schizophrenics suffer a mortality rate several times that of the general population. Risks of premature death in schizophrenia are due to accidents, suicide, and some medical illnesses, particularly respiratory disease.

107. The answer is E (all). (*Chapter 1 II D 2 b–e*) There are a number of projective tests used in psychological evaluations. These include the famous inkblot test or Rorschach Test, which attempts to elicit a patient's thinking patterns, the Thematic Apperception Test, which consists of pictures on which a patient projects his or her fears and feelings by telling a story about the pictures, the Sentence Completion Test, which consists of a series of incomplete sentences that are completed by a patient, eliciting the patient's associations, and the Draw-a-Person Test, which assumes that the drawing will represent, to some degree, the patient's view of him or herself.

108. The answer is B (1, 3). [*Chapter 8 V C 3 b (3)*] Orchiectomy causes erectile failure by reducing testosterone levels. Prostatectomy can disrupt autonomic nerve supply to the genitalia and, thus, impair erection. While patients with coronary artery disease may be concerned about sexual activity, the problem most commonly manifests as sexual avoidance rather than erectile failure. Systemic lupus erythematosus is not associated with erectile failure.

109. The answer is A (1, 2, 3). (*Chapter 10 II C 1*) Hospitalism is an extreme example of failure of any affective relationship to develop. No bond is established between the parent and child. It can cause severe inanition and susceptibility to infection. It is not, however, associated with jaundice. The syndrome develops in infants and is associated with a high mortality rate. Treatment consists of providing the infant with a figure with whom to attach. If parents are unavailable, surrogate parents should be provided.

110. The answer is B (1, 3). (*Chapter 10 VI A 2*) Night terrors are very common in early childhood, may be exacerbated by stress, and occur during deep sleep. They are characterized by their occurrence early in the sleep cycle, and by the inconsolability of the child during the event, the absence of recall of the content of the dream, and the lack of memory for the event the following day. Sedative-hypnotic medications, which suppress deep sleep, will treat the symptoms, though no treatment is usually indicated.

111. The answer is E (all). (*Chapter 7 I B 2 a*) The type A behavior pattern has been associated with the development of coronary artery disease; that is, men who have this personality type are at twice the risk for coronary artery disease as those who do not. Characteristics include competitiveness, ambition, drive for success, impatience, a sense of time urgency, abruptness of speech and gesture, and hostility.

112. The answer is E (all). (*Chapter 11 II B 1*) Cluster B personality disorders, including histrionic, narcissistic, antisocial, and borderline personality disorders, are problematic to treat. Affected individuals tend to use the defense mechanisms of dissociation (i.e., "forgetting" unpleasant feelings and associations), denial (i.e., the unconscious disavowal of thoughts, feelings, or wishes), splitting (i.e., dividing individuals into all good or all bad), and acting out (i.e., the motor expression of intolerable thoughts or feelings).

113. The answer is B (1, 3). (*Chapter 1 IV A–C*) As a result of the Epidemiologic Catchment Area (ECA) study, it is clear that 25%–40% of the population will suffer from 1 of 15 psychiatric disorders sometime during their lifetimes; thus, conservatively speaking, at least 25% of the population will suffer a psychiatric illness. Men and woman have about the same rates of psychiatric illness, but these disorders are expressed in different ways. Men appear to have more difficulty with substance abuse than women, and women have higher rates of depression than men.

114. The answer is B (1, 3). [*Chapter 8 V C 4 a (3)*] Although inhibited female orgasm is a common disorder, it is not always indicative of psychopathology. A lack of information about female sexual responsiveness and disturbed communication in the couple are common causes of inhibited female orgasm. Other causes include cultural restrictions, financial concerns, alcohol abuse, and extramarital affairs. Female orgasmic dysfunction is rarely related to the side effects of medications.

115. The answer is B (1, 3). (*Chapter 12 IV E 3 a, b*) Benzodiazepines are the treatment of choice for alcohol withdrawal. They can be used orally or intravenously. Amobarbital can also be used in acute withdrawal, although phenobarbital may be more useful because of its longer half life. Haloperidol, on the other hand, should be avoided because it may lower the seizure threshold. Lithium has no use in withdrawal syndromes.

116. The answer is E (all). (*Chapter 9 I C 1–3*) Theorists have postulated that anorexia nervosa represents psychosexual conflicts in which anorectic patients fear oral impregnation. Other theorists postulate that conflicted family relationships are etiologic. Anorectic individuals may be conflicted with controlling, intrusive, and competitive mothers. Sexual impulses can precipitate a conflict between an anoretic girl and her father. Other theorists postulate that anorexia nervosa represents the inability of the patient to regulate her own eating. She becomes dependent on her environment in a pervasive way for regulatory cues. Thus, lacking the ability to follow internal cues (i.e., satiety and hunger), anorectic girls depend on external regulation (i.e., strict diet, calorie counts, or intrusive parents).

117. The answer is E (all). (*Chapter 1 II C 3 c*) Positron emission tomography (PET) demonstrates specific areas of brain activity. For example, decreased activity in the frontal lobe has been demonstrated in patients with schizophrenia. However, the use of PET is limited by the necessity of a cyclotron to prepare labeled compounds used by the technique. Also, PET does not demonstrate detailed anatomy or very small lesions.

118. The answer is A (1, 2, 3). (*Chapter 7 II B 6*) Treatment of conversion disorder, which involves the unconscious conversion of a psychological conflict into a loss of physical functioning, involves psychotherapy and perhaps hypnosis. Confronting the patient about the psychological conflicts underlying the symptoms is counterproductive. However, education about the effects of stress, suggestions during hypnosis that the symptoms will improve, and reassurance about the prognosis allow the patient to "let go" of symptoms without losing face.

119. The answer is B (1, 3). (*Chapter 11 IV B 2*) The most important features of the borderline personality disorder are difficulties in regulation, including instability of self-image and impulsive behavior. A sense of entitlement and interpersonal exploitation are seen in the narcissistic personality disorder and are not prominent features of the borderline personality disorder.

120. The answer is D (4). (*Chapter 11 II A 3*) In families with a history of schizophrenia, there is also an increase in the number of relatives with schizotypal personality disorder, not schizoid, antisocial, or paranoid personality disorders. Not everyone who has a genetic vulnerability to schizophrenia becomes psychotic, and it is thought that some of these individuals may be diagnosed as having a schizotypal personality disorder.

121. The answer is E (all). (*Chapter 12 V B 1, 2*) Sexual abuse includes all forms of sexual contact, including intercourse. Although intercourse is more common with teenaged girls, grade-school girls may also be affected with a high incidence of vaginal trauma. Any perineal or vaginal trauma in young girls, and even infants, should indicate the need for an evaluation of sexual abuse. Sexual abuse is most common between father and daughter, and, regardless of how close their relationship is in other respects, the daughter usually experiences some shame and guilt. The feelings of shame and guilt may be increased by the father's threats or pressures to keep their behavior secret. Over one-half of female runaways give sexual abuse as the reason for leaving home.

122–124. The answers are: 122-B, 123-C, 124-A. (*Chapter 10 III A 4, C 2; XII B 1–8*) Autistic disorder almost certainly has a neurologic etiology. This etiology is supported by a high incidence of grand mal seizures, mental retardation, and abnormalities of auditory evoked potentials and vestibular stimulation.

Attention-deficit hyperactivity disorder may derive either from a reactive etiology or from a genetic/neurologic etiology. Some children appear to be constitutionally hyperactive, and there appears to be a family history of attention-deficit disorder. In other situations, it appears to be linked with neurologically based specific learning disabilities. A biologically based depression in some children may be expressed as an attention-deficit disorder. Certain medications (i.e., sedative-hypnotics) may cause hyperactivity in children. In other children, attention-deficit disorder represents a reaction to a variety of life stresses. Included among these are worries and anxieties, and dysfunction in the parent–child relationship, such as intrusive and overprotective parents or demanding, abusive or intolerant parents.

Symbiotic psychosis derives from a reactive etiology. It is a disorder characterized by obscure boundaries between the parent and child. Although the parent is usually the cause of the problem, the child usually manifests the symptoms.

125–130. The answers are: 125-C, 126-D, 127-A, 128-C, 129-D, 130-B. (*Chapter 9 I; II*) Cathartic abuse may be seen in both anorexia and bulimia nervosa as a means of weight regulation.

Male predominance is seen in neither anorexia nor bulimia nervosa. Both disorders have a marked female predominance.

Significant mortality of 5%–15% is seen only in anorexia nervosa. Mortality is seldom associated with bulimia nervosa.

Preoccupation with weight is observed in both anorexia and bulimia nervosa. Only in anorexia nervosa is extreme loss of body weight observed. Fluctuations on either side of ideal body weight may be seen in bulimia nervosa; however, extreme weight loss is not present.

Neither anorexia nor bulimia nervosa as primary conditions are pharmacologically treatable. In most cases, pharmacologic management is aimed at coexistent conditions, such as mood disorders.

Concomitant substance abuse is commonly seen among bulimics. It may represent an underlying disorder of self-regulation. It is not a common feature among anorectic patients.

131–135. The answers are: 131-A, 132-C, 133-B, 134-E, 135-D. (*Chapter 10 III A 6 c, B 3 b; VII C 3; XII C 2*) Childhood schizophrenia is a psychotic disorder of childhood. Low doses of antipsychotic medication, such as thioridazine, may be helpful. It should be kept in mind, however, that these medicines can cause serious side effects.

Methylphenidate is used to treat attention-deficit disorder. Hyperactivity may be a symptom of attention-deficit disorder. Side effects may include anorexia, growth retardation, tics, and excitation.

Imipramine may be used for the treatment of enuresis. It has anticholinergic properties, and it affects the central nervous system, both of which may be therapeutic in this condition. Side effects can be serious, the lethal dose ratio is low, and cardiac arrhythmias can develop. Consequently, imipramine should not be considered a first-line treatment for enuresis.

There is no medication that treats the primary dysfunction in autistic disorder. Autistic disorder is probably an organic (neurologic) condition. Stimulants or antipsychotic medications may be helpful in isolated individuals for specific target symptoms. In most cases, however, medication is not helpful.

Phenobarbital treats grand mal seizures. This drug, like other sedative-hypnotics, can cause paradoxic excitation and hyperactivity in children. When this occurs, it may necessitate a change of anticonvulsants.

136–140. The answers are: 136-C, 137-E, 138-B, 139-D, 140-A. (*Chapter 2 VIII B 1 a–e*) Benzodiazepines appear to alleviate both the negative and positive symptoms associated with a psychotic episode through some effect on the γ-aminobutyric acid (GABA) system in the brain. These effects may not be specific to schizophrenia as GABA abnormalities are also found in other psychiatric disorders.

For the last several decades, serotonin has been the subject of research in schizophrenia. The primary rationale for investigation of serotonin as a possible causative agent in schizophrenia involves hallucinogens, which produce schizophrenia-like symptoms. These hallucinogens appear to exert a major effect on serotoninergic systems in the brain.

Dopamine-β-hydroxylase is an enzyme that is involved in the synthesis of norepinephrine. It has been found not to be correlated with schizophrenia per se but with the level of psychosocial functioning; for example, good prognosis schizophrenics have low levels of dopamine-β-hydroxylase.

Dopamine is the neurotransmitter system most commonly associated with abnormalities of schizophrenia. Evidence for the involvement of dopamine in schizophrenia is extensive. Some of the best evidence may be the effectiveness of neuroleptics in managing schizophrenic symptoms. These medications appear to exert their primary effect through the blockade of dopamine receptors.

Included in the neuropeptides are the opioid peptides called endorphins. If initial reports of naloxone, a narcotic antagonist, to reverse schizophrenic symptomatology prove to be true, it would strongly suggest that endorphin systems of the brain are involved, either directly or indirectly, in the pathophysiology of schizophrenia.

141–145. The answers are: 141-E, 142-D, 143-A, 144-A, 145-C. (*Chapter 6 III C*) Antihistamines may be used as sleeping pills in the elderly, although they are not always as effective as other drugs. While addiction to benzodiazepines is rare when they are prescribed properly, they may produce abstinence syndromes if they are withdrawn too suddenly. Barbiturates, on the other hand, cause addiction and severe abstinence syndromes. Monoamine oxidase inhibitors are useful in the treatment of phobias and endogenous anxiety, but their potential adverse interactions preclude their use as a drug of first choice.

146–150. The answers are: 146-C, 147-B, 148-E, 149-D, 150-A. (*Chapter 7 II A 1, B 3, C 3 b, D 1, E 3*) In somatoform pain disorder, patients present with pain for which there is no demonstrable physical cause or that is excessive given the known organic pathology. This disorder may result in significant impairment and inability to function. One theory proposes that the catecholamine neurotransmitters, which appear to be involved in pain inhibition fibers in the brain stem, may be altered genetically, developmentally, or secondarily to stress, resulting in continued pain perception.

Patients with hypochondriasis are chronically preoccupied with fears that they have an illness despite thorough evaluation and reassurance from the physician that no organic etiology can be found. Normal physical sensations, such as sweating and bowel movements, are misinterpreted, and minor ailments, such as a cough or backache, are exaggerated. Impairment can range from mild to severe.

Conversion disorder involves the unconscious "conversion" of a psychological conflict into a loss of physical functioning. Conversion disorders are also seen in cases where there is real organic physical illness, and modeling, that is, the unconscious imitation of symptoms observed in a significant person in the patient's life, is common.

Body dysmorphic disorder is characterized by a preoccupation with some imagined defect in the body, usually of the face. Depressive mood and obsessive–compulsive traits are common. Psychotic disorders, such as delusional disorder or schizophrenia, must be ruled out.

Patients with somatization disorder present with a history of recurrent multiple physical complaints in many organ systems, beginning before the age of 30 years, generally in adolescence. The description of the symptoms is often vague, but the presentation is often dramatic.

151–155. The answers are: 151-E, 152-C, 153-A, 154-B, 155-D. (*Chapter 5 II A 3 a, B 4 f, C 4 b, E 4 b, F 3*) Narcotic-induced coma is reversed by naloxone, a narcotic antagonist. Anticholinergic-induced coma and fever may temporarily be improved by physostigmine. Nonsedating neuroleptics (e.g., haloperidol) may relieve amphetamine-induced psychosis and agitation. If the urine is alkalized maximally, excretion of barbiturates can be hastened by forced diuresis. Alcohol intoxication is treated with supportive care until the alcohol is metabolized.

156–159. The answers are: 156-E, 157-D, 158-B, 159-B. (*Chapter 4 III D; IV E; V E, F 1; IX E*) Progressive arteriosclerosis, involving cerebral vessels, may lead to frequent small infarctions. Multi-infarct dementia can develop as a result of this process.

Phencyclidine intoxication produces a classic picture of delirium. Acute symptoms include confusion, agitation, disorientation, apathy, hostility, and violence. The individual's condition fluctuates significantly as is typical in delirium.

Propranolol therapy, which is used to treat hypertension and arrhythmias, may lead to depression. Occasionally, severe depression or a psychosis with visual hallucinations may occur at high doses.

Mood disturbances have been observed in patients receiving high doses of prednisone or other corticosteroid treatment. Both depressive and manic syndromes occur, and psychosis may develop with delusions and hallucinations.

160–164. The answers are: 160-D, 161-C, 162-E, 163-A, 164-B. (*Chapter 6 II A, D, E, H, K*) Patients who are afraid of becoming too dependent upon or emotionally close to others may also be anxious about losing control. On the other hand, patients who become overly dependent may regress (i.e., adopt a psychological posture more appropriate to that of a child) and exhibit distress (separation anxiety) when they are left alone. Patients with a vulnerable self-esteem may attempt to make themselves seem more important by treating others as though they are less important. When a conflict of which a patient is unaware rises to the patient's consciousness, the anxiety (signal anxiety) may elicit psychological defenses to remove the conflict from the patient's consciousness. Anxiety that develops in a stressful situation may occur either while the stress is ongoing or long after the external stress has abated.

165–169. The answers are: 165-B, 166-A, 167-A, 168-C, 169-B. [*Chapter 3 IV A 1, 2 i, B 2 g; VIII A 3 a (2), 5*] Alterations in sleep architecture occur in more than 80% of severely depressed individuals. These changes include decreased rapid eye movement (REM) latency, increased density of REM sleep in the first half of the sleep cycle, and a decreased percentage of deep (stages III and IV) sleep.

Prolonged periods with little or no sleep are seen in bipolar individuals who go to bed late and are up early, often after only 2–4 hours of sleep. During mania, sleeplessness may continue for several days, ending only when exhaustion overcomes the individual.

Carbamazepine is a second-line drug for use in bipolar disorder. It is used for individuals who do not respond to or are unable to tolerate lithium carbonate. Side effects necessitate frequent monitoring.

Dysthymia is classified as primary or secondary, depending on whether or not the mood disturbance developed in the context of another condition. Chronic and debilitating illness are predisposing factors in the development of secondary dysthymia.

Many depressed individuals present with cognitive impairment, such as inability to concentrate or think clearly. However, in some depressed individuals, this impairment is severe enough to raise concerns about dementia (pseudodementia). Impairment is reversed with adequate antidepressant treatment.

170–175. The answers are: 170-D, 171-A, 172-C, 173-D, 174-E, 175-A. (*Chapter 8 III A; IV C 2, 5; V C 3 b; VIII*) An overindulgence in alcohol is often the initial cause of failure of erection; this event leads to anxiety about performance. Other sexual disorders, such as transvestism and exhibitionism, may also occur when a lack of impulse control is exacerbated by alcohol; however, paraphilias are not usually precipitated for the first time by drinking.

The etiology of transsexualism in males is thought to be associated with an excessively close physical and emotional relationship with the mother and with the absence of the father during childhood. Over 75% of transsexual males have a history of being crossdressed by their mothers in girls' clothing before the age of 4 years. Transvestites also dress in women's clothes; however, they do not have a history of doing so as early in life. Although these associations have also been postulated as causes of homosexuality, they are not consistent findings.

Men who expose themselves (usually to women and girls) in order to achieve sexual gratification often feel hostile towards their "victims" and wish to frighten them. They often do not take further action. Transsexuals wish to change their sex and are not necessarily hostile towards anyone. Transvestites are more concerned about wearing women's clothing to achieve sexual gratification than scaring women by this behavior.

Although anxiety is an issue in many of the sexual disorders, it is a primary cause of secondary erectile failure or impotence. Sympathetic nervous system arousal decreases the ability to have an erection, which is mediated by the parasympathetic nervous system. A man must relax in order to achieve erection, and anxiety interferes with this reaction.

The psychopathology of homosexuals is similar to that observed in heterosexuals, which is one of the reasons that homosexuality is no longer considered to be a mental illness. Exhibitionists may have concurrent and more pervasive personality disorders, including one that encompasses pedophilia. Transvestites, transsexuals, and patients with failure of erection may suffer other mental illnesses to varying degrees, but actual statistics are unknown.

176–180. The answers are: 176-D, 177-C, 178-A, 179-E, 180-E. (*Chapter 11 IV D 5 b; V C 2 c, 5 a, D 2 h; VI B 1*) Patients with a histrionic personality disorder are constantly seeking praise and reassurance and tend to be vain and overly concerned with their appearance. Illness can be seen as a threat to their physical attractiveness, as punishment for their thoughts and feelings, and occasionally, as a threat of castration.

Although sadistic personality disorder is not yet an official diagnosis, there appears to be a number of people with this character pathology, involving cruel and aggressive behavior towards others. Individuals with this disorder enjoy the suffering of others. Inflicting pain for sexual gratification is not considered sadistic personality disorder.

Individuals with passive–aggressive personality disorder hide their expressions of anger and aggression by being ineffective. They often resent authority and obstruct others by their poor performance as a way to express their anger.

Patients with an *obsessive–compulsive personality disorder*, which must be distinguished from *obsessive–compulsive disorder*, have a need to be in control. Illness is perceived by these patients as a threat to their control, particularly over their own impulses and feelings. These individuals tend to be inflexible and perfectionistic. They are preoccupied with details and rules and do not appreciate changes in routine. They are often reluctant to delegate work to others because they cannot control it, but because of their perfectionism, they are unable to complete the task themselves.

Index